Emerging Cancer Therapeutics

Jame Abraham, MD, FACP

Editor-in-Chief

Bonnie Wells Wilson Distinguished Professor and Eminent Scholar
Chief, Section of Hematology-Oncology
Medical Director, Mary Babb Randolph Cancer Center
West Virginia University
Morgantown, West Virginia

Editorial Board

Forthcoming Issues

Leukemia
Uday R. Popat, MD, Guest Editor
The University of Texas MD Anderson Cancer Center, Houston, Texas

Prostate Cancer
James L. Gulley, MD, PhD, Guest Editor
National Cancer Institute, Bethesda, Maryland

Emerging Cancer Therapeutics

VOLUME 2, ISSUE 1

Renal Cancer

Walter M. Stadler, MD, FACP
Guest Editor

Fred C. Buffett Professor of Medicine & Surgery
Sections of Hematology/Oncology & Urology
University of Chicago

demosMEDICAL
New York

Acquisitions Editor: Richard Winters
Cover Design: Joe Tenerelli
Compositor: Newgen Imaging
Printer: Hamilton Printing

Visit our website at www.demosmedpub.com

Emerging Cancer Therapeutics is published three times a year by Demos Medical Publishing.

Business Office. All business correspondence including subscriptions, renewals, and address changes should be sent to Demos Medical Publishing, 11 West 42nd Street, 15th Floor, New York, NY, 10036.

The ideas and opinions expressed in *Emerging Cancer Therapeutics* do not necessarily reflect those of the Publisher. The Publisher does not assume any responsibility for any injury and/or damage to persons or property arising out of or related to any use of the material contained in this periodical. The reader is advised to check the appropriate medical literature and the product information currently provided by the manufacturer of each drug to be administered to verify the dosage, the method and duration of administration, or contraindications. It is the responsibility of the treating physician or other health care professional relying on independent experience and knowledge of the patient, to determine drug dosages and the best treatment for the patient. Mention of any product in this issue should not be construed as endorsement by the contributors, editors, or the Publisher of the product or manufacturer's claims.

ISSN: 2151-4194
ISBN: 978-1-936287-20-8

Library of Congress Cataloging-in-Publication Data

Renal cancer / Walter M. Stadler, guest editor.
    p. ; cm. — (Emerging cancer therapeutics, ISSN 2151-4194 ; v. 2, issue 1)
  Includes bibliographical references and index.
  ISBN 978-1-936287-20-8
  1. Kidneys—Cancer. I. Stadler, Walter Michael. II. Series: Emerging cancer therapeutics ; v. 2, issue 1. 2151-4194
  [DNLM: 1. Kidney Neoplasms. WJ 358]
  RC280.K5R454 2011
  616.99'461—dc22   2011005050

Reprints. For copies of 100 or more of articles in this publication, please contact Reina Santana, Special Sales Manager.

Special discounts on bulk quantities of Demos Medical Publishing books are available to corporations, professional associations, pharmaceutical companies, health care organizations, and other qualifying groups. For details, please contact:

Reina Santana, Special Sales Manager
Demos Medical Publishing
11 W. 42nd Street
New York, NY 10036
Phone: 800–532–8663 or 212–683–0072
Fax: 212–941–7842
E-mail: rsantana@demosmedpub.com

Made in the United States of America
11 12 13   14   15   5 4 3 2 1

Contents

Foreword

Cancer treatment is one of the fastest growing specialties in modern medicine, with better understanding of the disease, improved diagnostic tools, better prognostic information, and ever-changing management options. The most important tool a clinician can have in the fight against cancer is access to current information.

The Emerging Cancer Therapeutics (ECAT) periodicals provide a thorough analysis of key clinical research related to cancer therapeutics, including a discussion and assessment of current evidence, current clinical best practice, and likely near future developments. The content is in the form of review articles, but the volume format will allow for much more in-depth discussion than the typical journal review article. As a periodical, the content can be dynamic and updated more frequently and regularly than the typical static textbook discussion. The goal is to provide for the practicing clinician a source of thorough ongoing analysis and translational assessment of "hot topics" and areas of rapidly emerging new data in cancer therapeutics with significant implications for clinical care.

Each ECAT issue is a valuable tool for practicing cancer specialists of all disciplines. It provides the most comprehensive evidence-based review of pathology, radiology, pharmacology, surgical oncology, radiation oncology, and medical oncology of the topic.

Renal Cancer provides a comprehensive approach in the pathophysiology, epidemiology, clinical features, diagnostic modalities, and current and future treatment options. Experts from across the United States and Canada contributed to this issue. This will be a valuable tool for clinicians, nurses, researchers, medical students, residents, and fellows.

Jame Abraham, MD, FACP
Editor-in-Chief

Bonnie Wells Wilson Distinguished Professor and Eminent Scholar
Chief, Section of Hematology-Oncology
Medical Director, Mary Babb Randolph Cancer Center
West Virginia University
Morgantown, West Virginia

Preface

It has been a distinct pleasure and honor to serve as the guest editor for this issue, *Renal Cancer*. The knowledge regarding renal cancer biology, pathology, and especially therapeutics has literally exploded in the last 5 to 10 years. It was not that long ago that renal cancer was classified as a single disease and the only "effective" therapies were interferon and interleukin-2, which provided limited benefit with associated high toxicity. The identification of VHL inactivation in familial renal cancer paved the way for development of multiple VEGF and mTOR pathway inhibitors for treatment of this disease. More recently, subtypes of each of the now "classic" renal cancer histologies have been identified and additional rare subtypes described. Simultaneously, improvements in imaging and surgical techniques have challenged our diagnostic and treatment paradigms. This issue represents a compilation of these remarkable advances, with a focus on the pragmatic aspects important for the clinical care of patients afflicted with this disease. Each article is written by an acknowledged expert in the field representing collectively decades of experience with this cancer. This book also provides a unique perspective not only on where the field currently stands, but also on the status of the remaining challenges to be addressed.

I trust that you will find the articles to be as enjoyable and informative as I have.

Walter M. Stadler, MD

Contributors

Lilyana Angelov, MD, FRCS(C)
Department of Neurosurgery
Cleveland Clinic Taussig Cancer Center
Cleveland, Ohio

Tatjana Antic, MD
Assistant Professor
Department of Pathology
The University of Chicago
Chicago, Illinois

Tessa Balach, MD
Fellow
Section of Orthopaedic Surgery
Department of Surgery
The University of Chicago
Chicago, Illinois

Steven C. Campbell, MD, PhD
Professor of Surgery
Center for Urologic Oncology
Glickman Urologic and Kidney Institute
Cleveland Clinic
Cleveland, Ohio

Daniel C. Cho, MD
Instructor of Medicine
Beth Israel Deaconess Medical center
Harvard Medical School
Boston, Massachusetts

Toni K. Choueiri, MD
Director
Kidney Cancer Center
Dana-Farber Cancer Institute/Brigham and
Women's Hospital and Harvard Medical School
Boston, Massachusetts

Steven Chmura, MD, PhD
Assistant Professor
Department of Radiation and
    Cellular Oncology
University of Chicago
Chicago, Illinois

Kevin D. Courtney, MD, PhD
Instructor of Medicine
Dana-Farber Cancer Institute
Harvard Medical School
Brookline, Massachusetts

C. Lance Cowey, MD
Genitourinary Oncology Program
Sammons Cancer Center
Baylor University Medical Center
Texas Oncology, PA
Dallas, Texas

Janice P. Dutcher, MD
Director of Immunotherapy
Division of Hematology/Oncology
Department of Medicine
St. Luke's Roosevelt Hospital Center,
    Continuum Cancer Centers
New York, New York

Scott E. Eggener, MD
Assistant Professor
Section of Urology
Department of Surgery
University of Chicago
Chicago, Illinois

Scott Haake, MD
Resident, Internal Medicine
Department of Medicine
University of North Carolina at Chapel Hill
Chapel Hill, North Carolina

Thomas E. Hutson, DO, PharmD
Genitourinary Oncology Program-Director
Sammons Cancer Center
Baylor University Medical Center
Texas Oncology, PA
Dallas, Texas

Gautam Jayram, MD
Resident
Department of Urology
University of Chicago
Chicago, Illinois

Byron Lee, MD, PhD
Glickman Urologic and Kidney Institute
Cleveland Clinic
Cleveland, Ohio

Rimas V. Lukas, MD
Assistant Professor
Department of Neurology
University of Chicago
Chicago, Illinois

David F. McDermott, MD
Clinical Director, Biologic Therapy Program
   Department of Medicine
Beth Israel Deaconess Medical Center
Assistant Professor of Medicine
Harvard Medical School
Boston, Massachusetts

Martin Kelly Nicholas, MD, PhD
Assistant Professor
Department of Neurology
University of Chicago
Chicago, Illinois

Terrance D. Peabody, MD
Professor
Section of Orthopaedic Surgery
Department of Surgery
The University of Chicago
Chicago, Illinois

W. Kimryn Rathmell, MD, PhD
Associate Professor
Division of Hematology and Oncology
Departments of Medicine and Genetics
University of North Carolina at
   Chapel Hill
Chapel Hill, North Carolina

Brian I. Rini, MD, FACP
Department of Solid Tumor Oncology
Cleveland Clinic Taussig Cancer Center
Cleveland, Ohio

Jacalyn Rosenblatt, MD, CM, MMSci
Attending Physician, Hematologic
   Malignancy and Bone Marrow
   Transplantation Program
Department of Medicine
Beth Israel Deaconess Medical Center
Instructor of Medicine
Harvard Medical School
Boston, Massachusetts

Jerome B. Taxy, MD
Professor
Department of Pathology
The University of Chicago
Chicago, Illinois

Michael W. Vannier, MD
Professor
Department of Radiology
The University of Chicago
Chicago, Illinois

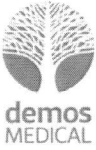

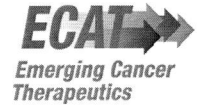

The Biology of Renal Cell Cancer

Scott Haake and W. Kimryn Rathmell*

University of North Carolina at Chapel Hill, Chapel Hill, NC

■ ABSTRACT

The intense efforts of a global community of scientists have extended immeasurably our understanding of renal cell carcinoma (RCC) tumor biology. The conventional histologic subtypes of RCC—clear cell, papillary (types 1 and 2), and chromophobe—are clearly distinct genetic and biological diseases, and warrant further discriminating analyses as we move toward biologically directed personalized therapy. The themes emerging, particularly in clear cell RCC of deregulation of hypoxia response signaling and specifically HIF-2α deregulation, provide a framework from which to understand critical steps in the path to invasive tumorigenesis and on which to support the future generations of molecularly targeted therapies.

Keywords: clear cell renal cell carcinoma, von Hippel-Lindau, hypoxia-inducible factor, Birt-Hogg-Dube, folliculin, fumarate hydratase

■ INTRODUCTION

It is estimated that 58,240 diagnoses of renal cancer will be made in 2010, making it the seventh most common cancer in the United States (1). The male:female ratio is approximately 2:1, for reasons that remain uncertain. The incidence of renal cell carcinoma (RCC) has been increasing by about 2% annually since the 1970s, partly due to an increase of incidentally detected lesions. However, the mortality attributed to renal cancer has also continued to rise, suggesting that increased imaging is not the only contributor (2). Understanding the root tumor biology of kidney cancer is important in determining the causes for these trends and taking steps forward for prevention, early detection, and effective therapy. Indeed, although patients who present with localized disease have a 90% survival rate at 5 years, unfortunately, up to 25% to 30% of patients present with metastatic disease (3) and the 5-year survival rate falls to 10% when distant

*Corresponding author, Department of Medicine, University of North Carolina at Chapel Hill, Lineberger Comprehensive Cancer Center, 450 West Dr, CB 7295, Chapel Hill, NC 27599
E-mail address: rathmell@med.unc.edu

Emerging Cancer Therapeutics 2:1 (2011) 1–20.
© 2011 Demos Medical Publishing LLC. All rights reserved.
DOI: 10.5003/2151–4194.2.1.1

demosmedpub.com/ecat

disease is present. Thus, major strides forward remain to be made as we unravel the molecular and genetic events that provide the driving force for this devastating cancer.

The collection of primary renal malignancies is a heterogenous group. Most renal tumors (92%) are renal carcinomas, with the remainder presenting as urothelial carcinomas arising in the renal pelvis (7%), Wilms tumor (1%), and several rare cancers, including renal medullary carcinoma; collecting duct carcinoma; primary renal lymphoma; and sarcomas (collectively < 1%). The tumor cell biology and molecular genetics of these tumors are outside the spectrum of this chapter. For the sake of clarity, this chapter will define RCC as one of a group of epithelial cancers arising from the renal parenchyma. These can be further subdivided into several histologically distinct subtypes whose unique biology has only recently become evident, including conventional (clear cell) (75%), papillary type 1 (5%), papillary type 2 (10%), chromophobe (5%), and the oncocytoma (5%) (4). This chapter overviews the molecular and genetic events associated with each of these tumor subtypes, using familial RCC as a paradigm and discussing available information on the tumor biology of sporadic RCC.

■ LESSONS FROM FAMILIAL RCC

Hereditary Clear Cell RCC

von Hippel-Lindau Disease
One of the classic genetic diseases, von Hippel-Lindau (VHL) disease is inherited in an autosomal dominant pattern. The incidence is 1 in 36,000 births with a high level of penetrance by the seventh decade of life (5). The disease affects a diverse but discrete list of organ systems. Among the more common features are retinal and central nervous system (CNS) hemangioblastomas (6). Indeed, it was the retinal angiomas that Eugen von Hippel first described in two patients in 1904 (7), and the hemangioblastomas of the cerebellum described by Arvid Lindau later in 1927 (8). The cerebellum is the most common site for the CNS

hemangioblastomas, followed by the spinal cord and brain stem. These tumors are histologically indistinguishable from the retinal lesions (9,10). Other features of VHL include pancreatic cysts and neoplasms, pheochromocytomas, and renal cysts and neoplasms, which are exclusively of the clear cell type. Clinically, VHL disease is divided by the presence (type 2) or absence (type 1) of pheochromocytomas, and a strong genotype/phenotype relationship exists with regard to this risk (11). Type 1 families typically inherit mutations, which produce a deleted, unstable, or severely truncated VHL protein, and they develop pheochromocytomas infrequently relative to type 2 families (12,13). They still manifest other aspects of the disease, including retinal and CNS hemangioblastomas and renal tumors. Type 2 families typically share a missense mutation in the VHL gene, are characterized by the risk for pheochromocytomas (~20% of families), and are further subdivided by their propensity to develop renal tumors. Type 2A families have low risk for renal cancer and 2B families have high risk. The only cancerous manifestation in 2C VHL patients is pheochromocytoma (5). These relative differences in rates of renal tumor development are important since kidney cancer is most common cause of death in VHL disease (14). Overall, 35% to 45% of patients with VHL develop kidney cancer (15). The histology is predominantly clear cell RCC (ccRCC) and is commonly associated with cystic architecture. The tumors are often bilateral and multifocal with any individual organ harboring 600 or more neoplasms (16).

The VHL gene was first mapped to the short arm of chromosome 3 in 1988 (17). Subsequently, it was isolated using a positional cloning strategy by an international collaboration between groups from the National Cancer Institute and Cambridge University (18). It is located at 3p25 and contains three exons. The gene encodes a 4.7 kb mRNA that is widely expressed in fetal and adult tissues (18–20). These tissues are diverse and do not exclusively include those affected by VHL disease (18,21). Alternative splicing exists and mRNAs have been isolated with or without exon 2, and the first 54 amino acids may be absent owing to an internal ATG start site (22). The role of exon 2 in tumor suppression remains openly debated, but the leading 54 residues appear to be uninvolved in the tumor suppressor activities of pVHL. Once the *VHL* gene was identified, it was possible to characterize the germ line mutations that are responsible for the disease. The mutations are diverse with nearly 500 kindreds identified, thanks to the dedicated efforts of Dr. Berton Zbar and his team (13,18,23–26). Various regions of the gene are affected with many predicted to affect the elongin-binding domain represented by codons 157–189 (12,27,28). The specific mutations are equally diverse and include deletions, missense, frameshift, and nonsense mutations. Across the described kindreds, there seem to be regions that are "hypermutable" and have a high rate of de novo mutations (29). In addition, a founder effect has been described for a missense mutation (C505T) in 14 German and 2 US families (30).

The *VHL* mRNA encodes a protein containing 213 amino acid residues (pVHL) and seems to be largely confined to the cytoplasm (20,31–33). Both sporadic and hereditary ccRCC display loss of heterozygosity, having mutated, silenced, or lost both copies of the *VHL* gene thus depriving them of any source of wild-type pVHL. The requirement that both copies be affected is consistent with the understanding that *VHL* acts as a tumor suppressor gene.

The function of pVHL in a normal cell is intimately associated with the cellular sensing of oxygen levels and the stability of hypoxia-induced factor (HIF), family of hypoxia responsive proteins. pVHL is the substrate recognition member of an E3 ubiquitin ligase complex, including elongins B and C, cullin 2, and Roc1, which targets the HIF-α proteins (HIF-1α and HIF-2α being the best characterized of the HIF family) for proteasome-mediated degradation (Figure 1) (34). The HIF family comprises a panel of highly regulated transcription factors that dimerize with the constitutively expressed HIF-β (also known as

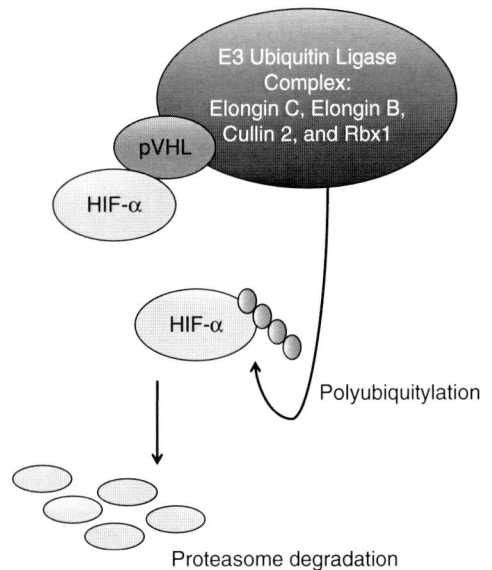

FIGURE 1

VHL-mediated regulation of HIF-α factors. VHL protein participates with elongin B, C, cullin 2, and rbx1 to form an E3 ubiquitin ligase complex. VHL engages proline hydroxylated HIF, facilitating the ubiquitylation modification, which marks HIF proteins for proteasomal degradation.

the aryl hydrocarbon nuclear transporter), which facilitates HIF-α translocation to the nucleus. The HIF heterodimer activates a host of genes, including those for vascular endothelial growth factor (VEGF), glucose transporter-1 (GLUT1), platelet-derived growth factor, transforming growth factor alpha, and erythropoietin (5). The transcriptional activation of these genes as a result of HIF-α stabilization comprises the cellular hypoxic response, and if inappropriately activated, contributes to carcinogenesis. Under conditions of normal oxygen, the HIF family members undergo a post-translational modification mediated by a family of prolyl hydroxylases. This hydroxylation occurs on one or more proline residues in the aptly named oxygen degradation domain and provides the structure necessary for binding by pVHL. This interaction ultimately leads to polyubiquitination and proteasome-mediated destruction of

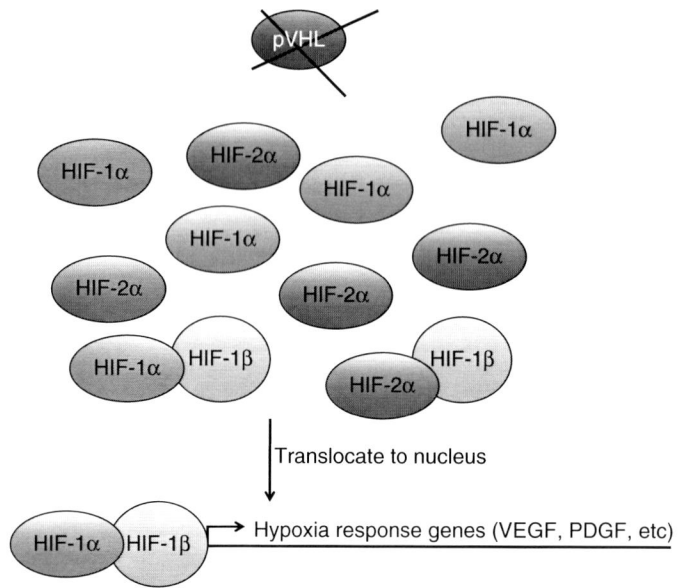

FIGURE 2
HIF stabilization promotes the hypoxia response as a result of VHL loss. In the setting of VHL loss, mutation or methylation, HIF-α factors are stabilized, heterodimerize with HIF-β, which facilitates translocation to the nucleus. This complex promotes the transcriptional activation of a broad panel of hypoxia response genes.

the HIF factors (35,36). Therefore, under hypoxic conditions, HIF-α is not hydroxylated, does not bind pVHL, and avoids degradation. This highly regulated oxygen response, therefore, mediates the transcriptional response to low oxygen. In the case of loss of VHL function, HIF-α levels are elevated regardless of oxygen tension and the aforementioned gene transcription ensues in an unregulated manner (Figure 2). The action of HIF, VHL, and the involved pathways will be discussed in more detail in later sections. These findings have tremendous implications for the management of sporadic ccRCC, as subsequent studies have demonstrated that VHL is lost, mutated, or methylated in the vast majority of ccRCC tumors (37).

Tuberous Sclerosis
Tuberous sclerosis (TS) is an autosomal dominant disorder characterized by hamartomatous growth in many organs, including development of benign and malignant tumors of the kidney (38,39). However, only one-third of cases of TS are familial with the remainder representing a high incidence of spontaneous germ line mutations as

well as a high incidence of parental mosaicism (40–42). These genetic features are important to consider when evaluating a patient with bilateral renal masses, but without a clear family history or syndromic constellation.

There are many renal manifestations of TS. The most common manifestation is the formation of angiomyolipomas (43–47). The angiomyolipomas are benign with varying amounts of mature tissues, including adipose tissue, smooth-walled blood vessels, and smooth muscle (48). Studies have shown that as many as 80% of TS patients will have some sort of renal manifestation (43,44,46,47). Both kidneys tend to be affected and the prevalence increases with age. The rate of ccRCC in TS patients is 1% to 2% (47,49).

Two genes make up the TS complex, labeled TS complex 1 (TSC1) and TSC2. TSC1 encodes the protein *hamartin* (50). TSC2 encodes the 200 kDa protein *tuberin* that contains a C-terminal GTPase-activating protein domain (GAP), which conveys the complex's activity (51,52). The TSC subunits combine to form a functioning heterodimer (53). Thus, in the absence of either partner, the TSC heterodimeric complex is inactive. The GAP activity of

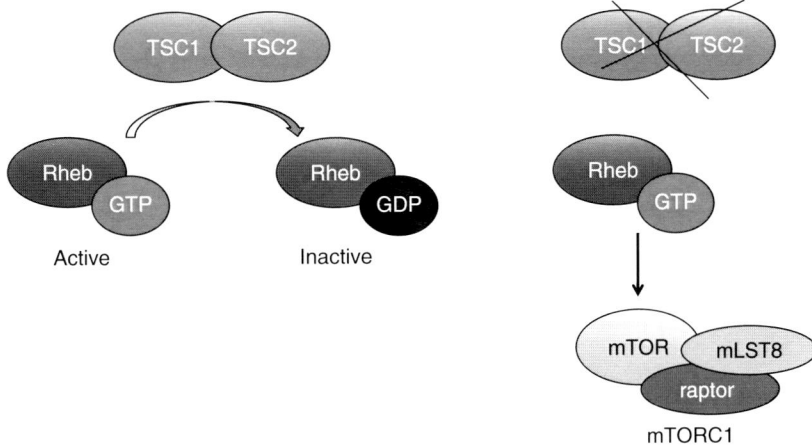

FIGURE 3

Tuberous sclerosis complex regulation of mTOR signaling. TSC1 and TSC2 form a heterodimer, which normally acts as a GAP protein to maintain Rheb in the GDP-bound, inactive state. In the absence of either member, the complex is ineffective, and Rheb is retained in active conformation to signal mTOR complex 1 activation.

hamartin/tuberin is strong and highly specific for Rheb (Ras homolog enriched in brain), a GTPase of the Ras superfamily (54–58). Rheb is highly active when in the GTP-bound form and is inactivated in the GDP form. Thus, in the absence of hamartin/tuberin, Rheb-GTP levels rise, resulting in increased activity (Figure 3) (57–60).

The most significant function of Rheb-GTP is its activation of mammalian target of rapamycin (mTOR). mTOR is a highly conserved ser/thr kinase, first identified as the target of inhibition of the immune suppressant rapamycin (61,62). mTOR is known to form two distinct complexes known as mTORC1 and mTORC2. mTORC2 is not thought to be affected by hamartin/tuberin and is involved in the regulation of the actin cytoskeleton (63–65). mTORC1 consists of mTOR and two other proteins (raptor and GbetaL) (64,66–69). It is activated by Rheb-GTP (61,62) and it activates two key targets: ribosomal S6 kinase and eukaryotic initiation factor 4E (eIF4E) (70–74), both of which function to promote specifically cap-dependent protein translation. The promotion of this activity results in cell growth and survival, and mTOR

pathway activation is a potent promoter of tumorigenesis. Unlike the situation with VHL, TSC disruption is not frequently encountered in sporadic renal cancers; however, the mTOR pathway is commonly deregulated and targeted by current therapeutic strategies and is instructive as such in considering the spectrum of molecular features of this cancer.

In an interesting twist on the VHL/HIF pathway discussed earlier, the production of HIF factor protein has been linked to mTOR-mediated cap-dependent translation (75). In particular, HIF-1α protein translation appears to be dependent on active mTORC1, and this mechanism of disrupting HIF signaling in RCC has been exploited in the therapeutic arena as discussed elsewhere. What remains less certain is the influence of mTOR signaling on HIF-2α translation. Recent evidence suggests that HIF-1α abundance can be influenced by both mTORC1 and mTORC2, but that HIF-2α translation is specifically regulated within the mTOR signaling pathway via mTORC2, a feature which may figure prominently in the activity of mTORC1-specific inhibitors in current clinical use (Figure 4) (76).

Growth Factor Activation

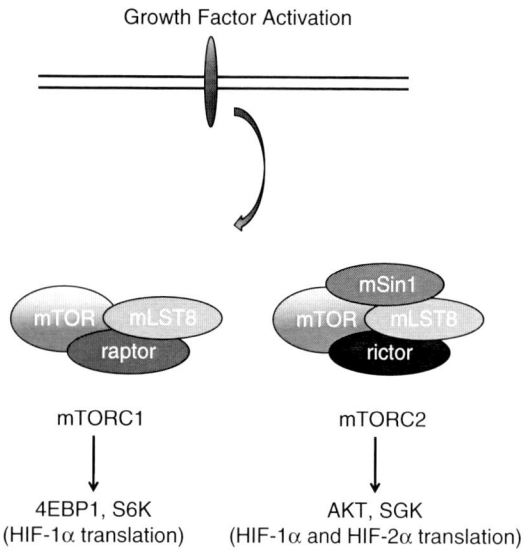

mTORC1

4EBP1, S6K
(HIF-1α translation)

mTORC2

AKT, SGK
(HIF-1α and HIF-2α translation)

FIGURE 4

mTORC1 versus mTORC2. mTOR protein participates in two distinct complexes, both of which can support HIF factor protein translation.

Hereditary Papillary RCC

Papillary renal cell cancer (PRCC) is a distinct pathologic variant of primary epithelial renal cancers. It is not as common as clear cell, accounting for only 7% 14% of primary epithelial renal cancers (77,78). Zbar et al. (79) described a family affected by kidney cancers with papillary renal cancer for three generations. This hereditary PRCC shared none of pathological or clinical manifestations of VHL disease, and mutations at 3p were not detected (11). As more families were identified certain traits became apparent. The syndrome was inherited in an autosomal dominant fashion and highly penetrant. Affected persons did not seem to be at a higher risk for other tumors and the renal tumors developed relatively late in life. Individuals had a life expectancy of 52 years (80). Since these initial studies, an early onset form has been described in which the disease presents in the second to third decade (81). Routine imaging would demonstrate multifocal bilateral tumors. In fact, pathological evaluation

would demonstrate as many as 3,000 microscopic papillary tumors per affected organ (82). According to current pathologic characterization, these are all considered type 1 tumors. Three years after the first description of this syndrome, after genetic linkage analyses eventually localized the gene to the long arm of chromosome 7, researchers identified the responsible gene at 7q31 (83,84).

The genetic defect responsible for hereditary papillary RCC is the proto-oncogene c-MET. c-MET codes for the cell surface receptor for hepatocyte growth factor (HGF) (85). Under normal signaling, c-MET is activated by its ligand HGF. Activation leads to increased activity of the tyrosine kinase activity of c-MET, which initiates multiple signal transduction pathways, including mitogenesis and migration (85,86). This is distinct from the loss-of-function nature of the mutations in VHL. The gain-of-function mechanism for carcinogenesis is supported by several observations. For example, missense mutations in the tyrosine kinase domain of the c-MET gene confer constitutive kinase activity. Furthermore, an analysis of 16 papillary tumors from two patients revealed a chromosome 7 trisomy, with nonrandom amplification of the chromosome bearing the mutated c-MET (87). Thus, whether due to increased constitutive activity of the c-MET tyrosine kinase or increased copies of the protein, the result is excessive stimulation of downstream pro-survival pathways mediated by mitogen-activated protein kinase (MAPK), paxillin, retinoblastoma protein, and the AKT/mTOR signaling pathways (Figure 5). Because the phenotype can be expressed with only one mutant allele and does not require loss-of-heterozygosity, it is an example of a proto-oncogene.

Of interest is whether sporadic PRCC involves this mechanism of carcinogenesis as this would provide a possible drug target. In support, trisomies of chromosome 7, which contain both the c-MET and HGF genes, occur in 95% of sporadic PRCCs (88). Indeed, similar missense mutations within the c-MET gene described earlier had been noted in some sporadic PRCCs (83). However,

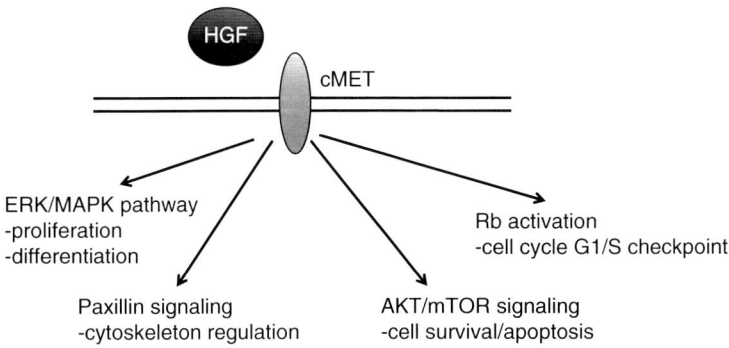

FIGURE 5
cMet signaling in cancer. cMet, the receptor for HGF ligand signaling, transmits this signal via MAPK, paxillin, AKT/mTOR, and Rb pathways to promote cell growth and survival.

further studies indicated that only 13% of sporadic RCCs contained identifiable c-MET mutations (89). Thus, it would seem that the molecular basis for carcinogenesis for most sporadic and hereditary PRCCs may indeed differ.

Hereditary Leiomyomatosis and Renal Cell Carcinoma

Hereditary leiomyomatosis and renal cell carcinoma (HLRCC) is a clinical syndrome inherited in an autosomal fashion in which individuals are at risk of developing leiomyomas of the skin and uterus, as well as kidney cancer, specifically of the papillary type 2 variety (90). Studies of affected kindreds started with identification of cutaneous and uterine leiomyomas inherited in an autosomal dominant fashion, known as multiple cutaneous and uterine leiomyomata or Reed syndrome (91). Subsequent analysis of the kindreds identified an association with the leiomyomas and type 2 PRCC (90). Later a region on chromosome 1 was identified, which eventually led to the identification of the culprit gene, fumarate hydratase (FH), at 1q42.3.

The cutaneous leiomyomata are benign though symptomatic. Patients often complain of pain, sensitivity to light touch, or paresthesias. The lesions arise from the smooth muscle associated with the erector pili apparatus. There is great variability in penetrance of this aspect of the phenotype as individuals with the germ line

mutation may have from 0 to 100 tumors (92,93). In contrast, the uterine leiomyomata aspect of the phenotype has tremendous penetrance. In the initial cohort of North American HLRCC, 98% of women who had cutaneous leimyomata also had the uterine tumors. In a different North American cohort 68% of women were discovered to have fibroids at age 30 or younger. Within this cohort, if the women required surgery for symptomatic relief from fibroids, 50% had the surgery by age 30 (93). The renal cancer associated with HLRCC is more aggressive than the other hereditary renal cancers discussed thus far in that it has a propensity to metastasize early even if the primary is small (94). As noted, the tumors of HLRCC are predominantly papillary type 2 histology, solitary, unilateral, and present early (4).

The FH gene contains 22 kb and 10 exons. Mutations have been found in 52 of 56 (93%) HLRCC kindreds identified at the National Cancer Institute. Thirty-one different germ line mutations have been identified. Of these, most (20% or 65%) were missense mutations involving a single nucleic acid substitution. Others include frameshift (3 insertions and 5 deletions), 2 nonsense, and 1 splice site (92,93). The gene product is an enzyme within the Krebs cycle and catalyzes the hydration of fumarate to form malate. Interestingly, FH was not the first gene whose gene product is a member of the Krebs cycle and also involved in a hereditary cancer syndrome. Succinate dehydrogenase catalyzes the conversion of succinate to fumarate, and germ line mutations have been detected in hereditary paragangliomas and pheochromocytomas (95–97). Loss of heterozygosity is observed frequently in HLRCC-associated kidney cancers (98). Furthermore, enzymatic FH activity has been noted to be low in affected cells (99). Thus, it appears that FH functions as a tumor suppressor gene.

The mechanism by which loss of heterozygosity of the FH gene and low levels of functional FH enzyme causes disease is similar to the pathogenesis of VHL disease. Both involve the transcription factor hypoxia-inducible factors HIF-1α and HIF-2α (5). As detailed earlier, under normal conditions, HIF is hydroxylated thus allowing it to bind pVHL, which eventually leads to polyubiquitination and degradation in the proteasome (100). However, under hypoxic conditions, HIF is not hydroxylated. Thus, it is unable to bind pVHL, which allows it to activate genes that could lead to carcinogenesis (5). In the setting of low enzymatic levels of FH, fumarate levels rise due to homeostatic mechanisms. It has been shown that high levels of fumarate leads to competitive inhibition of HIF prolyl hydroxylase (Figure 6) (101). Inhibition of HIF prolyl hydroxylase will lead to less hydroxylation of HIF. Thus, HIF will be unable to bind pVHL and it will not be degraded. HIF-α levels will rise due to stabilization. Indeed, HLRCC tumor specimens have been shown to have higher levels of HIF as well as higher expression of one HIF target gene, GLUT1, relative to adjacent renal epithelium. Thus, this is likely an example of a VHL gene–independent HIF-mediated carcinogenesis.

Hereditary Oncocytoma

Birt-Hogg-Dube Syndrome

In 1977, Birt, Hogg, and Dube described a constellation of skin findings in several family members including "fibrofolliculomas with trichodiscomas and acrochordons" (102). The skin lesions typically appeared after age 20 and were most commonly found on the nose and cheeks but can also be found on the neck, trunk, and ears (103). The fibrofolliculomas and trichodiscomas may represent a clinical spectrum and histologically are benign hair follicle tumors. The extent of the systemic manifestations was not appreciated until a patient with Birt-Hogg-Dube (BHD) syndrome was found to have bilateral renal cell cancers (104). Now the association of BHD and renal cell cancer is well accepted. Pavlovich and colleagues reported a series in which 34 of 127 individuals (27%) with BHD developed renal tumors (105,106). The mean age was 50.4 years though in other series persons as young as 20 have been reported with renal tumors (107). In another series of BHD patients,

FIGURE 6
Krebs cycle interaction with HIF regulation. As a result of fumarate hydratase muations, as seen in hereditary leimyoma and renal cell carcinoma, fumarate levels increase and inhibit the prolyl hydroxylases, which regulate HIF.

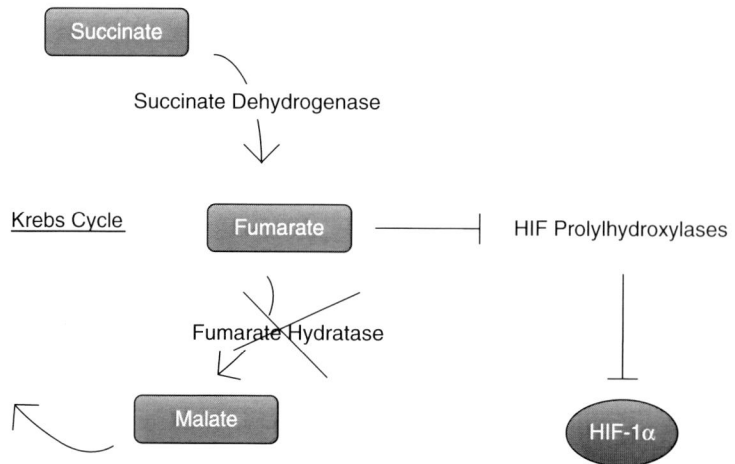

renal tumors were identified in 14% of affected individuals and only 2% of individuals in a control group of unaffected family members. When adjusted for age, the risk of renal tumors in the BHD arm was sevenfold higher (108). The histology of the renal tumors found in BHD patients is very different than other hereditary renal cancer syndromes. In one series, 50% of tumors from BHD patients were hybrid oncocytic tumors (features of both chromophobe kidney cancer and oncocytomas), 34% chromophobe kidney cancer, and another 9% were ccRCC (105). Interestingly, 58% of their patients had microscopic oncocytosis identified in the remaining macroscopically normal renal parenchyma.

Other features of the BHD phenotype include lung cysts. On CT examination of the chest, 80% of BHD patients have multiple cysts predominantly in the basal regions (109–112). The lung parenchyma is otherwise normal and patients generally have normal lung function (110). However, they are noted to have a 50-fold increase in the incidence of spontaneous pneumothorax, which is most likely secondary to the pleuropulmonary cysts. The BHD phenotype is extremely variable as patients may demonstrate only the renal or pulmonary manifestations and not the dermatological features.

Previous observations had established that BHD is inherited in an autosomal dominant fashion. Genetic linkage analysis eventually localized the *BHD* gene to chromosome 17p11.2 (113,114). Indeed, genetic testing has largely supplanted systems of major and minor criteria in the diagnosis of BHD. Currently, approximately 200 families worldwide have been identified with the BHD phenotype and *BHD* germ line mutation. The most common mutations observed in families are frameshift and nonsense mutations that lead to protein truncation (115,116). The most common site for mutations was a polycytosine tract within exon 11 consisting of eight cytosine residues. Variations of this polycytosine tract have distinct phenotypic manifestations. For example, cytosine-deletion mutations (i.e., seven cytosine residues)

have a much lower rate of kidney tumor development (6%) relative to cytosine-insertion mutations (i.e., nine cytosine residues, 33%) (117).

The *BHD* gene contains 14 exons and encodes for the protein folliculin. Northern blot analysis had demonstrated a wide distribution of the protein throughout the human body, including the skin, kidney, and lung (115). The protein consists of 579 amino acids and has no major homology to other known human proteins though it seems to be highly conserved across species, including mouse and *Drosophila* (118). While the function of the folliculin protein is still poorly understood, it does seem to harbor a tumor suppressor function. Loss-of-heterozygosity was observed in BHD-associated renal tumors (119). Furthermore, folliculin mRNA was not expressed in renal tumors of patients with BHD (120). Interestingly, the pathogenesis of the renal tumors seems to be distinct from that of the fibrofolliculomas. In the skin lesions, folliculin mRNA levels were high and loss-of-heterozygosity was not observed for the *BHD* gene (121).

One theory for the mechanism of tumorigenesis in BHD kidney tumors involves the loss-of-heterozygosity for the BHD gene, as well as the activation of mTOR signaling. Folliculin-interacting protein 1 (FNIP1) and FNIP2 have been shown to interact with both folliculin and another broadly important enzyme 5′AMP-activated protein kinase (AMPK). AMPK is known to be involved in the mTOR pathway as a stimulator of signaling complex formation (122–124). In one particular study of kidney-targeted BHD conditional knockout mice, the mTOR inhibitor rapamycin diminished kidney disease and increased survival (125,126). This would seem to suggest that folliculin acts as an mTOR inhibitor and mTOR over activity is the key step in tumorigenesis. This loss of mTOR inhibition is of course similar to the pathogenesis for TS. Studies have highlighted the overlap in clinical syndromes between BHD and TS (skin hamartomas, pulmonary cysts, pneumothorax, and renal tumors) (127,128). While much has been learned about the *BHD* gene and its protein product, much of

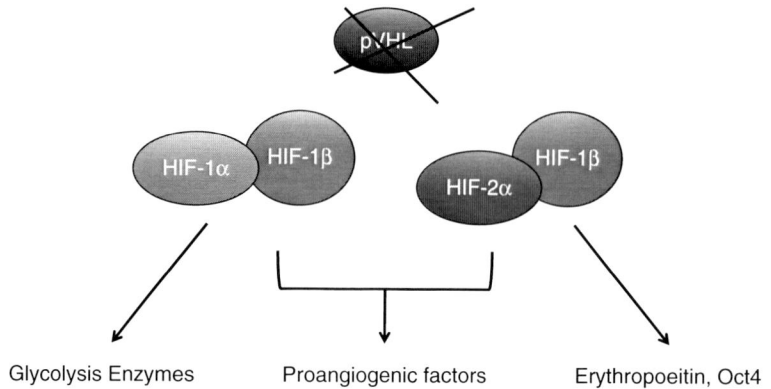

FIGURE 7
HIF transcriptional activation is not uniform. As a result of VHL loss, in vitro studies have shown that HIF-1α and HIF-2α have independent transcriptional targets, in addition to common targets of angiogenesis.

its interactions with signaling pathways, including mTOR, require further study.

■ UNDERSTANDING THE BIOLOGY OF SPORADIC RCC

Impact of VHL Mutation

ccRCC arising outside of the familial setting is the most frequently encountered manifestation of this disease. Fortunately, the lessons of heritable ccRCC are to sporadic tumors, which also harbor mutations, hypermethylation-based silencing, or allelic loss of the *VHL* gene. A recent study reported *VHL* mutation in 92% of tumors (37). Thus, the effects of constitutive activation of the hypoxia response pathway impact the vast majority of these tumors. Of note, *VHL* mutation or loss in ccRCC has differential effects on the stabilization of HIF-1α and HIF-2α. Specifically, HIF-2α is stabilized in all VHL-inactivated renal tumors, whereas HIF-1α is stabilized in only a subset (129). It has been recognized for some time that the transcriptional targets of HIF-1α and HIF-2α are largely, but not completely, overlapping. In particular, both factors promote the transcription of pro-angiogenic genes, such as VEGF. However, glycolytic and other metabolic regulatory enzymes are regulated exclusively by HIF-1α, whereas HIF-2α mediates the transcription of erythropoietin and Oct-4 to the exclusion of HIF-1α (Figure 7). Building on

the known tumor biology of *VHL* mutation to promote unequal stabilization of the two HIF factors, Gordan et al. sought to investigate the resulting molecular pathways affected by differential HIF-1α and HIF-2α expression (129).

In this analysis, ccRCC tumors were stratified based on their *VHL* mutation status and HIF-1α and HIF-2α expression patterns. Three groups were observed (Figure 8): ccRCCs with intact *VHL* (representing only about 10% of the total population), pVHL deficient ccRCCs expressing stabilized HIF-1α and HIF-2α (H1H2), and pVHL deficient ccRCCs expressing only stabilized HIF-2α (H2). An analysis of variance in tumor gene expression profiles across these three groups, using balanced representation of VHL wild type, H1H2, and H2, demonstrated distinct patterns in molecular pathway activation. As expected, all tumors with *VHL* disrupted and expressing any pattern of HIF stabilization displayed increased expression of angiogenic and common hypoxia-responsive gene targets. Consistent with prior reports from cell culture experiments, tumors displaying stabilized HIF-1α (H1H2 subtype) over-expressed genes involved in glycolytic metabolism relative to the H2 subtype, confirming the transcriptional specificity of this unique set of target genes (130). Specifically, the subgroup with intact *VHL* as well as the H1H2 subgroup displayed enhanced Akt/mTOR and ERK/MAPK signaling and the H2 subgroup exhibiting increased levels of

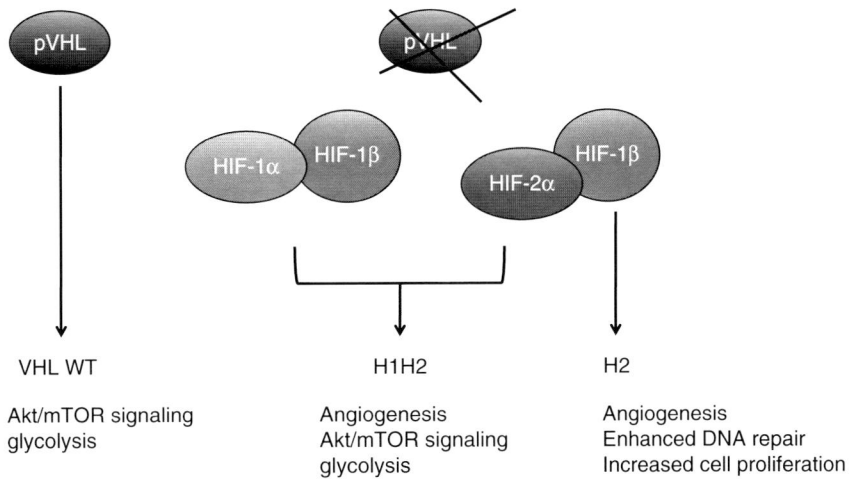

FIGURE 8
HIF defined subsets of clear cell renal cell carcinoma (ccRCC). ccRCC can be divided into those with wild-type VHL, and no stabilization of HIF factors, those that have VHL mutated and display stabilization of both HIF-1α and HIF-2α, and those with mutated VHL which only show HIF-2α stabilization. These tumors display highly distinct patterns of gene expression, and promote survival by divergent mechanisms.

cMyc activity and Ki-67 overexpression, resulting in enhanced proliferation and resistance to replication stress (129). The implications of this molecular subdivision remain an active area of investigation, and the mechanism (or mechanisms) that contribute to tumor cell adoption of these profiles remain uncertain. Since such remarkably different pathways are activated in this classification, it is predicted that subgroups would display varied responses to molecularly targeted therapies and such responses demand further exploration.

Tumor Gene Expression Profiles in RCC

The use of gene expression profiling to delineate the transcriptional repertoire of RCCs has reinforced the observations that clear cell and papillary tumors are highly distinct entities. The overriding transcriptional profile, which defines clear cell tumors, is that of the hypoxia response profile, including pro-angiogenic, metabolic, and growth factor signaling-related gene sets. These genes as a unit are tightly associated with clear cell tumors as

a result of VHL loss and activation of the hypoxia response pathway *in the presence of oxygen*, as discussed earlier. Non-clear cell histology tumors are highly divergent in this regard.

Within the ccRCC group, the use of gene expression profiling has been useful to classify ccRCC tumor subsets. Several studies have persistently demonstrated that ccRCC can be divided into at least two stable subsets by hierarchical clustering (131). One study of 177 clear cell tumors identified the existence of at least two subgroups and further demonstrated that these subsets imposed a clear association with survival (132). Further analysis of these gene expression clusters demonstrated that genes involved in wound healing and cell migration were more closely associated with the poor prognosis group, suggesting the acquisition of molecular changes that promote invasive features (133). The underlying changes that promote these features remain unknown. In a similar vein, a classification scheme for ccRCC was developed, which also defined two subsets based on a highly robust, stable, and manageable set of gene features labeled as ccA and ccB (131). Like other strategies to subdivide clear cell tumors, this scheme displays independent association with survival. ccA tumors, associated with a better prognosis, overexpress a more conventional hypoxia response pathway with a pro-angiogenic profile. While ccB tumors also display disruption in hypoxia response signals as compared to normal tissue, this subgroup also displays gene signatures indicative of a more immature and aggressive molecular phenotype with genes involved in epithelial to mesenchymal transition and cell cycle regulation (131). The underlying genetic or epigenetic events that contribute to these two subtypes of invasive carcinoma, relationship to the H1H2 subtypes discussed earlier, and confirmation of survival implications are an area of intense investigation.

In the largest analysis of its type, 931 tumors from the Cleveland Clinic were analyzed by RT-PCR for expression of 727 genes, identifying a signature of genes highly associated with the recurrence free interval for those patients (134). Generally speaking, a lower risk of recurrence was associated with gene signatures associated with angiogenesis, and higher recurrence risk with genes frequently associated with epithelial to mesenchymal transition. This strategy provides a tool for clinical decision-making and work to develop these gene signatures for clinical scenarios to assess risk for disease recurrence is underway. In particular, these recurrence/survival discriminatory gene sets belie biological diversity, which has to date eluded investigators.

Since these subgroups of ccRCC express such vastly different molecular profiles, it naturally follows that such differences may result in them responding differently to specific molecularly targeted therapies, including VEGF signaling pathway targeted agents such as bevacizumab, sunitinib, sorafenib, and pazopanib and mTORC1 disrupting agents such as everolimus and temsirolimus, as discussed in Chapters 8 and 9, respectively. The application of such a classification as a predictor of response to targeted therapies and selection of optimal therapy shows promise and is an active area of investigation.

Other Contributing Genetic and Epigenetic Events, ccRCC

Enhancing understanding of the root (genetic) causes of kidney cancers is essential for building robust and rational targeting strategies. The lessons we have learned from targeted therapy in diseases such as breast and lung cancer have revealed that identifying and targeting tumor cell-specific molecules provide the most effective methods of combating these cancers. This advancement will depend on exhaustive examination of the genome and epigenome of RCCs through systemic sequencing of the coding regions, copy number and single nucleotide polymorphism analysis, and genome-wide expression studies. Several recent studies have explored copy number variation and cancer exome sequencing using current-generation technologies in ccRCC (135–137). Encouragingly, trends are emerging which will enable future studies to focus on high-impact genetic regions. Specifically, in addition to the loss of chromosome 3p, tightly associated with *VHL* loss at 3p24, consistent losses of 4q, 6q, 8p, 9p, and 14 q and gains of 1q, 5q, and 7 have been observed. One group utilizing these methods to provide deep sequencing of over 3,000 known cancer-associated genes identified inactivating mutations in multiple genes that encode histone modification enzymes, including noted candidates *SETD2* and *JARID1C*, which were identified as mutational targets in multiple tumors in the study (136). The presence of mutations in histone modification enzymes could potentially alter gene expression due to the importance of histone function in DNA condensation and essential changes in chromatin structure. In this analysis, *NF2* mutations were also observed in tumors with intact *VHL*, suggesting some clues to the initiating events that can provide a surrogate for the tight association of ccRCC with *VHL* loss (136). The results of this study highlight the importance of broadening our exploration of RCC samples to genome-wide approaches.

To complete the extension of understanding RCC tumor biology from familial RCC, to sporadic disease, and back, a comparative study that used genome-wide approaches to explore the molecular classification of ccRCC analyzed genome-wide changes of copy number variations and gene expression profiles in both VHL-disease associated and sporadic ccRCC tumors was conducted (135). For copy number variation, 14 areas of nonrandom copy number change were observed, with equal incidence of deletion and amplification. When determining the relevant genes in these peaks, the analysis identified *VHL* deletion as a prevalent feature of both sets of tumors as expected. Interestingly, VHL disease-associated tumors were very homogeneous across tumor samples, suggesting that genetic divergence is less common among this tumor group. When compared to sporadic tumors, a subgroup was virtually indistinguishable from the familial set (135). This highlights the similarity of familial and sporadic forms of the disease. Further analysis remains to uncover important sources of somatic copy number change, but intriguingly, *CDKN2A* and *CDKN2B* were identified as potential genes in two of the deletion peaks commonly observed across familial and sporadic ccRCC tumors, and *MYC* was identified as the only gene in one amplification peak (135). Further studies of these datasets and the global efforts of many genome scientists are required to extend our understanding of the molecular pathogenesis of RCC.

Genetics of Non-Clear Cell Sporadic RCC Tumors

Because of the more limited prevalence of these tumors, our understanding of papillary and chromophobe tumors is comparably restrained. The application of modern genomic technologies to these tumor types does reinforce our appreciation of the highly dissimilar nature of these tumors from clear cell disease, but the genes involved in familial disease appear to more rarely contribute to sporadic tumors.

In understanding the genomic alterations that underlie chromophobe RCC, comparative studies have sought to distinguish this cancer from its histologically similar non-malignant cousin, oncocytoma. As discussed above, germ line inactivation of the BHD gene can contribute to the development of either of these cancers, but the participation of this gene in sporadic disease is largely unknown, although an initial evaluation suggests this event is not a common component of the sporadic disease (138). Comparative genomic studies, however, have identified high specificity of monosomies of chromosomes 1, 2, 6, 10, 13, 17, and 21 in the majority of chromophobe RCCs, while oncocytoma displayed more conservative losses limited to chromosome 1 and 14 (139). Similar cytogenetic studies using conventional karyotype analysis as well as microsatellite allelotyping have consistently demonstrated the abundant losses associated with this tumor (140,141), as well as the commonality of chromosome 1 loss with oncocytoma, suggesting these tumors may indeed share a common lineage. More recent single nucleotide polymorphism mapping further delineates the molecular divergence between these histologic subtypes (142).

In contrast, papillary RCCs have long been marked by copy number gains or trisomies, specifically in chromosomes 7 and 17 (143). An examination of genetic events associated with progression compared papillary renal adenomas, as a model of early stage disease, with papillary RCCs demonstrated that these invasive tumors displayed additional trisomies of 1q, 3q, 8q, 12q, 16q, and 20q (144). In particular, the acquisition of a 1q trisomy was thought to be synonymous with transition to invasive carcinoma, shedding light on a potentially important oncogene. The rarity of MET mutations in sporadic papillary renal cancer has already been noted. Further work combining expression profiling and genomic analysis has revealed common upregulation of myc gene expression in these tumors, although the underlying mechanisms have not been determined, and may be highly varied (145). Finally, the molecular determinants of the histologic type 1 and type 2 designations need to be identified.

■ SUMMARY

Clearly, the intense efforts of a global community of scientists have extended immeasurably our understanding of RCC tumor biology. The conventional histologic subtypes of RCC, clear cell, papillary (types 1 and 2), and chromophobe are clearly distinct genetic and biological diseases and warrant further discriminating analyses as we move toward biologically directed personalized therapy. The themes emerging, particularly in ccRCC of deregulation of hypoxia response signaling and specifically HIF-2α deregulation, provide a framework from which to understand critical steps in the path to invasive tumorigenesis and on which to support the future generations of molecularly targeted therapies.

■ REFERENCES

1. American Cancer Society. *Cancer Facts and Figures 2010*. Atlanta: American Cancer Society; 2010.
2. Chow WH, Devesa SS, Warren JL, Fraumeni JF Jr. Rising incidence of renal cell cancer in the United States. *JAMA* 1999;281(17):1628–1631.
3. Cohen HT, McGovern FJ. Renal-cell carcinoma. *N Engl J Med* 2005;353(23):2477–2490.
4. Linehan WM, Pinto PA, Bratslavsky G, et al. Hereditary kidney cancer: unique opportunity for disease-based therapy. *Cancer* 2009;115(10 suppl): 2252–2261.
5. Lonser RR, Glenn GM, Walther M, et al. von Hippel-Lindau disease. *Lancet* 2003;361(9374): 2059–2067.
6. Maher ER, Kaelin WG Jr. von Hippel-Lindau disease. *Medicine (Baltimore)* 1997;76(6):381–391.
7. Hippel EV. Ueber eine sehr seltene Erkrankung der Netzhaut. Klinische Beobachtungen. Klinische Beobachtungen. *Van Graefe's Archiv fuer Ophthalmologie* 1904;59:83.
8. Lindau A. Zur Frage der Angiomatosis Retinae und Ihrer Hirncomplikation. *Acta Ophthal* 1927; 4:193–226.
9. Grossniklaus HE, Thomas JW, Vigneswaran N, Jarrett WH 3rd. Retinal hemangioblastoma. A histologic, immunohistochemical, and ultrastructural evaluation. *Ophthalmology* 1992;99(1):140–145.
10. Filling-Katz MR, Choyke PL, Oldfield E, et al. Central nervous system involvement in Von Hippel-Lindau disease. *Neurology* 1991;41(1):41–46.
11. Sudarshan S, Linehan WM. Genetic basis of cancer of the kidney. *Semin Oncol* 2006;33(5):544–551.
12. Zbar B, Kishida T, Chen F, et al. Germline mutations in the Von Hippel-Lindau disease (VHL) gene in families from North America, Europe, and Japan. *Hum Mutat* 1996;8(4):348–357.
13. Chen F, Kishida T, Yao M, et al. Germline mutations in the von Hippel-Lindau disease tumor suppressor gene: correlations with phenotype. *Hum Mutat* 1995;5(1):66–75.
14. Maher ER, Yates JR, Harries R, et al. Clinical features and natural history of von Hippel-Lindau disease. *Q J Med* 1990;77(283):1151–1163.
15. Glenn GM, Choyke PL, Zbar B, et al. Von Hippel-Lindau disease: clinical review and molecular genetics. In: Anderson EE, ed. *Problems in Urologic Surgery: Benign and Malignant Tumors*. Philadelphia, PA: Lippincott; 1990:312.
16. Walther MM, Lubensky IA, Venzon D, Zbar B, Linehan WM. Prevalence of microscopic lesions in grossly normal renal parenchyma from patients with von Hippel-Lindau disease, sporadic renal cell carcinoma and no renal disease: clinical implications. *J Urol* 1995;154(6):2010–2014; discussion 2014.
17. Seizinger BR, Rouleau GA, Ozelius LJ, et al. Von Hippel-Lindau disease maps to the region of chromosome 3 associated with renal cell carcinoma. *Nature* 1988;332(6161):268–269.
18. Latif F, Tory K, Gnarra J, et al. Identification of the von Hippel-Lindau disease tumor suppressor gene. *Science* 1993;260(5112):1317–1320.
19. Renbaum P, Duh FM, Latif F, Zbar B, Lerman MI, Kuzmin I. Isolation and characterization of the full-length 3' untranslated region of the human von Hippel-Lindau tumor suppressor gene. *Hum Genet* 1996;98(6):666–671.
20. Iliopoulos O, Kibel A, Gray S, Kaelin WG Jr. Tumour suppression by the human von Hippel-Lindau gene product. *Nat Med* 1995;1(8):822–826.
21. Richards FM, Schofield PN, Fleming S, Maher ER. Expression of the von Hippel-Lindau disease tumour suppressor gene during human embryogenesis. *Hum Mol Genet* 1996;5(5):639–644.
22. Gnarra JR, Tory K, Weng Y, et al. Mutations of the VHL tumour suppressor gene in renal carcinoma. *Nat Genet* 1994;7(1):85–90.
23. Crossey PA, Richards FM, Foster K, et al. Identification of intragenic mutations in the von

Hippel-Lindau disease tumour suppressor gene and correlation with disease phenotype. *Hum Mol Genet* 1994;3(8):1303–1308.

24. Maher ER, Webster AR, Richards FM, et al. Phenotypic expression in von Hippel-Lindau disease: correlations with germline VHL gene mutations. *J Med Genet* 1996;33(4):328–332.

25. Richards FM, Crossey PA, Phipps ME, et al. Detailed mapping of germline deletions of the von Hippel-Lindau disease tumour suppressor gene. *Hum Mol Genet* 1994;3(4):595–598.

26. Whaley JM, Naglich J, Gelbert L, et al. Germ-line mutations in the von Hippel-Lindau tumor-suppressor gene are similar to somatic von Hippel-Lindau aberrations in sporadic renal cell carcinoma. *Am J Hum Genet* 1994;55(6):1092–1102.

27. Kibel A, Iliopoulos O, DeCaprio JA, Kaelin WG Jr. Binding of the von Hippel-Lindau tumor suppressor protein to Elongin B and C. *Science* 1995;269(5229):1444–1446.

28. Kishida T, Stackhouse TM, Chen F, Lerman MI, Zbar B. Cellular proteins that bind the von Hippel-Lindau disease gene product: mapping of binding domains and the effect of missense mutations. *Cancer Res* 1995;55(20):4544–4548.

29. Richards FM, Payne SJ, Zbar B, Affara NA, Ferguson-Smith MA, Maher ER. Molecular analysis of de novo germline mutations in the von Hippel-Lindau disease gene. *Hum Mol Genet* 1995;4(11):2139–2143.

30. Brauch H, Kishida T, Glavac D, et al. Von Hippel-Lindau (VHL) disease with pheochromocytoma in the Black Forest region of Germany: evidence for a founder effect. *Hum Genet* 1995;95(5):551–556.

31. Corless CL, Kibel AS, Iliopoulos O, Kaelin WG Jr. Immunostaining of the von Hippel-Lindau gene product in normal and neoplastic human tissues. *Hum Pathol* 1997;28(4):459–464.

32. Lee S, Chen DY, Humphrey JS, Gnarra JR, Linehan WM, Klausner RD. Nuclear/cytoplasmic localization of the von Hippel-Lindau tumor suppressor gene product is determined by cell density. *Proc Natl Acad Sci USA* 1996;93(5):1770–1775.

33. Los M, Jansen GH, Kaelin WG, Lips CJ, Blijham GH, Voest EE. Expression pattern of the von Hippel-Lindau protein in human tissues. *Lab Invest* 1996;75(2):231–238.

34. Kamura T, Brower CS, Conaway RC, Conaway JW. A molecular basis for stabilization of the von Hippel-Lindau (VHL) tumor suppressor protein by components of the VHL ubiquitin ligase. *J Biol Chem* 2002;277(33):30388–30393.

35. Jaakkola P, Mole DR, Tian YM, et al. Targeting of HIF-alpha to the von Hippel-Lindau ubiquitylation complex by O2-regulated prolyl hydroxylation. *Science* 2001;292(5516):468–472.

36. Ivan M, Kondo K, Yang H, et al. HIFalpha targeted for VHL-mediated destruction by proline hydroxylation: implications for O2 sensing. *Science* 2001;292(5516):464–468.

37. Nickerson ML, Jaeger E, Shi Y, et al. Improved identification of von Hippel-Lindau gene alterations in clear cell renal tumors. *Clin Cancer Res* 2008;14(15):4726–4734.

38. Osborne JP, Fryer A, Webb D. Epidemiology of tuberous sclerosis. *Ann N Y Acad Sci* 1991;615:125–127.

39. Levy M, Feingold J. Estimating prevalence in single-gene kidney diseases progressing to renal failure. *Kidney Int* 2000;58(3):925–943.

40. Rose VM, Au KS, Pollom G, Roach ES, Prashner HR, Northrup H. Germ-line mosaicism in tuberous sclerosis: how common? *Am J Hum Genet* 1999;64(4):986–992.

41. Kwiatkowska J, Wigowska-Sowinska J, Napierala D, Slomski R, Kwiatkowski DJ. Mosaicism in tuberous sclerosis as a potential cause of the failure of molecular diagnosis. *N Engl J Med* 1999;340(9):703–707.

42. Verhoef S, Bakker L, Tempelaars AM, et al. High rate of mosaicism in tuberous sclerosis complex. *Am J Hum Genet* 1999;64(6):1632–1637.

43. Casper KA, Donnelly LF, Chen B, Bissler JJ. Tuberous sclerosis complex: renal imaging findings. *Radiology* 2002;225(2):451–456.

44. Ewalt DH, Sheffield E, Sparagana SP, Delgado MR, Roach ES. Renal lesion growth in children with tuberous sclerosis complex. *J Urol* 1998;160(1):141–145.

45. Stillwell TJ, Gomez MR, Kelalis PP. Renal lesions in tuberous sclerosis. *J Urol* 1987;138(3):477–481.

46. O'Callaghan FJ, Noakes MJ, Martyn CN, Osborne JP. An epidemiological study of renal pathology in tuberous sclerosis complex. *BJU Int* 2004;94(6):853–857.

47. Rakowski SK, Winterkorn EB, Paul E, Steele DJ, Halpern EF, Thiele EA. Renal manifestations of tuberous sclerosis complex: Incidence, prognosis, and predictive factors. *Kidney Int* 2006;70(10):1777–1782.

48. van Baal JG, Smits NJ, Keeman JN, Lindhout D, Verhoef S. The evolution of renal angiomyolipomas in patients with tuberous sclerosis. *J Urol* 1994;152(1):35–38.

49. Shepherd CW, Gomez MR, Lie JT, Crowson CS. Causes of death in patients with tuberous sclerosis. *Mayo Clin Proc* 1991;66(8):792–796.

50. Orlova KA, Crino PB. The tuberous sclerosis complex. *Ann N Y Acad Sci* 2010;1184:87–105.

51. Kandt RS, Haines JL, Smith M, et al. Linkage of an important gene locus for tuberous sclerosis to a chromosome 16 marker for polycystic kidney disease. *Nat Genet* 1992;2(1):37–41.

52. Maheshwar MM, Cheadle JP, Jones AC, et al. The GAP-related domain of tuberin, the product of the TSC2 gene, is a target for missense mutations in tuberous sclerosis. *Hum Mol Genet* 1997;6(11):1991–1996.

53. van Slegtenhorst M, Nellist M, Nagelkerken B, et al. Interaction between hamartin and tuberin, the TSC1 and TSC2 gene products. *Hum Mol Genet* 1998;7(6):1053–1057.

54. Saucedo LJ, Gao X, Chiarelli DA, Li L, Pan D, Edgar BA. Rheb promotes cell growth as a component of the insulin/TOR signalling network. *Nat Cell Biol* 2003;5(6):566–571.

55. Stocker H, Radimerski T, Schindelholz B, et al. Rheb is an essential regulator of S6K in controlling cell growth in Drosophila. *Nat Cell Biol* 2003;5(6):559–565.

56. Zhang Y, Gao X, Saucedo LJ, Ru B, Edgar BA, Pan D. Rheb is a direct target of the tuberous sclerosis tumour suppressor proteins. *Nat Cell Biol* 2003;5(6):578–581.

57. Garami A, Zwartkruis FJ, Nobukuni T, et al. Insulin activation of Rheb, a mediator of mTOR/S6K/4E-BP signaling, is inhibited by TSC1 and 2. *Mol Cell* 2003;11(6):1457–1466.

58. Inoki K, Li Y, Xu T, Guan KL. Rheb GTPase is a direct target of TSC2 GAP activity and regulates mTOR signaling. *Genes Dev* 2003;17(15):1829–1834.

59. Tee AR, Manning BD, Roux PP, Cantley LC, Blenis J. Tuberous sclerosis complex gene products, Tuberin and Hamartin, control mTOR signaling by acting as a GTPase-activating protein complex toward Rheb. *Curr Biol* 2003;13(15):1259–1268.

60. Castro AF, Rebhun JF, Clark GJ, Quilliam LA. Rheb binds tuberous sclerosis complex 2 (TSC2) and promotes S6 kinase activation in a rapamycin- and farnesylation-dependent manner. *J Biol Chem* 2003;278(35):32493–32496.

61. Martin DE, Hall MN. The expanding TOR signaling network. *Curr Opin Cell Biol* 2005;17(2):158–166.

62. Tee AR, Blenis J. mTOR, translational control and human disease. *Semin Cell Dev Biol* 2005;16(1):29–37.

63. Sarbassov DD, Guertin DA, Ali SM, Sabatini DM. Phosphorylation and regulation of Akt/PKB by the rictor-mTOR complex. *Science* 2005;307(5712):1098–1101.

64. Sarbassov DD, Ali SM, Kim DH, et al. Rictor, a novel binding partner of mTOR, defines a rapamycin-insensitive and raptor-independent pathway that regulates the cytoskeleton. *Curr Biol* 2004;14(14):1296–1302.

65. Jacinto E, Loewith R, Schmidt A, et al. Mammalian TOR complex 2 controls the actin cytoskeleton and is rapamycin insensitive. *Nat Cell Biol* 2004;6(11):1122–1128.

66. Loewith R, Jacinto E, Wullschleger S, et al. Two TOR complexes, only one of which is rapamycin sensitive, have distinct roles in cell growth control. *Mol Cell* 2002;10(3):457–468.

67. Hara K, Maruki Y, Long X, et al. Raptor, a binding partner of target of rapamycin (TOR), mediates TOR action. *Cell* 2002;110(2):177–189.

68. Kim DH, Sarbassov DD, Ali SM, et al. mTOR interacts with raptor to form a nutrient-sensitive complex that signals to the cell growth machinery. *Cell* 2002;110(2):163–175.

69. Kim DH, Sarbassov DD, Ali SM, et al. GbetaL, a positive regulator of the rapamycin-sensitive pathway required for the nutrient-sensitive interaction between raptor and mTOR. *Mol Cell* 2003;11(4):895–904.

70. Fingar DC, Blenis J. Target of rapamycin (TOR): an integrator of nutrient and growth factor signals and coordinator of cell growth and cell cycle progression. *Oncogene* 2004;23(18):3151–3171.

71. Nobukini T, Thomas G. The mTOR/S6K signalling pathway: the role of the TSC1/2 tumour suppressor complex and the proto-oncogene Rheb. *Novartis Found Symp* 2004;262:148–54; discussion 154.

72. Pan D, Dong J, Zhang Y, Gao X. Tuberous sclerosis complex: from Drosophila to human disease. *Trends Cell Biol* 2004;14(2):78–85.

73. Findlay GM, Harrington LS, Lamb RF. TSC1–2 tumour suppressor and regulation of mTOR signalling: linking cell growth and proliferation? *Curr Opin Genet Dev* 2005;15(1):69–76.

74. Inoki K, Corradetti MN, Guan KL. Dysregulation of the TSC-mTOR pathway in human disease. *Nat Genet* 2005;37(1):19–24.

75. Thomas GV, Tran C, Mellinghoff IK, et al. Hypoxia-inducible factor determines sensitivity to inhibitors of mTOR in kidney cancer. *Nat Med* 2006;12(1):122–127.

76. Toschi A, Lee E, Gadir N, Ohh M, Foster DA. Differential dependence of hypoxia-inducible factors 1 alpha and 2 alpha on mTORC1 and mTORC2. *J Biol Chem* 2008;283(50):34495–34499.

77. Amin MB, Amin MB, Tamboli P, et al. Prognostic impact of histologic subtyping of adult renal epithelial

neoplasms: an experience of 405 cases. *Am J Surg Pathol* 2002;26(3):281–291.

78. Cheville JC, Lohse CM, Zincke H, Weaver AL, Blute ML. Comparisons of outcome and prognostic features among histologic subtypes of renal cell carcinoma. *Am J Surg Pathol* 2003;27(5):612–624.

79. Zbar B, Tory K, Merino M, et al. Hereditary papillary renal cell carcinoma. *J Urol* 1994;151(3):561–566.

80. Zbar B, Glenn G, Lubensky I, et al. Hereditary papillary renal cell carcinoma: clinical studies in 10 families. *J Urol* 1995;153(3 Pt 2):907–912.

81. Schmidt LS, Nickerson ML, Angeloni D, et al. Early onset hereditary papillary renal carcinoma: germline missense mutations in the tyrosine kinase domain of the met proto-oncogene. *J Urol* 2004;172(4 Pt 1):1256–1261.

82. Mukhopadhyay D, Knebelmann B, Cohen HT, Ananth S, Sukhatme VP. The von Hippel-Lindau tumor suppressor gene product interacts with Sp1 to repress vascular endothelial growth factor promoter activity. *Mol Cell Biol* 1997;17(9):5629–5639.

83. Schmidt L, Duh FM, Chen F, et al. Germline and somatic mutations in the tyrosine kinase domain of the MET proto-oncogene in papillary renal carcinomas. *Nat Genet* 1997;16(1):68–73.

84. Schmidt L, Junker K, Weirich G, et al. Two North American families with hereditary papillary renal carcinoma and identical novel mutations in the MET proto-oncogene. *Cancer Res* 1998;58(8):1719–1722.

85. Linehan WM, Vasselli J, Srinivasan R, et al. Genetic basis of cancer of the kidney: disease-specific approaches to therapy. *Clin Cancer Res* 2004;10(18 Pt 2):6282S–6289S.

86. Michalopoulos GK, DeFrances MC. Liver regeneration. *Science* 1997;276(5309):60–66.

87. Zhuang Z, Park WS, Pack S, et al. Trisomy 7-harbouring non-random duplication of the mutant MET allele in hereditary papillary renal carcinomas. *Nat Genet* 1998;20(1):66–69.

88. Kovacs G. Molecular cytogenetics of renal cell tumors. *Adv Cancer Res* 1993;62:89–124.

89. Schmidt L, Junker K, Nakaigawa N, et al. Novel mutations of the MET proto-oncogene in papillary renal carcinomas. *Oncogene* 1999;18(14):2343–2350.

90. Launonen V, Vierimaa O, Kiuru M, et al. Inherited susceptibility to uterine leiomyomas and renal cell cancer. *Proc Natl Acad Sci USA* 2001;98(6):3387–3392.

91. Reed WB, Walker R, Horowitz R. Cutaneous leiomyomata with uterine leiomyomata. *Acta Derm Venereol* 1973;53(5):409–416.

92. Toro JR, Nickerson ML, Wei MH, et al. Mutations in the fumarate hydratase gene cause hereditary leiomyomatosis and renal cell cancer in families in North America. *Am J Hum Genet* 2003;73(1):95–106.

93. Wei MH, Toure O, Glenn GM, et al. Novel mutations in FH and expansion of the spectrum of phenotypes expressed in families with hereditary leiomyomatosis and renal cell cancer. *J Med Genet* 2006;43(1):18–27.

94. Grubb RL 3rd, Franks ME, Toro J, et al. Hereditary leiomyomatosis and renal cell cancer: a syndrome associated with an aggressive form of inherited renal cancer. *J Urol* 2007;177(6):2074–9; discussion 2079.

95. Baysal BE, Ferrell RE, Willett-Brozick JE, et al. Mutations in SDHD, a mitochondrial complex II gene, in hereditary paraganglioma. *Science* 2000;287(5454):848–851.

96. Niemann S, Müller U. Mutations in SDHC cause autosomal dominant paraganglioma, type 3. *Nat Genet* 2000;26(3):268–270.

97. Astuti D, Latif F, Dallol A, et al. Gene mutations in the succinate dehydrogenase subunit SDHB cause susceptibility to familial pheochromocytoma and to familial paraganglioma. *Am J Hum Genet* 2001;69(1):49–54.

98. Mazzone M, Basilico C, Cavassa S, et al. An uncleavable form of pro-scatter factor suppresses tumor growth and dissemination in mice. *J Clin Invest* 2004;114(10):1418–1432.

99. Tomlinson IP, Alam NA, Rowan AJ, et al.; Multiple Leiomyoma Consortium. Germline mutations in FH predispose to dominantly inherited uterine fibroids, skin leiomyomata and papillary renal cell cancer. *Nat Genet* 2002;30(4):406–410.

100. Kaelin WG. Proline hydroxylation and gene expression. *Annu Rev Biochem* 2005;74:115–128.

101. Isaacs JS, Jung YJ, Mole DR, et al. HIF overexpression correlates with biallelic loss of fumarate hydratase in renal cancer: novel role of fumarate in regulation of HIF stability. *Cancer Cell* 2005;8(2):143–153.

102. Birt AR, Hogg GR, Dubé WJ. Hereditary multiple fibrofolliculomas with trichodiscomas and acrochordons. *Arch Dermatol* 1977;113(12):1674–1677.

103. Menko FH, van Steensel MA, Giraud S, et al.; European BHD Consortium. Birt-Hogg-Dubé syndrome: diagnosis and management. *Lancet Oncol* 2009;10(12):1199–1206.

104. Roth JS, Rabinowitz AD, Benson M, Grossman ME. Bilateral renal cell carcinoma in the Birt-Hogg-Dubé syndrome. *J Am Acad Dermatol* 1993;29(6):1055–1056.

105. Pavlovich CP, Walther MM, Eyler RA, et al. Renal tumors in the Birt-Hogg-Dubé syndrome. *Am J Surg Pathol* 2002;26(12):1542–1552.

106. Pavlovich CP, Grubb RL 3rd, Hurley K, et al. Evaluation and management of renal tumors in the Birt-Hogg-Dubé syndrome. *J Urol* 2005;173(5):1482–1486.

107. Souza CA, Finley R, Müller NL. Birt-Hogg-Dubé syndrome: a rare cause of pulmonary cysts. *AJR Am J Roentgenol* 2005;185(5):1237–1239.

108. Zbar B, Alvord WG, Glenn G, et al. Risk of renal and colonic neoplasms and spontaneous pneumothorax in the Birt-Hogg-Dubé syndrome. *Cancer Epidemiol Biomarkers Prev* 2002;11(4):393–400.

109. Toro JR, Wei MH, Glenn GM, et al. BHD mutations, clinical and molecular genetic investigations of Birt-Hogg-Dubé syndrome: a new series of 50 families and a review of published reports. *J Med Genet* 2008;45(6):321–331.

110. Toro JR, Pautler SE, Stewart L, et al. Lung cysts, spontaneous pneumothorax, and genetic associations in 89 families with Birt-Hogg-Dubé syndrome. *Am J Respir Crit Care Med* 2007;175(10):1044–1053.

111. Sahn SA, Heffner JE. Spontaneous pneumothorax. *N Engl J Med* 2000;342(12):868–874.

112. Grant LA, Babar J, Griffin N. Cysts, cavities, and honeycombing in multisystem disorders: differential diagnosis and findings on thin-section CT. *Clin Radiol* 2009;64(4):439–448.

113. Khoo SK, Bradley M, Wong FK, Hedblad MA, Nordenskjöld M, Teh BT. Birt-Hogg-Dubé syndrome: mapping of a novel hereditary neoplasia gene to chromosome 17p12-q11.2. *Oncogene* 2001;20(37):5239–5242.

114. Schmidt LS, Warren MB, Nickerson ML, et al. Birt-Hogg-Dubé syndrome, a genodermatosis associated with spontaneous pneumothorax and kidney neoplasia, maps to chromosome 17p11.2. *Am J Hum Genet* 2001;69(4):876–882.

115. Nickerson ML, Warren MB, Toro JR, et al. Mutations in a novel gene lead to kidney tumors, lung wall defects, and benign tumors of the hair follicle in patients with the Birt-Hogg-Dubé syndrome. *Cancer Cell* 2002;2(2):157–164.

116. Schmidt LS, Nickerson ML, Warren MB, et al. Germline BHD-mutation spectrum and phenotype analysis of a large cohort of families with Birt-Hogg-Dubé syndrome. *Am J Hum Genet* 2005;76(6):1023–1033.

117. Ren HZ, Zhu CC, Yang C, et al. Mutation analysis of the FLCN gene in Chinese patients with sporadic and familial isolated primary spontaneous pneumothorax. *Clin Genet* 2008;74(2):178–183.

118. Gunji Y, Akiyoshi T, Sato T, et al. Mutations of the Birt Hogg Dube gene in patients with multiple lung cysts and recurrent pneumothorax. *J Med Genet* 2007;44(9):588–593.

119. Vocke CD, Yang Y, Pavlovich CP, et al. High frequency of somatic frameshift BHD gene mutations in Birt-Hogg-Dubé-associated renal tumors. *J Natl Cancer Inst* 2005;97(12):931–935.

120. Warren MB, Torres-Cabala CA, Turner ML, et al. Expression of Birt-Hogg-Dubé gene mRNA in normal and neoplastic human tissues. *Mod Pathol* 2004;17(8):998–1011.

121. van Steensel MA, Verstraeten VL, Frank J, et al. Novel mutations in the BHD gene and absence of loss of heterozygosity in fibrofolliculomas of Birt-Hogg-Dubé patients. *J Invest Dermatol* 2007;127(3):588–593.

122. Baba M, Hong SB, Sharma N, et al. Folliculin encoded by the BHD gene interacts with a binding protein, FNIP1, and AMPK, and is involved in AMPK and mTOR signaling. *Proc Natl Acad Sci USA* 2006;103(42):15552–15557.

123. Hasumi H, Baba M, Hong SB, et al. Identification and characterization of a novel folliculin-interacting protein FNIP2. *Gene* 2008;415(1–2):60–67.

124. Takagi Y, Kobayashi T, Shiono M, et al. Interaction of folliculin (Birt-Hogg-Dubé gene product) with a novel Fnip1-like (FnipL/Fnip2) protein. *Oncogene* 2008;27(40):5339–5347.

125. Baba M, Furihata M, Hong SB, et al. Kidney-targeted Birt-Hogg-Dube gene inactivation in a mouse model: Erk1/2 and Akt-mTOR activation, cell hyperproliferation, and polycystic kidneys. *J Natl Cancer Inst* 2008;100(2):140–154.

126. Chen J, Futami K, Petillo D, et al. Deficiency of FLCN in mouse kidney led to development of polycystic kidneys and renal neoplasia. *PLoS ONE* 2008;3(10):e3581.

127. van Slegtenhorst M, Khabibullin D, Hartman TR, Nicolas E, Kruger WD, Henske EP. The Birt-Hogg-Dube and tuberous sclerosis complex homologs have opposing roles in amino acid homeostasis in Schizosaccharomyces pombe. *J Biol Chem* 2007;282(34):24583–24590.

128. Hartman TR, Nicolas E, Klein-Szanto A, et al. The role of the Birt-Hogg-Dubé protein in mTOR activation and renal tumorigenesis. *Oncogene* 2009;28(13):1594–1604.

129. Gordan JD, Lal P, Dondeti VR, et al. HIF-alpha effects on c-Myc distinguish two subtypes of sporadic VHL-deficient clear cell renal carcinoma. *Cancer Cell* 2008;14(6):435–446.

130. Hu CJ, Wang LY, Chodosh LA, Keith B, Simon MC. Differential roles of hypoxia-inducible factor 1alpha (HIF-1alpha) and HIF-2alpha in hypoxic gene regulation. *Mol Cell Biol* 2003;23(24):9361–9374.

131. Brannon AR, Rathmell WK. Renal cell carcinoma: where will the state-of-the-art lead us? *Curr Oncol Rep* 2010;12(3):193–201.

132. Zhao H, Ljungberg B, Grankvist K, Rasmuson T, Tibshirani R, Brooks JD. Gene expression profiling predicts survival in conventional renal cell carcinoma. *PLoS Med* 2006;3(1):e13.

133. Zhao H, Zongming Ma, Tibshirani R, Higgins JP, Ljungberg B, Brooks JD. Alteration of gene expression signatures of cortical differentiation and wound response in lethal clear cell renal cell carcinomas. *PLoS ONE* 2009;4(6):e6039.

134. Rini BI, Zhou M, Aydin H, et al. Identification of prognostic genomic markers in patients with localized clear cell renal cell carcinoma (ccRCC). *J Clin Oncol* 2010;28:15s.

135. Beroukhim R, Brunet JP, Di Napoli A, et al. Patterns of gene expression and copy-number alterations in von-Hippel-Lindau disease-associated and sporadic clear cell carcinoma of the kidney. *Cancer Res* 2009;69(11):4674–4681.

136. Dalgliesh GL, Furge K, Greenman C, et al. Systematic sequencing of renal carcinoma reveals inactivation of histone modifying genes. *Nature* 2010;463(7279):360–363.

137. Pei J, Feder MM, Al-Saleem T, et al. Combined classical cytogenetics and microarray-based genomic copy number analysis reveal frequent 3;5 rearrangements in clear cell renal cell carcinoma. *Genes Chromosomes Cancer* 2010;49(7):610–619.

138. Nagy A, Zoubakov D, Stupar Z, Kovacs G. Lack of mutation of the folliculin gene in sporadic chromophobe renal cell carcinoma and renal oncocytoma. *Int J Cancer* 2004;109(3):472–475.

139. Yusenko MV, Kuiper RP, Boethe T, Ljungberg B, van Kessel AG, Kovacs G. High-resolution DNA copy number and gene expression analyses distinguish chromophobe renal cell carcinomas and renal oncocytomas. *BMC Cancer* 2009;9:152.

140. Nagy A, Buzogany I, Kovacs G. Microsatellite allelotyping differentiates chromophobe renal cell carcinomas from renal oncocytomas and identifies new genetic changes. *Histopathology* 2004;44(6):542–546.

141. Bugert P, Kovacs G. Molecular differential diagnosis of renal cell carcinomas by microsatellite analysis. *Am J Pathol* 1996;149(6):2081–2088.

142. Tan MH, Wong CF, Tan HL, et al. Genomic expression and single-nucleotide polymorphism profiling discriminates chromophobe renal cell carcinoma and oncocytoma. *BMC Cancer* 2010;10:196.

143. Balint I, Szponar A, Jauch A, Kovacs G. Trisomy 7 and 17 mark papillary renal cell tumours irrespectively of variation of the phenotype. *J Clin Pathol* 2009;62(10):892–895.

144. Szponar A, Zubakov D, Pawlak J, Jauch A, Kovacs G. Three genetic developmental stages of papillary renal cell tumors: duplication of chromosome 1q marks fatal progression. *Int J Cancer* 2009;124(9):2071–2076.

145. Furge KA, Chen J, Koeman J, et al. Detection of DNA copy number changes and oncogenic signaling abnormalities from gene expression data reveals MYC activation in high-grade papillary renal cell carcinoma. *Cancer Res* 2007;67(7):3171–3176.

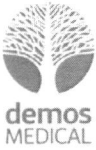

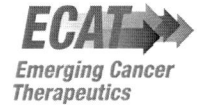

Renal Cell Carcinoma: Current Concepts of Morphologic Subclassification and Clinical Relevance

Tatjana Antic* and Jerome B. Taxy

The University of Chicago, Chicago, IL

■ ABSTRACT

The classification of renal tumors was initiated by Konig in 1826. The current concepts of renal cell carcinoma (RCC) have progressed from the "hypernephroma" proposed by Grawitz to a multitiered classification still evolving. The present classification relies heavily on conventional H&E morphology, although the WHO integrates cytogenetic and molecular findings. Although the histologic subclassification and grading of RCC has clinical relevance, many authors still emphasize stage as the most important prognostic factor. The present review will summarize the current histologic and ancillary features of each major and some less frequent variants of RCC. Since the first nephrectomy by Simon in 1869 demonstrating that patients could live with only one kidney, surgery remains the major treatment option for RCC. The more frequent incidental discovery of small renal tumors has resulted in the increasing use of partial nephrectomy and tumor ablation in place of the standard radical nephrectomy without compromising survival. Newly discovered RCCs with specific chromosomal translocations have offered hope that targeted therapies may be available and especially applicable to patients with metastatic disease.

Keywords: renal cell carcinoma, histologic subtypes, immunohistochemical stains

*Corresponding author, Department of Pathology, The University of Chicago, 5841 S. Maryland Ave, P-631, MC 6101, Chicago, IL 60637
   E-mail address: tatjana.antic@uchospitals.edu

Emerging Cancer Therapeutics 2:1 (2011) 21–36.
DOI: 10.5003/2151–4194.2.1.21

■ INTRODUCTION

Renal cell carcinoma (RCC; renal adenocarcinoma) is ranked as the 14th most common malignancy worldwide (1), accounting for 3% of all adult malignancies and is the most common renal tumor (2). The incidence of RCC in the United States continues to rise, possibly reflecting incidental discoveries during imaging workups for nonspecific abdominal symptoms. Kidney cancer mortalities have leveled, also possibly due to early detection of incidental, often early-stage tumors (3).

The classification of RCC, first proposed by Konig in 1826 (4), has progressed from a monomorphic concept to an appreciation of a histologically heterogeneous group of tumors that is principally subclassified according to cell type by standard hematoxylin and eosin morphology. Ancillary techniques currently supplement the standard approach and include immunohistochemistry, cytogenetics, and molecular studies. The effort to encompass all this data is reflected in the current World Health Organization (WHO) renal tumor classification (5). The three dominant, commonly recognized, and WHO-accepted entities include conventional (clear cell), papillary, and chromophobe. Less frequent histologic types are collecting duct and medullary, mucinous, tubular and spindle cell, translocation, and RCC associated with neuroblastoma. In addition,

new RCC variants have been described, that is, tubulocystic; acquired cystic disease-associated; papillary clear cell, oncocytic papillary, and thyroid-like follicular RCC (Table 1). Each of these entities exhibits characteristic microscopic features and some possess specific cytogenetic and molecular signatures.

As a practical matter, the diagnosis in most RCC is based on standard histomorphology. In this context, it is now recognized that sarcomatoid transformation, once thought to represent a specific tumor cell type, is a potential histologic feature of all cell types of RCC. Although numerous immunohistochemical stains are available to study RCC, their true diagnostic utility is exceptional, possibly restricted to TFE3 and TFEB. Nonetheless, the various immunohistochemical stains do support and confirm the original standard histological impression. Infrequently, molecular techniques are required.

This new era in RCC classification is influenced by and parallels the development of new therapies. For example, from the time of the first nephrectomy by Simon in 1869, demonstrating that patients could live with one kidney, radical nephrectomy has been the standard of surgical therapy. With smaller, incidentally discovered tumors and increasing numbers of patients with renal insufficiency, partial nephrectomy has become popular with no apparent deleterious consequences (6,7).

TABLE 1 Renal cell carcinoma classification

WHO-Accepted RCC Types	Newly Described RCC Types Not Included in WHO
Clear cell RCC	Tubulocystic RCC
Multilocular clear cell RCC	Oncocytic papillary RCC
Papillary RCC	Acquired cystic disease-related RCC
Chromophobe RCC	Clear cell papillary RCC
Carcinoma of the collecting ducts of Bellini	Thyroid follicular carcinoma-like RCC
Renal medullary carcinoma	
Xp11 translocation carcinomas	
Carcinoma associated with neuroblastoma	
Mucinous tubular and spindle cell carcinoma	

RCC, renal cell carcinoma.

In addition, based on respective gene signatures, targeted chemotherapy and immunotherapy for certain RCCs are becoming available. Different histologic types, sometimes associated with certain clinical parameters, may imply prognostic significance (8), possibly insufficiently conveyed through the traditional TNM system (9,10). In current practice, given ongoing treatment developments and the inherent communication demands among physicians caring for RCC patients, the subclassification of RCC has become essential for the surgical pathologist in the reporting of these tumors, both the common and newly described types. The degree to which a diagnosis may require study or confirmation by ancillary techniques has not yet become a major treatment issue. The subclassification of RCC will be the focus of this review.

■ CONVENTIONAL/CLEAR CELL RCC

The first description of what is now recognized as conventional (clear cell) RCC was by Grawitz, who believed that the tumor arose from heterotopic adrenal rests in the kidney. RCC has been historically referred to as a "Grawitz tumor," and as a result of his concept of tumor origin, the unfortunate term "hypernephroma" was employed for many years. It is now generally accepted that RCC is a tumor of the renal cortex, possibly representing a neoplasm of proximal tubular epithelium. The cytoplasmic clarity responsible for the term "clear cell" represents a fixation and processing artifact, removing the abundant intracytoplasmic lipid and glycogen characteristic of this variant, leaving "empty" cytoplasm. In addition, ultrastructurally clear cell carcinoma in metastatic sites has the capacity to recreate the organized microvilli of the proximal tubular brush border (11). Clear cell carcinoma also encompasses or coexists with cells having dense, granular eosinophilic cytoplasm. The term "conventional" was proposed to include both cell types.

Clear cell RCC is the most common histologic type and accounts for more than 70% of all RCCs. Most cases occur in adults older than 40 years of age; men are affected more frequently than women (a ratio of approximately 1.5:1). The connection of clear RCC with a genetic abnormality is well established and best studied in patients with the von Hippel-Lindau (VHL) syndrome caused by the germline mutations in the VHL tumor suppressor gene. VHL inactivation is involved in the development of either sporadic or hereditary forms (12). One of the effects of VHL inactivation is activated angiogenesis due to an accumulation of hypoxia-inducible-factor (HIF-α), causing upregulation of vascular endothelial growth factor (VEGF) and other factors (see Chapter 1). In addition to correlating with the well-recognized histologic vascularity of RCC, these growth factors have been used to develop VEGF pathway-specific therapies (see Chapter 8).

Grossly, most sporadic clear cell RCCs are solitary, solid tumors, occasionally extensively cystic or hemorrhagic and necrotic, randomly localized in the renal cortex (Figure 1). Only 4% are multicentric. The presence of bilateral and multifocal tumors in patients less than 40 years of age suggests a hereditary origin. The tumors are commonly yellow due to lipid content. Depending on size, tumors are localized to the kidney or protrude into the perinephric or renal sinus adipose tissue with or without renal vein involvement. All of these parameters are important for staging purposes and together with Fuhrman nuclear grading (13) form the basis for prognosis.

Histologically, clear cell RCC exhibits growth as solid nests in alveolar, tubular, or acinar arrangements, composed of polygonal cells with sharp cell outlines and clear to variably granular cytoplasm (Figure 2). The characteristic rich vascularity consists of thin-walled blood vessels. Papillary or pseudopapillary architecture is rare. Fibrosis, hyalinization, and occasional osseous metaplasia may be present in large, low-grade tumors. Conventional morphology is the most important tool to distinguish this tumor type from other RCCs. Numerous immunohistochemical studies have shown a variety of antigens being positive in clear cell RCC.

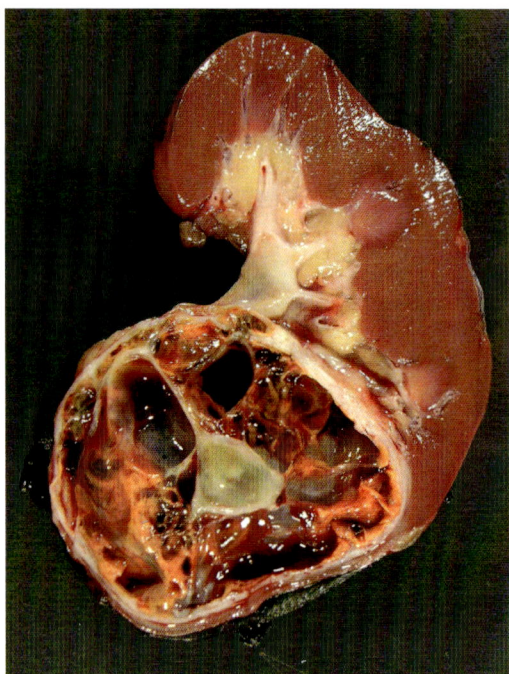

FIGURE 1
Extensively cystic and loculated typically orange-yellow clear cell renal cell carcinoma, involving cortex and renal pelvis.

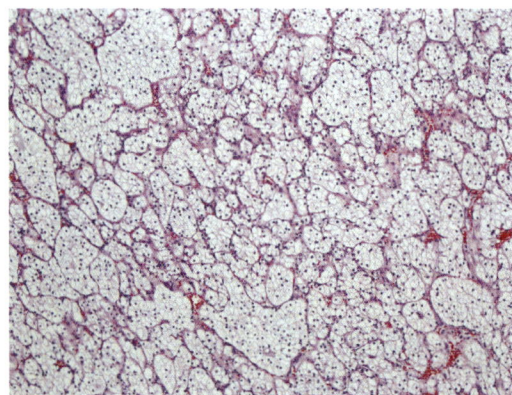

FIGURE 2
Clear cell renal cell carcinoma showing acinar arrangement. A plethora of thin-walled capillaries divide nests of tumor cells with low-grade nuclear features.

The most diagnostically helpful may be a combination of pankeratin (AE1/AE3, Cam 5.2) and vimentin; CK7, P504S (racemase), and TFE3 are typically absent. EMA, CD10, CA-IX, and RCC are also commonly positive; however, their additional value to the immunohistochemical profile is questionable.

Multilocular cystic RCC is considered a subtype of clear cell RCC with an excellent prognosis (5). The well-defined morphologic features include the septations of the cyst locules lined by the typical polygonal cells with flattened shapes, clear to pale cytoplasm. The thin septae may contain varying sized aggregates of clear tumor cells which do not form a tumor mass. The tumor nuclei are typically of Fuhrman grade 1. In support of these tumors being considered a clear cell variant is a recent report in which 74% of multilocular cystic RCCs had chromosome 3p deletions (14). However, there are no reports of recurrent or metastatic behavior, perhaps raising the issue of the validity of classifying these cystic lesions as malignant.

■ PAPILLARY RCC

The currently recognized specific morphologic, immunohistochemical, cytogenetic, and molecular features of papillary renal cell carcinoma (PRCC) (15–17) have followed its initial recognition in 1976 as a separate entity in the study by Mancilla-Jimenez et al. who described 34 cases (18). PRCC accounts for 10% to 15% of RCCs. It is more often multifocal and bilateral than other subtypes. In cytogenetic studies, it is characterized by polysomies, especially trisomies of chromosomes 7 and 17. The hereditary form of PRCC has a germline mutation of the proto-oncogene MET at 7q31 (19). In one study, trisomy of chromosome 7 (containing the MET gene and its ligand hepatocyte growth factor) was found in 75% of sporadic PRCC. However, since trisomy of chromosome 7 is found in otherwise normal renal tubular cells, benign prostatic hyperplasia as well as in prostatic and bladder cancer, perhaps only trisomy 17 may be regarded as specific. Gains of chromosomes 12, 16, and 20 are also common (15,20–23); the loss of the Y chromosome is found in male patients.

Grossly, its soft consistency correlates with hemorrhage and necrosis, which on preoperative imaging studies suggest a hypovascular, nonenhancing mass sometimes interpreted as hemorrhage within a benign cyst. Necrosis, while diagnostically important, may not be as clinically significant in this tumor type as in clear cell or chromophobe types.

The histomorphology of PRCC includes two types (24), both of which exhibit predominant papillary architecture that may coexist with tubular and solid sheet-like growth. In type I tumors, the papillary projections display a monolayer of low cuboidal cells with uniform, bland, low-grade nuclei, and scant rims of amphophilic cytoplasm (Figure 3). The stroma often exhibits intervening clusters of benign foamy histiocytes. In type II tumors, the cells are larger and often pseudostratified around the papillary cores (Figure 4). The nuclei are more vesicular with coarse chromatin and prominent nucleoli. The cytoplasm is abundant and densely eosinophilic. Histiocyte clusters,

while present, are less prominent. The two types may coexist in the same tumor. Fuhrman nuclear grading of PRCC is probably not clinically relevant. In any event, nuclear grade seems to correlate with tumor subtype: type I being more low grade and type II more high grade. Immunohistochemically, type I tumors are commonly positive for vimentin, strongly and diffusely positive for CK7 and P504S (racemase); type II tumors rarely show strong, diffuse CK7 positivity, often being entirely negative or focally positive. In reviews of the cytogenetic and molecular abnormalities in PRCC, there is disagreement regarding the two histologic types as separate, distinct entities (25,26) or type I giving rise to type II (27). The histologic distinction of type I and type II tumors may have a prognostic value since type II tumors may have poorer clinical outcome (24,27).

In 2006, Lefèvre et al. (28) published a series of 10 oncocytic renal papillary tumors with abundant eosinophilic cytoplasm and nuclear features resembling the nuclei of oncocytoma. All tumors were limited to the kidney and no metastasis was found in a median follow up of 62 months. None of the cases had trisomy 7 or 17. Three additional

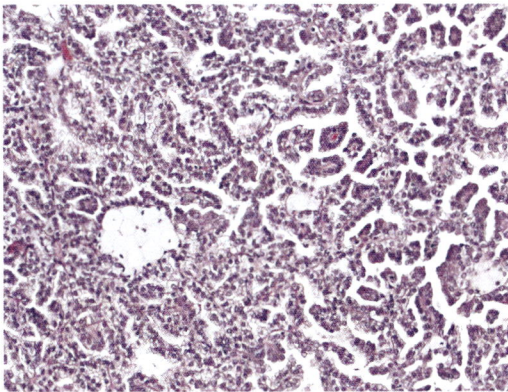

FIGURE 3
Papillary renal cell carcinoma type I. Fibrovascular cores lined by a monolayer of low-grade cuboidal cells with small amounts of amphophilic cytoplasm. Clusters of foamy macrophages are present in the interstitium.

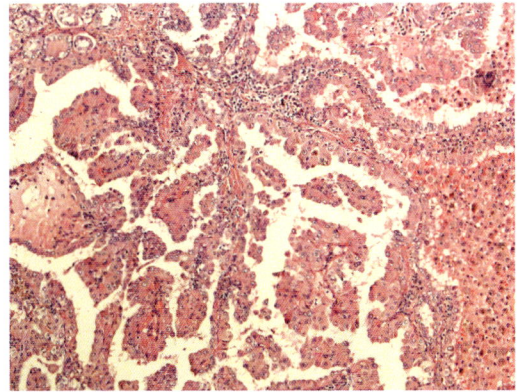

FIGURE 4
Papillary renal cell carcinoma type II. Pseudostratified cells with high-grade nuclei and abundant dense eosinophilic cytoplasm over delicate fibrovascular cores. Foamy macrophages and necrosis are common findings.

series published to date describe similar tumors predominantly found in male patients (87%) in a wide age range (40–80 years) (29–31). Usually, the tumors are of small size and limited to the kidney. Trisomy 7 and 17 were found in 13 and 14 of 19 cases, respectively, showing that these tumors are similar to the rest of PRCC. The importance of this observation is the possibility of mistaking this tumor subtype for oncocytoma or PRCC type II. Although the oncocytic cells of this tumor resemble oncocytoma cells, papillary structures are not features of oncocytoma. In addition, necrosis and foam cells are characteristic of PRCC. The presence of vimentin, CD10, RCC, and P504S (racemase) staining in oncocytic PRCC is helpful in making the distinction between it and oncocytoma. The immunohistochemical study does not have a role in distinguishing PRCC type II and oncocytic PRCC since they share the same immunohistochemical profile. The histomorphology shows much more nuclear stratification and higher nuclear grade in PRCC type II.

■ CHROMOPHOBE RCC

Chromophobe RCC was first recognized by Bannasch et al. in rats exposed to nitrosomorpholine (32). Subsequently, this tumor type was described in humans and considered less aggressive than conventional RCC (33,34). Chromophobe RCC constitutes about 5% of all RCCs and is seldom multifocal. Cytogenetic examinations have shown multiple and complex losses of chromosomes Y, 1, 2, 6, 10, 13, 17 and 21 (35–37).

Grossly, it is typically tan-brown and well circumscribed, features it shares with benign oncocytoma with which it is also occasionally confused microscopically. Necrosis is rare unless the tumor is large. Histologically, there are broad sheets of cells divided by thin vascular septae. The tumor cell nuclei are pleomorphic with occasional binucleation and nucleoli, giving a high-grade appearance. The nuclear membranes are "raisinoid" and characteristically show a perinuclear halo-simulating koilocytes. The cells immediately adjacent to

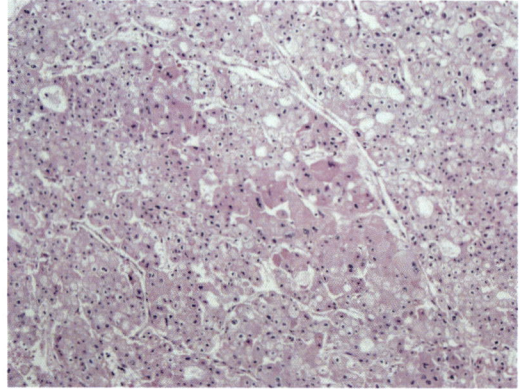

FIGURE 5
Chromophobe renal cell carcinoma. Solid sheets of cells divided by occasional thin-walled vessels. The cells are variable in size with oncocytic type cytoplasm, raisinoid nuclei with occasional binucleation. Perinuclear halo and well-defined cell borders are prominent features of this renal cell carcinoma variant.

the vascular septae often demonstrate clear cytoplasm; granular cytoplasmic accumulations occur further away from the septae. Cell borders are well defined (Figure 5). Some authors have found that sarcomatoid change occurs more commonly in chromophobe compared to clear cell and papillary types (38,39). An eosinophilic variant of this tumor is recognized as the cytoplasm assumes uniformly, dense granular properties. The differential diagnosis in this instance includes oncocytoma, which is in difficult cases only excluded by cytogenetics (40).

Chromophobe RCC is not subject to Fuhrman nuclear grading, which does not correlate with the typical indolent clinical course of these tumors. New attempts to develop a meaningful grading system for chromophobe RCC have used nuclear features coupled with cellularity, necrosis, and sarcomatoid transformation as key points (41). The most important and diagnostic features of chromophobe RCC are on routine histologic examination by H&E staining. In the past, chromophobe RCC was alleged to react characteristically with colloidal iron, a histochemical stain difficult to control and inconsistent in its reactive cytoplasmic pattern. Colloidal iron is no longer applied to this tumor. Although chromophobe RCC does not have a specific immunohistochemical profile, a negative vimentin reaction with a strong, diffuse CK7 stain may help to identify this tumor type.

■ CARCINOMA OF THE COLLECTING DUCTS OF BELLINI/ COLLECTING DUCT CARCINOMA

Collecting duct carcinoma (CDC), the least common major RCC variant, is regarded as a highly aggressive neoplasm presumed to arise from the collecting duct epithelium. The tumor affects an older adult population (mean age 55 years) with 2:1 male predominance. Cytogenetic findings are variable (42) and often overlap with other RCCs as well as urothelial carcinomas (43,44).

The gross appearance of the tumor is infiltrative, poorly circumscribed, shows variable colors, and, in instances of smaller tumors, a central location in the renal medulla. Grossly, these features are also those of urothelial carcinoma of the renal pelvis, especially high-grade variants. Histologically, CDC demonstrates papillary and/or tubular arrangements of pleomorphic epithelial cells often with high-grade, hobnail nuclei and prominent nucleoli (Figure 6). Mitotic figures are easily seen. The infiltrative growth often uses the pre-existing tubular framework of the renal collecting system, in addition to direct parenchymal stromal invasion. There is prominent desmoplasia and a frequent inflammatory infiltrate. Tumor cells often contain intracytoplasmic mucin, which is not a feature of other RCCs. These histologic features are also common to high-grade urothelial carcinoma, which often remains a diagnostic consideration. The finding of urothelial carcinoma in situ excludes CDC. There is no characteristic or diagnostic immunohistochemical profile for this tumor; however, absence of CD10, RCC (renal cell carcinoma marker), and P504S (racemase) staining may be useful.

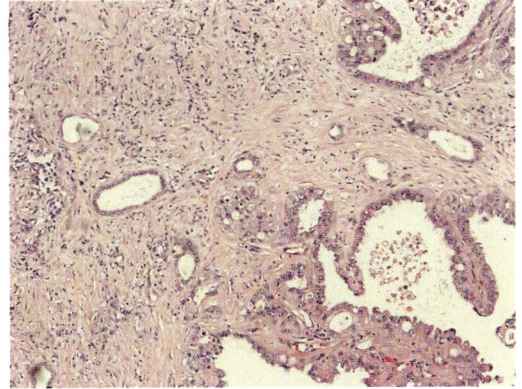

FIGURE 6
Collecting duct carcinoma. Papillary and tubular arrangement of pleomorphic high-grade nuclei with prominent nucleoli and desmoplastic stroma.

■ RENAL MEDULLARY CARCINOMA

This newly recognized primary RCC occurs in a younger patient population (mean age of 19 years) in the specific clinical setting of sickle cell trait (45). There is 2:1 male predominance; however, in the pediatric population (less than 10 years of age) the ratio increases to 5:1 (46). Although tumor size at presentation varies, even small tumors may progress quickly with metastatic disease to distant clinical sites. About 95% of patients have metastases at the time of presentation. Yang et al. have reported that the gene expression profile of renal medullary carcinoma closely resembles that of urothelial carcinoma (47).

Grossly, the tumor is poorly circumscribed with obvious necrosis and hemorrhage. The histologic features are variable and include solid, papillary, and rhabdoid forms (Figure 7); INI1 staining is uniformly negative in both rhabdoid and nonrhabdoid tumors (48). There is usually pronounced acute inflammatory infiltrate. The cells show high-grade nuclear features and numerous mitotic figures. All tumors express cytokeratin AE1/AE3, EMA, and vimentin. The other immunohistochemical stains are variably expressed (i.e., CK7, CEA, and high molecular weight cytokeratin).

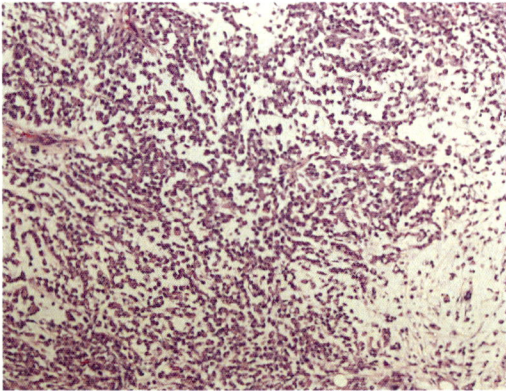

FIGURE 7
Renal medullary carcinoma. Discohesive cells with rhabdoid morphology in mucoid background.

TABLE 2 Translocation renal cell carcinoma

Genes Involved	Chromosomal Translocations
ASPL-TFE3	t(X;17)(p11.2;q25)
PRCC-TFE3	t(X;1)(p11.2;q21)
PSF-TFE3	t(X;1)(p11.2;q34)
NonO-TFE3	inv(X)(p11;q12)
CLTC-TFE3	t(X;17)(p11.2;q23)
Unknown	t(X;3)(p11;q23)
Unknown	t(X;10)(p11.2;q23)
Alpha-TFEB	t(6;11)(p21;q12)

■ XP11 TRANSLOCATION CARCINOMAS/TRANSLOCATION RCC

The first reports on what is now appreciated as translocation RCC concerned a pediatric population of papillary cancers with novel translocations (49,50). The first described chromosomal breakpoint in this newly recognized tumor (Xp11.2) is identical to those identified in alveolar soft part sarcoma, a rare soft tissue sarcoma in children and young adults (51). Subsequently, various translocations involving chromosome Xp11.2 have been described (49–55) involving the TFE3 transcription factor gene (Table 2). Nuclear immunohistochemical labeling of these tumors with TFE3 identifies them (56). In addition to Xp11.2 another pediatric renal tumor was described that also has a specific translocation t(6;11)(p21.1;q12) (57). This tumor is characterized by expression of melanocytic markers and nuclear labeling with TFEB. Both TFE3 and TFEB tumors are members of the MITF family of tumors that also include PEComas and melanomas (58). The pediatric connection has given a wide age range for TFE3 carcinomas (52–54) and in this population, translocation RCC often shows an indolent course despite lymph node metastasis (54) compared to the adult population where the tumors often present in advanced stage and are rapidly progressive (59–61).

However, there has not been enough clinical data to demonstrate prognostic difference between pediatric and adult TFE3 renal carcinomas mostly due to late tumor recurrence and the short follow-up in most studies.

TFE3 translocation carcinoma does not show a specific gross appearance. Histologically, there is either a papillary or nested architecture of cells with abundant eosinophilic or clear cytoplasm (Figure 8). The histologic resemblance to alveolar soft part sarcoma is often striking. The nuclei have prominent nucleoli corresponding to Fuhrman nuclear grade 2 or 3. Psammomatous calcification is present ranging from minimal to abundant. Spindle cells with focally bland features, myxoid stroma, and multinucleated giant cells are also found (60). The tumors uniformly express TFE3 nuclear staining, best expressed in well-fixed areas (Figure 9). Since the tumors have overlapping morphology with papillary and clear cell RCCs, TFE3 immunostaining is crucial for the diagnosis. Rarely, the specific translocation has been found by cytogenetic and molecular studies despite negative TFE3 staining (61). Underexpression of vimentin and cytokeratins is also a common finding; CD10, P504S (racemase), and RCC are commonly expressed. In some cases, melanocytic markers are expressed (60,61) and in some cases there is frank melanin production (55,58) confirmed by Fontana-Mason stain as well as with permanganate bleaching.

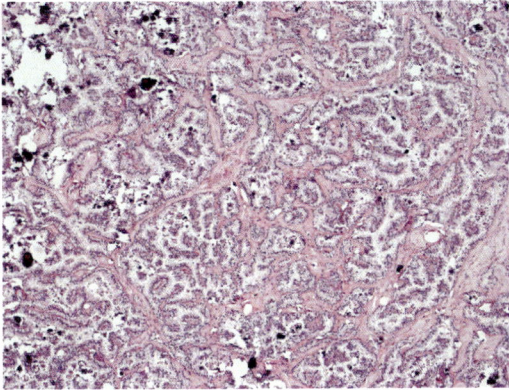

FIGURE 8

Translocation renal cell carcinoma. Variable nests of tumor composed of low-grade cells with abundant clear cytoplasm. Numerous calcifications are also present.

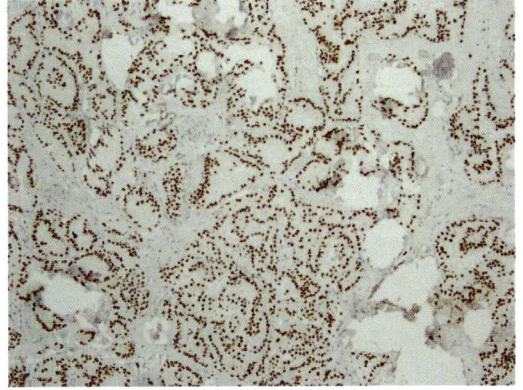

FIGURE 9

Translocation renal cell carcinoma with strong and diffuse nuclear reactivity for the immunohistochemical stain TFE-3.

TFEB RCC shows nests and tubules of polygonal cells that are separated by thin capillaries. The cells have low-grade nuclei. There is also a second population of small dark cells clustered around a hyalinized basement membrane. Although this morphology was considered specific for TFEB RCC, the subsequent report by Argani et al. (60) showed that there are cases of TFE3 RCCs with similar morphology.

It was recently demonstrated in vitro that the ASPL-TFE3 fusion protein activates a MET promoter (62). This could potentially play a role in developing targeted therapy for translocation RCC through use of the MET pathway inhibitors.

■ RCC ASSOCIATED WITH NEUROBLASTOMA

In 2003, Eble (63) summarized previously published cases of RCCs in neuroblastoma survivors. Although some cases were clear cell RCC, others had an unusual histology not consistent with any previously known subtype. It was postulated that radiation therapy was a contributing factor; however, some of the patients received only chemotherapy and some did not receive any additional treatment. No molecular studies are reported to date.

Eight cases published by Medeiros (64) and Koyle (65) describe tumors with papillary and solid growth with abundant oncocytic cells. Some tumors show high nuclear grade with prominent nucleoli. There is no specific immunohistochemical profile for these tumors, although reportedly tumor cells are positive for Cam5.2, EMA, and vimentin.

■ MUCINOUS TUBULAR AND SPINDLE CELL RCC

Mucinous tubular and spindle cell RCC (MTS) is the newest addition to the WHO 2004 classification (5). This tumor occurs predominantly in women (female to male ratio 4:1) and is of low pathologic stage at the time of surgery. Previously considered in the spectrum of "low-grade collecting duct carcinoma," "tumor derived from cells of the loop of Henle" or even PRCCs, it is now recognized as a separate entity with specific clinical, pathologic, and cytogenetic features. By comparative genomic hybridization, the tumor has multiple genetic alterations of which losses of chromosomes 1, 4, 6, 8, 9, 13, 14, 15, 16, and 22 are common (66,67).

Grossly, the tumors are circumscribed, yellow-tan, and rarely hemorrhagic and necrotic. Histologically, the tumor is variable. In some areas, there are tightly packed elongated tubules and abundant extracellular basophilic mucin (Figure 10), which is positive with Alcian blue at pH 2.5. In other areas, the tubules are lined by low nuclear grade cuboidal cells and focal aggregates of spindle cells. Recent reports have described a mucin-poor variant with neuroendocrine differentiation (68,69). Although MTS RCC has an overlapping immunohistochemical profile with PRCC (70), the specific chromosomal losses and absence of commonly found cytogenetic abnormalities of PRCC suggest that this is a distinctive subtype. The majority of these tumors have an indolent clinical course and a good prognosis, with rare patients developing distant metastasis. However, there are recently reported cases of sarcomatoid change in which two of four patients have developed metastases (71,72).

■ TUBULOCYSTIC RCC

The first description of tubulocystic RCC was by Pierre Masson in 1956 (73). Farrow grouped this "low-grade collecting duct carcinoma" together with mucinous, tubular, and spindle cell RCC (74). Tubulocystic RCC is now separately recognized. It has a strong male preponderance with a ratio of 7:1 (75–77). These tumors are typically incidental findings in subcapsular, cortical or medullary locations, are well circumscribed, spongy and range from 0.5 to 17.0 cm (mean 4.0 cm). Imaging studies often interpret this tumor as a cystic lesion, Bosniak type II or III. Although tubulocystic RCC is considered a distinctive subtype (76,77) some of the findings are shared with PRCC, which peculiarly can be found in the same kidney either as a separate tumor or admixed with tubulocystic RCC (76).

Histologically, tubulocystic RCC is composed of cystically dilated tubules lined by polygonal cells with eosinophilic cytoplasm and hobnail nuclei with prominent nucleoli corresponding to Fuhrman nuclear grade 3 (Figure 11). Although the cytologic features are of high-grade carcinoma, most tumors are stage T1. In the three major published series only four patients had metastatic disease (75–77). The stroma between the tubules is fibrotic. Immunohistochemical studies have failed to define specific markers and in many cases have shown overlapping features with other RCCs, especially papillary carcinomas (76,77).

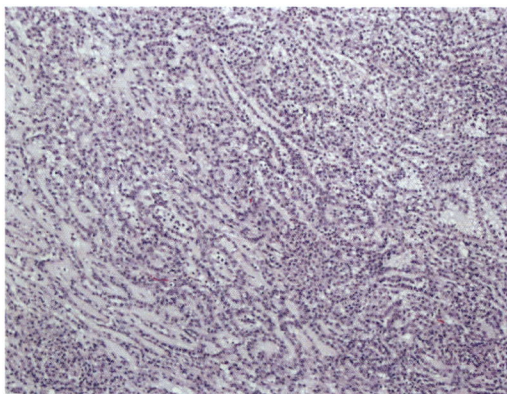

FIGURE 10
Mucinous tubular and spindle cell renal cell carcinoma represented by tightly packed elongated tubules and abundant extracellular amphophilic mucin.

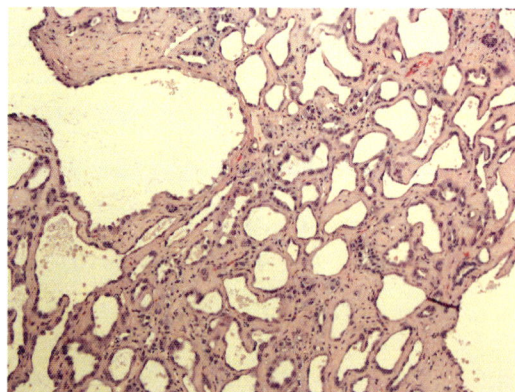

FIGURE 11
Tubulocystic renal cell carcinoma. Numerous small and large cysts lined by cells with dense eosinophilic cytoplasm and focally hobnail nuclei.

Ultrastructural analysis has shown that tubulo-cystic carcinoma shows features of both proximal convoluted tubules and intercalated cells of the collecting ducts (77).

■ ACQUIRED CYSTIC DISEASE-ASSOCIATED RCC

Patients on long-term hemodialysis with acquired cystic kidney disease have an increased risk of developing RCC (78). PRCC is the most commonly described tumor in this clinical setting; however, some tumors are histologically distinctive and hard to classify. The first is designated "acquired cystic disease-associated RCC" and the second is "clear cell PRCC" (79,80). The first type is exclusively seen in patients with acquired renal cystic disease related to hemodialysis (79,80). The second type is also described in patients with end-stage kidney disease with or without acquired renal cystic disease (80). The two largest series "acquired cystic disease-associated RCC" show that most of tumors were pT1 stage. Of 29 patients only one died of widespread metastasis and two had lymph node metastasis at presentation (79,80). Some authors have found correlation between the duration of

hemodialysis and the specific tumor type (81). Rare molecular studies by FISH have demonstrated that some tumors have gains of chromosomes 1, 2, 6, and 10, while others do not show any gains or losses (82).

Acquired cystic disease-associated RCC is typically well circumscribed, often arising within a cyst, commonly bilateral or multifocal. Histologically, acquired cystic disease-associated RCC shows cribriform, papillary, tubulocystic, and solid architecture. The cells have abundant eosino-philic cytoplasm and nuclei with Fuhrman nuclear grade 3 (Figure 12). Hemorrhage and necrosis are common findings. The variable presence of intra-tumoral oxalate crystals (Figure 13) is postulated to play a role in tumorigenesis (79,80). There is an extensive fibrohistiocytic reaction around the tumor. No specific immunohistochemical pro-file is reported for these tumors, although Sule et al. (79) reported that they express markers of proximal tubules, that is, RCC and CD10. Their characteristic morphology obviates the need for immunohistochemistry.

The second distinctive tumor type in this clin-ical setting is clear cell PRCC. This tumor has been described in end-stage kidney disease with or with-out acquired cystic disease as well as in otherwise

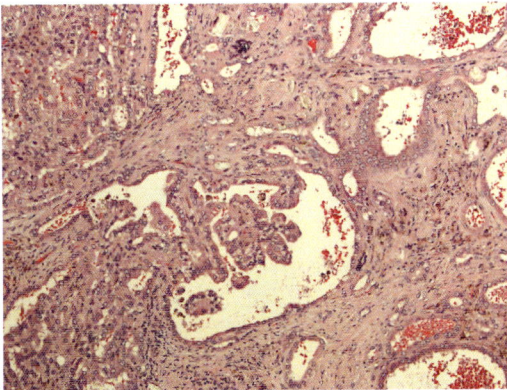

FIGURE 12
Acquired cystic disease renal cell carcinoma with papillary features arising in a cyst. The tumor cells have dense eosinophilic cytoplasm and high-grade nuclei with prominent nucleoli.

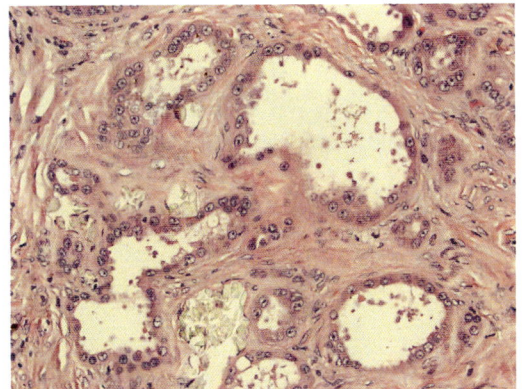

FIGURE 13
Acquired cystic disease renal cell carcinoma with oxalate crystals in the interstitium.

normal kidneys (83). These tumors do not have cytogenetic abnormalities of either PRCC or clear cell RCC (83). Histologically, there are cysts and thin fibrovascular cores lined by a single layer of clear cells with low-grade nuclei. Tumor cells are positive for CK7 and CA-IX and negative for P504S (racemase), CD10, and TFE3. None of the patients developed recurrence or metastasis in follow-up time of 1 to 48 months (mean 24 months) (83).

■ THYROID FOLLICULAR CARCINOMA-LIKE TUMOR

This recently described tumor (84,85) is so designated because it resembles "thyroidization" of the kidney, the well-recognized diffuse change in the renal parenchyma in end-stage kidney disease. It affects a wide age range and both genders equally. The nature of the tumor is considered to be of low malignant potential. It was found, albeit in a single case, that the genetic abnormalities are distinct from those known in any other subtype of RCC (84). In a larger study, it was found that the tumors overexpressed cell cycle regulatory genes, specifically MLL/trithorax located on chromosome 12q23, which is a recurring translocation site for hematologic malignancies (85). Although the presence of the MLL/trithorax is a poor prognostic sign in hematologic malignancies, the significance of this finding is unknown in this low malignant potential RCC.

Grossly, all reported tumors were well circumscribed; tan to brown and without necrosis or hemorrhage. Histologically, the tumor closely resembles a follicular thyroid neoplasm composed of variably sized follicular structures with colloid-like material. Although none of the tumors were positive for TTF-1 or thyroglobulin, it is still important to clinically exclude a primary thyroid lesion. There has been a report of a thyroid appearing renal neoplasm that did not express TTF-1 or thyroglobulin; however, a subsequent lung metastasis showed expression of thyroid tissue immuno-markers (86).

■ REFERENCES

1. Ferlay J, Bray F, Pisani P, Parkin DM. *GLOBOCAN 2002: Cancer Incidence, Mortality, and Prevalence Worldwide.* Lyon, France: IARC Press; 2004.
2. Jemal A, Tiwari RC, Murray T, et al. Cancer statistics, 2004. *CA Cancer J Clin* 2004;54:8–29.
3. Chow WH, Dong LM, Devesa SS. Epidemiology and risk factors for kidney cancer. *Nat Rev Urol* 2010;7(5):245–257.
4. Konig G. *Practical Treatment of Diseases of the Kidney as Explained by Case Histories* (in German). Leipzig, Germany: C.Cnobloch; 1826.
5. Eble JN, Sauter G, Epstein JI, et al. *World Heath Organization Classification of Tumours. Pathology and Genetics. Tumours of the Urinary System and Male Genital Organs.* Lyon, France: IARC Press; 2004.
6. Uzzo RG, Novick AC. Nephron sparing surgery for renal tumors: indications, techniques and outcomes. *J Urol* 2001;166(1):6–18.
7. Pahernik S, Roos F, Hampel C, Gillitzer R, Melchior SW, Thüroff JW. Nephron sparing surgery for renal cell carcinoma with normal contralateral kidney: 25 years of experience. *J Urol* 2006;175(6):2027–2031.
8. Leibovich BC, Lohse CM, Crispen PL, et al. Histological subtype is an independent predictor of outcome for patients with renal cell carcinoma. *J Urol* 2010;183(4):1309–1315.
9. Patard JJ, Leray E, Rioux-Leclercq N, et al. Prognostic value of histologic subtypes in renal cell carcinoma: a multicenter experience. *J Clin Oncol* 2005;23(12):2763–2771.
10. Karakiewicz PI, Briganti A, Chun FK, et al. Multi-institutional validation of a new renal cancer-specific survival nomogram. *J Clin Oncol* 2007;25(11):1316–1322.
11. Taxy JB. Renal adenocarcinoma presenting as a solitary metastasis: contribution of electron microscopy to diagnosis. *Cancer* 1981;48(6):1381–1391.
12. Hadaczek P, Podolski J, Toloczko A, et al. Losses at 3p common deletion sites in subtypes of kidney tumours: histopathological correlations. *Virchows Arch* 1996;429(1):37–42.
13. Fuhrman SA, Lasky LC, Limas C. Prognostic significance of morphologic parameters in renal cell carcinoma. *Am J Surg Pathol* 1982;6(7):655–663.

14. Halat S, Eble JN, Grignon DJ, et al. Multilocular cystic renal cell carcinoma is a subtype of clear cell renal cell carcinoma. *Mod Pathol* 2010;23(7):931–936.

15. Kovacs G. Papillary renal cell carcinoma. A morphologic and cytogenetic study of 11 cases. *Am J Pathol* 1989;134(1):27–34.

16. Corless CL, Aburatani H, Fletcher JA, Housman DE, Amin MB, Weinberg DS. Papillary renal cell carcinoma: quantitation of chromosomes 7 and 17 by FISH, analysis of chromosome 3p for LOH, and DNA ploidy. *Diagn Mol Pathol* 1996;5(1):53–64.

17. Delahunt B, Eble JN. Papillary renal cell carcinoma: a clinicopathologic and immunohistochemical study of 105 tumors. *Mod Pathol* 1997;10(6):537–544.

18. Mancilla-Jimenez R, Stanley RJ, Blath RA. Papillary renal cell carcinoma: a clinical, radiologic, and pathologic study of 34 cases. *Cancer* 1976;38(6):2469–2480.

19. Schmidt L, Duh FM, Chen F, et al. Germline and somatic mutations in the tyrosine kinase domain of the MET proto-oncogene in papillary renal carcinomas. *Nat Genet* 1997;16(1):68–73.

20. Presti JC Jr, Rao PH, Chen Q, et al. Histopathological, cytogenetic, and molecular characterization of renal cortical tumors. *Cancer Res* 1991;51(5):1544–1552.

21. Kovacs G, Fuzesi L, Emanual A, Kung HF. Cytogenetics of papillary renal cell tumors. *Genes Chromosomes Cancer* 1991;3(4):249–255.

22. Dal Cin P, Gaeta J, Huben R, Li FP, Prout GR Jr, Sandberg AA. Renal cortical tumors. Cytogenetic characterization. *Am J Clin Pathol* 1989;92(4):408–414.

23. Kovacs G, Wilkens L, Papp T, de Riese W. Differentiation between papillary and nonpapillary renal cell carcinomas by DNA analysis. *J Natl Cancer Inst* 1989;81(7):527–530.

24. Delahunt B, Eble JN, McCredie MR, Bethwaite PB, Stewart JH, Bilous AM. Morphologic typing of papillary renal cell carcinoma: comparison of growth kinetics and patient survival in 66 cases. *Hum Pathol* 2001;32(6):590–595.

25. Jiang F, Richter J, Schraml P, et al. Chromosomal imbalances in papillary renal cell carcinoma: genetic differences between histological subtypes. *Am J Pathol* 1998;153(5):1467–1473.

26. Sanders ME, Mick R, Tomaszewski JE, Barr FG. Unique patterns of allelic imbalance distinguish type 1 from type 2 sporadic papillary renal cell carcinoma. *Am J Pathol* 2002;161(3):997–1005.

27. Gunawan B, von Heydebreck A, Fritsch T, et al. Cytogenetic and morphologic typing of 58 papillary renal cell carcinomas: evidence for a cytogenetic evolution of type 2 from type 1 tumors. *Cancer Res* 2003;63(19):6200–6205.

28. Lefevre M, Couturier J, Sibony M, et al. Adult papillary renal tumor with oncocytic cells. *Am J Surg Pathol* 2005;29(12):1576–1581.

29. Masuzawa N, Kishimoto M, Nishimura A, Shichiri Y, Yanagisawa A. Oncocytic renal cell carcinoma having papillotubular growth: rare morphological variant of papillary renal cell carcinoma. *Pathol Int* 2008;58(5):300–305.

30. Kunju LP, Wojno K, Wolf JS Jr, et al. Papillary renal cell carcinoma with oncocytic cells and nonoverlapping low grade nuclei: expanding the morphologic spectrum with emphasis on clinicopathologic, immunohistochemical and molecular features. *Hum Pathol* 2008;39:96–101.

31. Hes O, Brunelli M, Michal M, et al. Oncocytic papillary renal cell carcinoma: a clinicopathologic, immunohistochemical, ultrastructural, and interphase cytogenetic study of 12 cases. *Ann Diagn Pathol* 2006;10(3):133–139.

32. Bannasch P, Schnacht U, Storch E. Morphogenese und Mikromorphologie epithelialier Nierentumoren bei Nitrosomorpholin-vergifteten Ratt. I Induktion und Histologie der Tumoren. *Z Krebsforsch* 1974;81:311–331.

33. Thoenes W, Störkel S, Rumpelt HJ. Human chromophobe cell renal carcinoma. *Virchows Arch, B, Cell Pathol* 1985;48(3):207–217.

34. Thoenes W, Störkel S, Rumpelt HJ, Moll R, Baum HP, Werner S. Chromophobe cell renal carcinoma and its variants—a report on 32 cases. *J Pathol* 1988;155(4):277–287.

35. Kovacs G. Molecular differential pathology of renal cell tumours. *Histopathology* 1993;22(1):1–8.

36. Kovacs G. Molecular cytogenetics of renal cell tumors. *Adv Cancer Res* 1993;62:89–124.

37. Kovacs A, Kovacs G. Low chromosome number in chromophobe renal cell carcinomas. *Genes Chromosomes Cancer* 1992;4(3):267–268.

38. Akhtar M, Tulbah A, Kardar AH, Ali MA. Sarcomatoid renal cell carcinoma: the chromophobe connection. *Am J Surg Pathol* 1997;21(10):1188–1195.

39. de Peralta-Venturina M, Moch H, Amin M, et al. Sarcomatoid differentiation in renal cell carcinoma: a study of 101 cases. *Am J Surg Pathol* 2001;25(3):275–284.

40. Brunneli M, Eble JN, Zhang S, et al. Eosinophilic and classic chromophobe renal cell carcinomas have similar frequent losses of multiple chromosomes from among chromosomes 1,2,6,10, and 17, and this

pattern of genetic abnormality is not present in renal oncocytoma. *Mod Pathol* 2004;18:161–169.

41. Paner GP, Amin MB, Alvarado-Cabrero I, et al. A novel tumor grading scheme for chromophobe renal cell carcinoma: prognostic utility and comparison with Fuhrman nuclear grade. *Am J Surg Pathol* 2010;34(9):1233–1240.

42. Füzesi L, Cober M, Mittermayer C. Collecting duct carcinoma: cytogenetic characterization. *Histopathology* 1992;21(2):155–160.

43. Chao D, Zisman A, Pantuck AJ, et al. Collecting duct renal cell carcinoma: clinical study of a rare tumor. *J Urol* 2002;167(1):71–74.

44. Schoenberg M, Cairns P, Brooks JD, et al. Frequent loss of chromosome arms 8p and 13q in collecting duct carcinoma (CDC) of the kidney. *Genes Chromosomes Cancer* 1995;12(1):76–80.

45. Davis CJ Jr, Mostofi FK, Sesterhenn IA. Renal medullary carcinoma. The seventh sickle cell nephropathy. *Am J Surg Pathol* 1995;19(1):1–11.

46. Simpson L, He X, Pins M, et al. Renal medullary carcinoma and ABL gene amplification. *J Urol* 2005;173(6):1883–1888.

47. Yang XJ, Sugimura J, Tretiakova MS, et al. Gene expression profiling of renal medullary carcinoma: potential clinical relevance. *Cancer* 2004;100(5):976–985.

48. Cheng JX, Tretiakova M, Gong C, Mandal S, Krausz T, Taxy JB. Renal medullary carcinoma: rhabdoid features and the absence of INI1 expression as markers of aggressive behavior. *Mod Pathol* 2008;21(6):647–652.

49. Sidhar SK, Clark J, Gill S, et al. The t(X;1)(p11.2;q21.2) translocation in papillary renal cell carcinoma fuses a novel gene PRCC to the TFE3 transcription factor gene. *Hum Mol Genet* 1996;5(9):1333–1338.

50. Clark J, Lu YJ, Sidhar SK, et al. Fusion of splicing factor genes PSF and NonO (p54nrb) to the TFE3 gene in papillary renal cell carcinoma. *Oncogene* 1997;15(18):2233–2239.

51. Argani P, Antonescu CR, Illei PB, et al. Primary renal neoplasms with the ASPL-TFE3 gene fusion of alveolar soft part sarcoma: a distinctive tumor entity previously included among renal cell carcinomas of children and adolescents. *Am J Pathol* 2001;159(1):179–192.

52. Argani P, Antonescu CR, Couturier J, et al. PRCC-TFE3 renal carcinomas: morphologic, immunohistochemical, ultrastructural, and molecular analysis of an entity associated with the t(X;1)(p11.2;q21). *Am J Surg Pathol* 2002;26(12):1553–1566.

53. Argani P, Lui MY, Couturier J, Bouvier R, Fournet JC, Ladanyi M. A novel CLTC-TFE3 gene fusion in pediatric renal adenocarcinoma with t(X;17) (p11.2;q23). *Oncogene* 2003;22(34):5374–5378.

54. Geller JI, Argani P, Adeniran A, et al. Translocation renal cell carcinoma: lack of negative impact due to lymph node spread. *Cancer* 2008; 112(7):1607–1616.

55. Chang IW, Huang HY, Sung MT. Melanotic Xp11 translocation renal cancer: a case with PSF-TFE3 gene fusion and up-regulation of melanogenetic transcripts. *Am J Surg Pathol* 2009;33(12):1894–1901.

56. Argani P, Lal P, Hutchinson B, Lui MY, Reuter VE, Ladanyi M. Aberrant nuclear immunoreactivity for TFE3 in neoplasms with TFE3 gene fusions: a sensitive and specific immunohistochemical assay. *Am J Surg Pathol* 2003;27(6):750–761.

57. Argani P, Hawkins A, Griffin CA, et al. A distinctive pediatric renal neoplasm characterized by epithelioid morphology, basement membrane production, focal HMB45 immunoreactivity, and t(6;11) (p21.1;q12) chromosome translocation. *Am J Pathol* 2001;158(6):2089–2096.

58. Argani P, Aulmann S, Karanjawala Z, Fraser RB, Ladanyi M, Rodriguez MM. Melanotic Xp11 translocation renal cancers: a distinctive neoplasm with overlapping features of PEComa, carcinoma, and melanoma. *Am J Surg Pathol* 2009;33(4):609–619.

59. Meyer PN, Clark JL, Flanigan RC, et al. Xp11.2 translocation renal cell carcinoma with very aggressive course in five adult patients. *Mod Pathol* 2006;19(S1)50A.

60. Argani P, Olgac S, Tickoo SK, et al. Xp11 translocation renal cell carcinoma in adults: expanded clinical, pathologic, and genetic spectrum. *Am J Surg Pathol* 2007;31(8):1149–1160.

61. Camparo P, Vasiliu V, Molinie V, et al. Renal translocation carcinomas: clinicopathologic, immunohistochemical, and gene expression profiling analysis of 31 cases with a review of the literature. *Am J Surg Pathol* 2008;32(5):656–670.

62. Tsuda M, Davis IJ, Argani P, et al. TFE3 fusions activate MET signaling by transcriptional up-regulation, defining another class of tumors as candidates for therapeutic MET inhibition. *Cancer Res* 2007;67(3):919–929.

63. Eble JN. Mucinous tubular and spindle cell carcinoma and post-neuroblastoma carcinoma: newly recognised entities in the renal cell carcinoma family. *Pathology* 2003;35(6):499–504.

64. Medeiros LJ, Palmedo G, Krigman HR, Kovacs G, Beckwith JB. Oncocytoid renal cell carcinoma after neuroblastoma: a report of four cases of a

distinct clinicopathologic entity. *Am J Surg Pathol* 1999;23(7):772–780.

65. Koyle MA, Hatch DA, Furness PD 3rd, Lovell MA, Odom LF, Kurzrock EA. Long-term urological complications in survivors younger than 15 months of advanced stage abdominal neuroblastoma. *J Urol* 2001;166(4):1455–1458.

66. Rakozy C, Schmahl GE, Bogner S, Störkel S. Low-grade tubular-mucinous renal neoplasms: morphologic, immunohistochemical, and genetic features. *Mod Pathol* 2002;15(11):1162–1171.

67. Ferlicot S, Allory Y, Compérat E, et al. Mucinous tubular and spindle cell carcinoma: a report of 15 cases and a review of the literature. *Virchows Arch* 2005;447(6):978–983.

68. Fine SW, Argani P, DeMarzo AM, et al. Expanding the histologic spectrum of mucinous tubular and spindle cell carcinoma of the kidney. *Am J Surg Pathol* 2006;30(12):1554–1560.

69. Kuroda N, Nakamura S, Miyazaki E, et al. Low-grade tubular-mucinous renal neoplasm with neuroendocrine differentiation: a histological, immunohistochemical and ultrastructural study. *Pathol Int* 2004;54(3):201–207.

70. Paner GP, Srigley JR, Radhakrishnan A, et al. Immunohistochemical analysis of mucinous tubular and spindle cell carcinoma and papillary renal cell carcinoma of the kidney: significant immunophenotypic overlap warrants diagnostic caution. *Am J Surg Pathol* 2006;30(1):13–19.

71. Dhillon J, Amin MB, Selbs E, Turi GK, Paner GP, Reuter VE. Mucinous tubular and spindle cell carcinoma of the kidney with sarcomatoid change. *Am J Surg Pathol* 2009;33(1):44–49.

72. Simon RA, di Sant'agnese PA, Palapattu GS, et al. Mucinous tubular and spindle cell carcinoma of the kidney with sarcomatoid differentiation. *Int J Clin Exp Pathol* 2008;1(2):180–184.

73. Masson P. *Tumeurs Humaines 1955. Human Tumors, Histology, Diagnosis and Technique.* Detroit: Wayne State University Press; 1970.

74. Murphy W, Beckwith BJ, Farrow GM. *Tumors of the Kidney and Bladder.* Washington, DC: Armed Forces Institute of Pathology; 1994.

75. Azoulay S, Vieillefond A, Paraf F, et al. Tubulocystic carcinoma of the kidney: a new entity among renal tumors. *Virchows Arch* 2007;451(5):905–909.

76. Yang XJ, Zhou M, Hes O, et al. Tubulocystic carcinoma of the kidney: clinicopathologic and molec-

ular characterization. *Am J Surg Pathol* 2008;32(2):177–187.

77. Amin MB, MacLennan GT, Gupta R, et al. Tubulocystic carcinoma of the kidney: clinicopathologic analysis of 31 cases of a distinctive rare subtype of renal cell carcinoma. *Am J Surg Pathol* 2009;33(3):384–392.

78. Basile JJ, McCullough DL, Harrison LH, Dyer RB. End stage renal disease associated with acquired cystic disease and neoplasia. *J Urol* 1988;140(5):938–943.

79. Sule N, Yakupoglu U, Shen SS, et al. Calcium oxalate deposition in renal cell carcinoma associated with acquired cystic kidney disease: a comprehensive study. *Am J Surg Pathol* 2005;29(4):443–451.

80. Tickoo SK, dePeralta-Venturina MN, Harik LR, et al. Spectrum of epithelial neoplasms in end-stage renal disease: an experience from 66 tumor-bearing kidneys with emphasis on histologic patterns distinct from those in sporadic adult renal neoplasia. *Am J Surg Pathol* 2006;30(2):141–153.

81. Nouh MA, Kuroda N, Yamashita M, et al. Renal cell carcinoma in patients with end-stage renal disease: relationship between histological type and duration of dialysis. *BJU Int* 2010;105(5):620–627.

82. Cossu-Rocca P, Eble JN, Zhang S, Martignoni G, Brunelli M, Cheng L. Acquired cystic disease-associated renal tumors: an immunohistochemical and fluorescence in situ hybridization study. *Mod Pathol* 2006;19(6):780–787.

83. Gobbo S, Eble JN, Grignon DJ, et al. Clear cell papillary renal cell carcinoma: a distinct histopathologic and molecular genetic entity. *Am J Surg Pathol* 2008;32(8):1239–1245.

84. Jung SJ, Chung JI, Park SH, Ayala AG, Ro JY. Thyroid follicular carcinoma-like tumor of kidney: a case report with morphologic, immunohistochemical, and genetic analysis. *Am J Surg Pathol* 2006;30(3):411–415.

85. Amin MB, Gupta R, Ondrej H, et al. Primary thyroid-like follicular carcinoma of the kidney: report of 6 cases of a histologically distinctive adult renal epithelial neoplasm. *Am J Surg Pathol* 2009;33(3):393–400.

86. William S, Irmgard V, Michael G, et al. Thyroid follicular carcinoma-like tumor: a case report with morphologic, immunophenotypic, cytogenetic, and scintigraphic studies. *Virchows Arch* 2009;452:91–95.

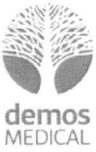

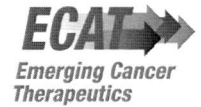

Imaging Renal Carcinoma

Michael W. Vannier*

University of Chicago Medical Center, Chicago, IL

■ ABSTRACT

Imaging is essential for the diagnosis, staging, treatment, and follow-up of renal cancer. All common imaging modalities have some role in renal cancer evaluation, including computed radiography, x-ray computed tomography (CT), ultrasonography (US), magnetic resonance imaging (MRI), positron emission tomography, and single-photon emission computed tomography (SPECT). Renal carcinoma is often first detected and characterized with imaging. US can separate solid versus cystic renal masses, but cannot further characterize solid tumors and stage malignancy. CT and MRI are the most common modalities used for diagnosis, staging, and surveillance of renal cancers. Specific renal carcinoma protocols demonstrate different imaging characteristics of histological subtypes, based on variations in dynamic contrast enhancement, MR weighting, and diffusion sequences, but are insufficiently reliable for clinical decision making in most cases. Cystic renal masses are evaluated with standardized diagnostic criteria that predict the likelihood of malignancy. Ionizing radiation from frequent CT imaging may cause secondary malignancy, and intravenous CT/MRI contrast agents have greatest risk when renal function is compromised. Standard imaging protocols and evaluation criteria have been developed to evaluate serial examinations and determine response to therapy.

Keywords: renal cell cancer, imaging, computed tomography, magnetic resonance imaging, ultrasonography

*Corresponding author, University of Chicago Medical Center, Chicago, IL 60637
  E-mail address: mvannier@uchicago.edu

Emerging Cancer Therapeutics 2:1 (2011) 37–56.
DOI: 10.5003/2151–4194.2.1.37
demosmedpub.com/ecat

■ INTRODUCTION

Ultrasonography (US), computed tomography (CT), and magnetic resonance imaging (MRI) are used to diagnose renal masses and monitor treatment of established renal carcinomas. Imaging modalities (US, CT, MRI, and positron emission tomography [PET]/single-photon emission computed tomography [SPECT]) have specific advantages and disadvantages, so study selection depends on the specific question to be addressed (1). Imaging of renal cell carcinoma is very common in clinical radiology and has been the topic of recent reviews and books (2,3).

Kidney cancers account for about 3% of all cancer cases, as well as about 3% of all cancer deaths. About 38,890 new diagnoses and 12,840 deaths were expected in 2006 with US$1.9 billion spent in the United States each year on treatment. Renal carcinoma is the 13th most common cancer worldwide, accounting for more than 208,000 new diagnoses and 102,000 deaths per year. Although not all of the difference is due to increased use of abdominal imaging, renal carcinoma incidence in North America has increased by 2% per year. Small renal masses (enhancing masses 4 cm or less in size on abdominal imaging) are more frequently detected, and most are carcinomas (4). The risk of malignancy varies from approximately 50% in tumors less than 1 cm in size to around 95% in tumors larger than 7 cm. Approximately one third of patients present with metastatic disease at the time of diagnosis. Another 30% will develop metastases at a later stage of their disease (2,5).

As noted in Chapter 2, most renal tumors arise from the renal parenchyma, with a much smaller number arising from the urothelium of the renal collecting system (urothelial carcinoma or transitional cell carcinoma) or the mesenchyma (e.g., angiomyolipoma [AML], leiomyoma, liposarcoma). Benign renal parenchymal tumors include renal oncocytoma (5%) and the rarer metanephric adenoma, metanephric adenofibroma, and papillary renal cell adenoma (6).

Common symptoms that lead to the detection of a renal mass are hematuria, flank mass, and flank pain. Many renal masses are found incidentally on CT, US, or MRI scans obtained for other purposes. Less frequently, patients present with signs or symptoms resulting from metastatic disease, such as bone pain, adenopathy, and pulmonary symptoms.

■ KIDNEY TUMOR DETECTION, DIAGNOSIS, AND STAGING

CT, MR imaging, and US are now performed in place of traditional diagnostic imaging tests, such as intravenous (IV) urography and angiography. Among these diagnostic tools, CT is the modality of choice for detection and diagnosis of renal cortical tumors, with MR imaging and ultrasound serving as problem-solving tools or when contrast-enhanced CT is contraindicated. Up to 70% of renal tumors are discovered incidentally, with a median size of less than 5 cm.

CT is the gold standard for the evaluation of a suspicious renal mass; protocols include pre-contrast images as well as images obtained at multiple times after contrast administration. CT is an effective staging modality that can assess lymphadenopathy, metastatic disease, adrenal gland involvement, and response to systemic therapy. US is rarely used alone to evaluate a solid renal mass; contrast-enhanced renal US is not yet approved in the United States but can assess vascularity of lesions without radiation. MRI does not employ ionizing radiation, can often differentiate benign and malignant lesions, and detect vascular tumor thrombus. Cystic renal masses require classification to determine the likelihood of malignancy; MRI can usually differentiate benign from malignant cysts.

Characterization of complex renal lesions is based on the presence or absence of enhancement on contrast-enhanced computed tomographic and magnetic resonance (MR) images. Contrast enhancement suggests the presence of carcinoma (excluding AMLs and oncocytomas). With MR dynamic contrast-enhanced (DCE) imaging, signal intensity changes can be measured or evaluated visually. Recently, risk of nephrogenic systemic fibrosis has precluded DCE-MRI in cases of renal insufficiency. As a result, nonenhanced imaging with CT, MR, and US have grown in importance.

■ TREATMENT MONITORING

For decades, treatment options for patients with metastatic renal cancer were very limited, with interferon-α and/or interleukin-2 being the most common systemic therapy. In the past 5 years, VEGF and mTOR-directed therapy have emerged as dominant treatment modalities (see Chapters 8 and 9) (7).

Notably, targeted therapy for metastatic renal cancer may result in disease stabilization rather than substantial tumor regression. Imaging measurements to assess early tumor response are being developed and tested. Imaging response evaluation criteria used for evaluating metastatic renal carcinoma therapy include Response Evaluation Criteria in Solid Tumors (RECIST), the Choi criteria, the modified Choi criteria, Morphology, Attenuation, Size and Structure (MASS) criteria, and the size and attenuation CT (SACT) criteria. Functional imaging such as dynamic contrast-enhanced CT (DCE-CT), dynamic contrast-enhanced MRI (DCE-MRI), dynamic contrast-enhanced US (DCE-US), and PET are also sometimes used.

The following sections describe some of the advantages and limitations of the various available imaging modalities for diagnosis, staging, and monitoring of systemic therapy response.

■ COMPUTED TOMOGRAPHY

CT is not always the first imaging modality used to detect renal parenchymal masses, but virtually all patients with renal carcinoma undergo one or more CT scans. Overall, approximately 85% of renal masses resected via radical or partial nephrectomy that were diagnosed as a carcinoma on preoperative CT are confirmed as such at nephrectomy. Guidelines from the American College of Radiology, American Urological Association, and European Association of Urology endorse CT as the preferred modality for diagnosing and characterizing renal masses (8).

CT Evaluation of a Renal Mass

CT scans for evaluation of a renal mass typically consists of three imaging series performed during breath hold: 1) Precontrast images are essential for evaluation of the presence of calcifications and provide a baseline density measurement for evaluating the degree and pattern of enhancement in cystic or solid renal masses; 2) Corticomedullary images (typical scan delay 70–85 seconds after injection) are performed for assessment of lesion vascularity, renal vascular anatomy, and tumor involvement of venous structures and; 3) Excretory phase images with a scan delay of 5 to 10 minutes may show tumor involvement of the renal collecting system. Generally, the presence of calcifications in a solid renal mass suggests malignancy. Rarely, a malignant renal tumor may be diffusely calcified (9). The nephrographic phase is usually best for detection of renal masses (10).

A CT urogram examination typically includes the multiphase contrast enhancement of the kidneys plus abdominopelvic scan of the kidneys, ureters, and bladder. These may be reconstructed with special MPR and 3D views on an independent workstation. Urologists often find the excretory-phase assessment of the collecting system, ureters, and bladder to be valuable, especially in non-routine cases (11).

Dual energy CT (DECT) scanning is now available and can characterize non-contrast- and contrast-enhanced examinations. Without contrast, DECT may provide quantitative information on lesion attenuation. After contrast enhancement, the VNC or "virtual no-contrast" view can be derived by combining dual energy scans to eliminate the iodine signal (12,13).

CT Pitfalls

Apparent and real enhancement may be found in multiphase renal CT exams, so small renal lesions can measure higher in attenuation relative to surrounding normal renal parenchyma. Local beam hardening and partial volume effects can produce "pseudoenhancement," so evaluation of local tissue properties using CT has known limitations and should be viewed with caution. If the slice thickness is too large, averaging of local attenuators with surrounding structures can change the mean value, while slices that are too thin result in excess noise. Calibration standards are tested in CT daily quality control scans, and they provide the basis for quantitative attenuation measurements (14–19).

Renal Mass Types

Classification of renal masses detected on CT as benign or malignant and prediction of histologic subtype are insufficiently reliable for clinical decision making. Size alone is a good, but imperfect, predictor of malignancy. At a size of less than 1 cm, 46% of tumors were benign; by contrast, 20% to 22% of tumors of 1 to 4 cm and less than 10% of masses greater than 4 cm were benign (20,21). The most consistent and valuable parameter for imaging characterization of renal mass types is the degree of enhancement, and this may further distinguish some histological subtypes. Renal mass lesions that enhance by 20 Hounsfield unit (HU) or more are clearly solid and vascular and likely malignant, but lesser degrees of enhancement may be indeterminate. It is essential to compare the same target lesion on the unenhanced and enhanced scans, especially in heterogeneous or small masses. MRI DCE and diffusion-weighted imaging parameters provide complementary information (Figure 1). The presence of calcification is not useful for distinguishing between pathologic subtypes (22).

Despite the fact that biopsy, or pathologic evaluation of the resected specimen, is still required for definitive diagnosis, the various benign lesions and renal cancer subtypes have been reported to have different imaging characteristics on CT scanning.

Clear Cell Carcinoma

Clear cell renal carcinomas are the most vascular among all malignant renal cortical tumors and enhance with IV contrast to a greater degree than other subtypes, especially papillary carcinomas. In addition, papillary renal carcinomas are typically homogeneous (23–25), and cystic degeneration is more evident in the clear cell subtype than in the other subtypes (26). A mixed enhancement pattern containing enhancing solid soft tissue and low-attenuation areas that may represent cystic or necrotic changes is most predictive of the clear cell type.

More specifically, 49% of clear cell renal carcinomas are hypervascular, as compared with only 15% of papillary renal carcinoma and 4% of chromophobe cancer. Heterogeneous enhancement alone has a positive predictive value of 67% for clear cell renal carcinoma. Avid enhancement, defined as greater than 140 HU, also predicted clear cell carcinoma well; 90% of these tumors were avidly enhancing (27).

Oncocytoma

Oncocytoma, a benign renal epithelial neoplasm, is indistinguishable from renal carcinoma by imaging alone; however, this neoplasm can have a characteristic central stellate scar on CT in up to one-third of cases. Segmental enhancement inversion during the corticomedullary phase and early excretory phase of biphasic MDCT could be used to differentiate small renal carcinoma from oncocytoma (28). Oncocytomas may overlap with clear cell renal carcinoma in terms of imaging features and degree of enhancement. On CT scans, the diagnosis of oncocytoma may be suggested if a central stellate scar is identified within an otherwise homogeneous tumor (27,29–33).

Papillary Renal Carcinoma

Papillary renal carcinomas are typically less vascular compared to other renal tumors and most

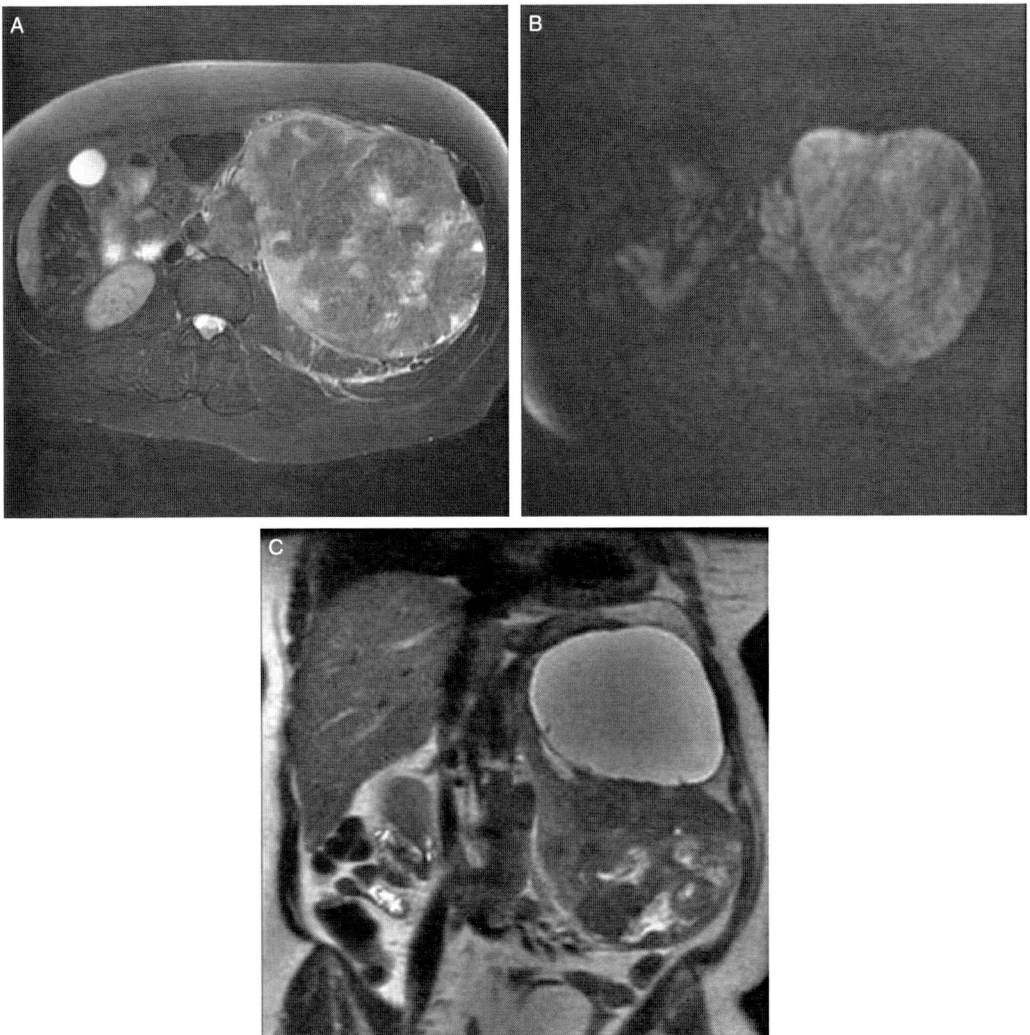

FIGURE 1

MRI of a 61-year-old woman with a large renal cell carcinoma. (A) T2 axial image shows a heterogeneous 15 cm mass filling the left hemiabdomen. (B) Diffusion-weighted image shows increased signal in the mass. (C) Coronal T2 image shows enlarged left renal vein with extensive tumor thrombus and a large upper pole uniloculated cyst.

commonly show homogeneous or peripheral enhancement. Contrast-enhanced CT during the renal parenchymal phase shows mild enhancement in peripherally distributed soft tissue. No enhancement is identified in the central low-attenuation region. Chromophobe and papillary tumors tend to be homogeneous. Avid enhancement is seen in 25% of chromophobe carcinomas but only 2% of papillary cancers (9,27).

Angiomyolipoma

Evidence of macroscopic fat on unenhanced images is highly predictive of AML, an important benign lesion that mimics renal cell carcinoma. Some

AMLs are fat-poor, so this diagnosis can be difficult. Subjective evaluation by an expert radiologist,
combined with pixel analysis that reveals more than
20 pixels with attenuation less than –20 HU and
more than 5 pixels with attenuation less than –30
HU, enables reliable prediction of AML. AMLs
with minimal fat have homogeneous enhancement
and a prolonged enhancement pattern compared
to size-matched renal carcinoma. Homogeneous
high attenuation on unenhanced CT images and
homogeneous enhancement on contrast-enhanced
CT images suggest an AML containing abundant
muscle and minimal fat.

CT for Tumor Staging

Staging of renal carcinoma is essential for surgical
planning, prognosis, and surveillance of systemic
therapies before or after cytoreductive nephrectomy. Invasion of contiguous structures (stage T4)
on CT is important in determining resectability.
Invasion of adjacent organs such as the liver, pancreas, or psoas muscle may preclude resection. The
presence of a discrete mass in the perinephric space
on CT has a specificity of up to 98% for predicting extension of tumor into the perirenal fat (stage
T3a). Most pathologically confirmed extrarenal
disease is not identified during preoperative CT

imaging. Tumor thrombus in the renal vein or
inferior vena cava (stage T3b–c) can be detected
on CT.

Multifocality, upper pole lesions and renal
vein involvement predict adrenal gland involvement. CT staging of regional lymph nodes is based
on size criteria, although all enlarged nodes do not
harbor metastases. Clinical node-negative patients
with renal masses rarely have metastatic disease in
their lymph nodes.

Contrast-enhanced CT may determine if
nephron-sparing surgery is possible, and facilitate
surgical planning. CT urography is used to assess
involvement of the renal collecting system, ureters,
and bladder so the choice between a partial or radical nephrectomy or nephroureterectomy can be
made. It may not be possible to separate urothelial
and renal cell cancer using CT. If urothelial cancer
is suspected, the surgical approach changes from
radical nephrectomy to nephroureterectomy.

Cystic Renal Tumors on CT

Bosniak classification system grades cystic renal
masses for the likelihood of malignancy based on
the complexity of these lesions (Table 1). When
any solid-enhancing component is present, the cystic renal mass is graded as a Bosniak type 4 lesion,

TABLE 1   Bosniak classification of renal cysts

Category I	Simple benign cyst with (1) enhanced through transmission, (2) no echoes within the cyst, (3) sharply, marginated smooth wall. This lesion requires no surgery.
Category II	Benign appearance with septation, minimal calcification, or high attenuation (CT). No internal blood flow or enhancement. This lesion requires no surgery.
Category II F	Calcification in cyst wall is thicker and more nodular than in category II, the septa have minimal enhancement, especially those with calcium. Follow-up is required, but not immediate surgery.
Category III	Calcification in cyst wall is thicker and more nodular than in category II, the septa have minimal enhancement, especially those with calcium. Follow-up is required, but not immediate surgery.
Category IV	Clearly malignant lesion with large cystic components, irregular margins; solid vascular elements; internal contrast enhancement and/or blood flow. These lesions require surgical removal.

highly suspicious for malignancy. Cystic tumors with thin walls and septations without solid components in an adult may represent benign cystic nephroma, multilocular cystic renal carcinoma, or cystic hamartoma of the renal pelvis (18,34–37).

Ionizing Radiation and CT

Dedicated renal CT protocols for study of renal masses involve multiple abdominal and pelvic scans before and at multiple time points after IV contrast administration. CT scan of a renal cortical mass includes pre-contrast, nephrographic, and delayed phases at a minimum, which requires a relatively high radiation dose, particularly in the case of repeated imaging during surveillance or follow-up. No specific prospective studies have detailed the role of CT in the development of cancer. Instead, estimation of cancer risk from medical radiation exposure is largely based on the estimated radiation exposure and recorded rates of cancer among survivors of the atomic bomb explosions in Japan in 1945. Attributable lifetime cancer risks from a single scan are related to both age and dose. Radiation dose reduction techniques have been introduced recently for cardiac, abdominopelvic, and other CT examinations (38–42).

IV Contrast Media

Contrast enhancement aids renal mass identification on CT, but the contrast agents have significant risk in patients with renal insufficiency. Iodinated contrast agents used in CT may induce contrast-induced nephropathy (CIN), a multifactorial and often irreversible renal function deterioration that occurs in up to 25% of patients with diabetes mellitus or pre-existing renal insufficiency. CIN is defined as an increase in serum creatinine level of at least 25%, or an absolute increase of at least 0.5 mg/dL (44 μmol/L) after the administration of contrast media, typically within 2 to 3 days.

Iodinated contrast agents can induce renal hemodynamic changes and ischemic injury through hyperosmolarity and effects on vasoactive substances, as well as through direct toxic effects on renal epithelium. Common CIN risk factors are diabetes mellitus and pre-existing renal dysfunction, which can be ameliorated with vigorous hydration, and the use of vasodilators and antioxidants. Hydration with normal saline has been shown in prospective trials to decrease the incidence of contrast nephropathy. Contrast media are contraindicated in patients with documented hypersensitivity reactions to previous administration, but IV steroid prophylaxis is sometimes used when there is sufficient clinical justification (43–46).

■ MAGNETIC RESONANCE IMAGING

The major advantage of MRI is lack of ionizing radiation. MRI provides high signal-to-noise tissue characterization of necrosis, hemorrhage, fat, and intracystic architecture. Renal MRI has been limited to cases when US or CT are inconclusive, iodinated contrast medium is contraindicated, or tumor thrombus is suspected. MR imaging is advantageous for detection and staging of renal neoplasms, due to the intrinsically high soft tissue contrast, direct multiplanar imaging capabilities, and availability of non-nephrotoxic, renally excreted contrast agents. Typical MR sequences used for renal mass imaging include: 1) T1 in and out of phase gradient echo—for identification of macroscopic and microscopic fat in a renal tumor; 2) T2-FSE in axial or coronal planes—for evaluating the overall anatomy, renal collecting system, and complexity of a cystic renal lesion; and 3) dynamic contrast-enhanced T1-weighted fat-suppressed sequence—for evaluation of the presence and pattern of enhancement in a renal mass. New MR sequences for diffusion weighted and other types of imaging have been introduced and tested in evaluation of renal masses.

MRI of small renal masses provides superior soft tissue contrast, whereas CT can be indeterminate due to pseudoenhancement. Because of its intrinsic multiplanar capability, MR imaging may be superior to CT for determining the origin of a renal mass. Non-contrast MR imaging can be performed safely in patients with renal failure and used for evaluation of renal tumors in these patients, an advantage for many patients with renal masses.

MRI Evaluation of a Renal Mass

Simple cysts are typically hypointense on T1 and hyperintense on T2. Some complex cysts may show a higher T1 signal and lower T2 signal owing to hemorrhage, debris, or proteinaceous material; there should be no enhancement in cysts after administration of contrast. Solid renal masses are typically isointense or moderately hypointense. In T2-weighted imaging, clear cell renal carcinoma is typically hyperintense; by contrast, AML with minimal fat and papillary renal carcinoma are typically hypointense on T2-weighted imaging.

Importantly, MRI can detect both macroscopic and microscopic fat. The detection of macroscopic fat within a renal tumor is highly suggestive of AML; renal carcinoma is devoid of macroscopic fat in almost all cases. However, 4.5% of AMLs have been reported to have minimal macroscopic fat. On MRI, AMLs with minimal fat are typically hypointense on T2-weighted imaging. Although the presence of macroscopic fat is diagnostic of AML, the presence of microscopic fat is not; both clear cell renal carcinoma and papillary renal carcinoma can contain microscopic fat deposits. When such a lesion is noted, percutaneous biopsy may be necessary.

As not all enhancing solid renal tumors are malignant, imaging techniques capable of differentiating cancers from benign neoplasms have been investigated. In CT studies, attenuation measurements in HU are used to quantify contrast enhancement. In MRI studies, gadolinium enhancement can be defined either qualitatively (presence versus absence) or quantitatively (percentage of enhancement) (Figure 2). Subtraction images can also be used on dynamic contrast-enhanced MRI; these are particularly useful when enhancement is subtle. In this technique, the signal intensity of the pre-contrast image is digitally subtracted from the post-contrast image; thus, any high signal intensity on the final image can be attributed to genuine lesion enhancement (47).

Role of MRI in Tumor Staging

After the identification of a mass as a likely renal carcinoma, the most important role of imaging is correct staging. MRI has been shown to have 84% sensitivity, 95% specificity, and a positive predictive value of 91% for differentiating pT3a renal carcinoma (tumor with perirenal extension) from localized disease. Tumor invasion into renal vein and inferior vena cava and the cephalad extent of tumor thrombus can be determined before surgery. MRI has replaced venacavography for evaluation of renal tumor extension into the inferior vena cava. MRI can discriminate blood from thrombus without contrast in most cases, which is advantageous if the patient has renal failure. However, MDCT is comparable to MRI for tumor thrombus detection when IV contrast is used.

Diffusion-Weighted MR Imaging

Diffusion-weighted (DW) MRI is routinely performed for neuroimaging, particularly in acute stroke, intracranial tumors, and demyelinating diseases; however, its use in renal imaging has been limited because of artifacts associated with respiratory motion, cardiac movement, and bowel peristalsis. With the development of echo-planar breath-hold imaging techniques, DW MRI of the abdomen was introduced, leading to reports on the clinical utility of the apparent diffusion coefficient (ADC) across a range of applications. ADC is a quantitative parameter calculated from DW MR images. By defining cutoff values in ADCs, separation of diseased and normal tissues can be achieved. DW MRI senses the diffusion of water between cells related to cell density and can differentiate renal lesions. This technique can be useful for discriminating cystic renal carcinoma from benign cysts and for characterizing renal carcinoma subtypes (48). The kidney

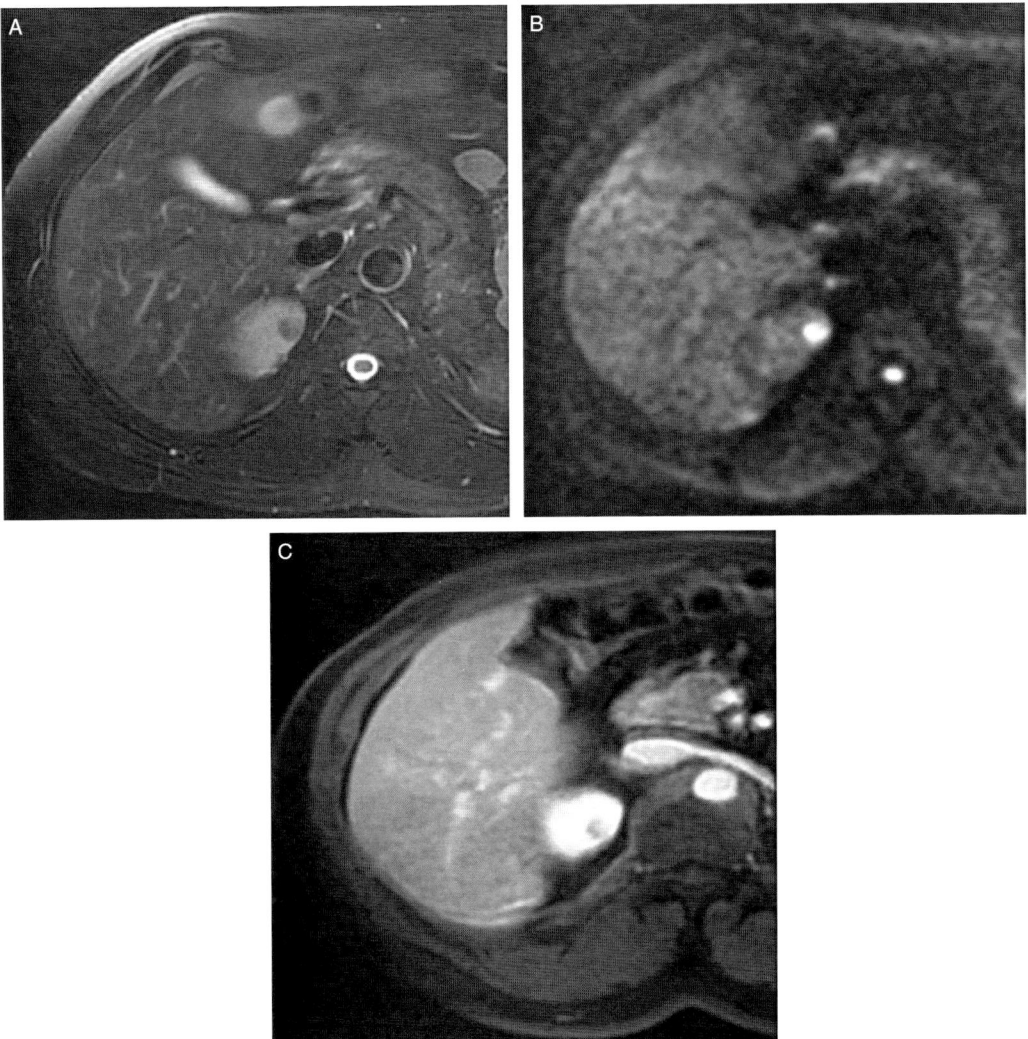

FIGURE 2
MRI of a 55-year-old man with a small renal cell carcinoma. (A) Axial T2 image shows that the signal within a 1.2 cm mass is lower than the CSF surrounding the spinal cord, so this is not a simple cyst. (B) Diffusion-weighted axial image shows high signal within the lesion. (C) Axial T1 image after contrast shows enhancement in this small solid lesion.

is a particularly suitable organ to study with DW imaging because of its high blood flow and water transport functions.

The potential utility of DW imaging for the characterization of renal lesions for the diagnosis of solid renal masses in particular comes from significantly lower ADCs in renal carcinomas, indicative of restricted diffusion, than in simple or mildly complex cysts and oncocytomas. These results are similar to findings of focal liver lesions, which, if malignant, generally exhibit decreased ADCs compared with the ADCs of liver hemangiomas and cysts. The restricted diffusion in renal neoplasms is probably multifactorial. It is possibly related to tissue cellularity (as in brain and breast tumors) and degree of cell membrane integrity.

Cystic renal carcinomas have higher ADCs owing to their cystic or necrotic components. In addition, ADCs reflect the combined effects of capillary perfusion and diffusion, and the decreased perfusion in papillary renal carcinomas, which have been shown to be hypovascular compared with clear cell carcinomas, could partially explain their decreased ADC. The decreased ADC of AMLs can be explained by muscle and fat components that restrict diffusion (49).

The accurate identification of the histologic subtypes of renal carcinoma with MR imaging is of clinical interest, as papillary renal carcinomas generally have a better prognosis than do nonpapillary renal carcinomas. Clear cell renal carcinomas demonstrated higher ADCs than papillary renal carcinomas and chromophobic renal carcinomas. One illustrative study evaluated the diagnostic performance of DW MR imaging in comparison to contrast-enhanced (CE) MR imaging to assess the ability to characterize renal lesions, with MR follow-up and histopathologic analysis as the reference standards (50). DW imaging was able to characterize renal lesions; however, when compared with CE MR imaging, it was overall less accurate in distinguishing benign from malignant masses. DW imaging was, however, able to differentiate solid renal carcinomas from oncocytomas and had utility for characterizing histologic subtypes (Figure 3).

In sum, breath-hold DW imaging can be easily added to a routine renal MR imaging protocol, is an accurate method for renal lesion characterization, and may yield useful information additional to that obtained with contrast-enhanced MR imaging.

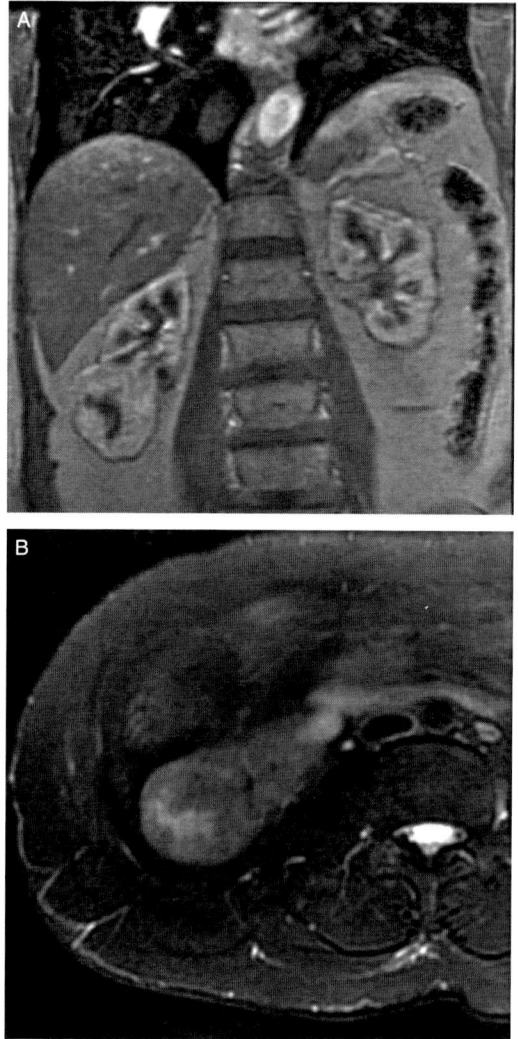

FIGURE 3
MRI of a 69-year-old woman with oncocytoma. (A) The 5 cm right lower pole mass has a central low signal region in a coronal T1 image. (B) The central scar has a higher signal than the surrounding parenchyma on T2 axial imaging.

■ ULTRASONOGRAPHY

US diagnosis and characterization of renal masses is rarely the sole imaging study, especially if a solid mass or complex cystic mass is identified. Since population-based screening for renal cell cancer is not justified, US is most often used for other applications that may lead to incidental renal mass detection. In general, US is most useful for characterization of renal lesions as cystic or solid. Benign cysts are typically completely anechoic, have a thin imperceptible wall, posterior enhancement, a round or oval shape, and are avascular. A benign cyst can become complex due to hemorrhage or infection and could mimic a solid lesion. If a lesion does not meet criteria for a simple cyst, a CT or MR examination (typically with and without IV contrast) will be recommended. Features suggesting a malignant cystic lesion include a thickened cystic wall, numerous septations, thickened or nodular septations, irregular or central calcifications, and the presence of blood flow in the septations or cystic wall on Doppler imaging. Most renal carcinomas are solid on US. Small, 3 cm or less, renal masses are more likely to be hyperechoic than larger tumors. Vascular flow within a renal mass, identified by color and power Doppler, is strongly associated with clear cell carcinoma. US can help characterize masses for which CT findings are indeterminate. US is particularly useful for determining whether a lesion is likely to be cystic and benign in cases of a hyperdense cyst found on CT in which enhancement cannot be assessed because contrast media is contraindicated.

There have been many changes since the European Association of Urology introduced Guidelines for Diagnosis, Therapy and Follow-Up of Renal Cell Carcinoma Patients in 2001 (51). US is limited by body habitus and bowel gas and is operator-dependent, so the American Urological Association (8) and American College of Radiology (52,53) rate CT much more favorably than US for investigating renal carcinoma.

Contrast-enhanced US (CEUS) uses microbubble US contrast agents together with specialized imaging techniques to enhance vascular elements within tissue. Microbubble contrast agents are not nephrotoxic and can be used in patients with any level of renal function. Despite such US contrast agents being used in Europe and Asia, they are not approved for radiology imaging by the FDA in the United States. Lack of FDA approval and reimbursement for US contrast agents impede their acceptance in the United States (2,54–59).

Cystic Masses

Renal cysts are prevalent in older adults; more than 50% of patients aged over 60 years have cysts on CT scans. The Bosniak classification system of renal cysts is universally accepted (Table 1). Simple cysts typically have clearly defined margins, thin

walls, and a lack of enhancement, septa, and calcification. Any septation, calcification, or ill-defined margin classifies a cyst as complex; these signs can range from a solitary septation with very low malignant potential to the presence of enhancing mural nodules that indicate malignancy with high specificity (18,34–37) (Figure 4).

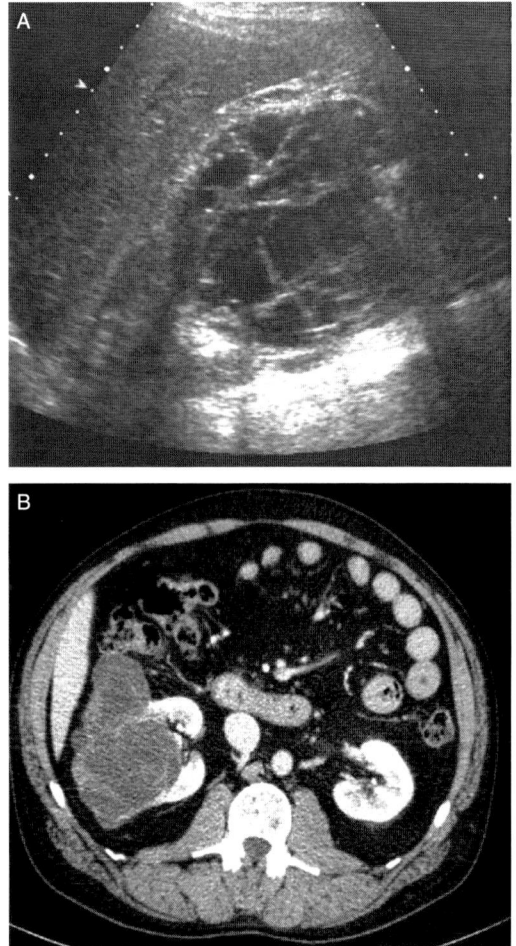

FIGURE 4

Ultrasound and CT of a 50-year-old man with a cystic renal cell carcinoma. (A) Longitudinal sonogram shows the right kidney is replaced by an 8-cm-diameter multiloculated cyst with thickened septations. Bosniak III lesion. (B) Contrast-enhanced CT axial image shows right midpole lesion suspicious for malignancy.

Classification of incidentally detected cysts and follow-up of complex cysts is often required. MRI can detect cyst fluids of varying densities; for example, protein or blood versus simple cyst fluid. On MRI, simple cysts are typically hypointense on T1-weighted and hyperintense on T2-weighted images. Complex cysts with hemorrhage or debris will not enhance. In the MRI assessment of complex cysts, mural irregularity, masses or nodules, increased mural thickness, and intense mural enhancement predict malignancy. In general, complex cystic renal masses should be evaluated with unenhanced and contrast-enhanced images since the presence of enhancement is the critical determinant used to differentiate surgical lesions (Bosniak classes III and IV) from non-surgical cases (Bosniak classes I and II).

■ EMISSION TOMOGRAPHY—SPECT AND PET

Nuclear medicine employs radioisotope tracers incorporated in small molecules that are imaged by mapping radioactive decay processes. Commonly used radioactive isotope agents may emit gamma ray photons (e.g., iodine-131, technitium-99m) or positrons (e.g., fluorine-18). Depending on the isotope chosen, an SPECT system or PET system may be used to create images.

SPECT systems are typically less expensive but more widely available, usually employed in cardiac emission tomography. But the same instrument may be used for other applications, for example, to acquire functional images of the urinary tract. SPECT is sometimes used for oncologic applications (60).

PET systems are established as a major asset for oncologic imaging, especially integrated with x-ray CT in PET-CT scanners. The PET-CT unit provides localization of functional activity detected by PET in the morphologic framework provided by CT. The x-ray CT component of a PET-CT system provides local x-ray attenuation maps used to correct the emission data and achieve quantitatively accurate image reconstructions. The CT component of PET-CT scans is not equivalent to dedicated renal CT scans since the former are obtained without IV or enteric contrast, and using minimal x-ray dose resulting in low contrast relatively noisy images (27). Expectation maximization iterative image reconstruction and 3D visualization are often used in SPECT and PET imaging.

SPECT systems used in oncology typically image Tc99m-based agents (technetium 99m half-life of 6 hours), whereas PET systems are used for F18-deoxyglucose imaging (fluorine-18 half-life is approximately 110 min) (61). Other agents have been developed and tested, but may require on-site radiochemistry facilities for synthesis and a nearby cyclotron to generate short-lived isotopes based upon carbon-11 (half-life of 20.38 min) (62,63) and oxygen-15 (half-life of 122 seconds) (64,65). Some promising PET agents include 18F-fluoroethylcholine (66), 11C-acetate (62,67,68), and many others. Such isotopes and unique tracers have impressive capabilities, but high cost of facilities, operations, and lack of reimbursement hinder their widespread acceptance and use.

SPECT is sometimes used for staging of complex renal masses and for evaluation of recurrent masses (60,69). PET has been applied to renal cancer detection, characterization, staging, and to evaluate therapy, usually with 18F-deoxyglucose (61,70–74). There are numerous case reports of SPECT and PET applied for problem solving in unusual cases, but sensitivity and specificity remain problematic and there is no specific recommendation for routine use of these modalities.

■ IMAGE-GUIDED TARGETED THERAPY

Antiangiogenic drugs, including bevacizumab, sorafenib, sunitinib, axitinib, and pazopanib, have demonstrated significant efficacy in renal carcinoma. The response to oncologic therapy is usually assessed by RECIST (75), the most widely used measurement system in clinical trials. However, RECIST may underestimate drug effect during targeted therapy, as it is only based on the sum of the longest diameters of the appointed target lesions in the transversal plane and does not account for other drug-induced morphological changes (7) Other imaging evaluation criteria for assessment of drug-induced tumor response in renal carcinoma patients include the Choi criteria (59), the modified Choi criteria, the SACT criteria, and the MASS criteria (Table 2). Functional imaging modalities, such as DCE-CT, DCE-MRI, DCE-US, and PET, have potential value as markers for treatment response (7).

Response Evaluation Criteria in Solid Tumors—CT

Assessment of morphological changes, that is, changes in tumor size burden, is an important evaluation method to determine the effect of anticancer drugs (Table 2). As noted, RECIST is the most commonly used measurement system. RECIST is a one-dimensional method and is based on the sum of the longest diameters of the appointed target lesions in the transverse (axial) plane. To determine tumor response accurately, target lesions (≥ 10 mm) are usually identified on CT or MRI.

RECIST provides four classes to determine the objective tumor response. Briefly, complete response is defined as disappearance of all target lesions, whereas a partial response (PR) requires a decrease in the sum of diameters of at least 30%, taking as reference the sum of the diameters at baseline. The appearance of new lesions or at least a 20% increase in the sum of the diameters is classified as PD, taking as reference the smallest sum during treatment. When the changes in the sum of the diameters are not sufficient to qualify for PR or PD, the objective response is defined as stable disease (SD).

Recently, RECIST has been updated and version 1.1 has been introduced. Changes include a reduction in the number of target lesions to be assessed per patient (from a maximum of 10 to a maximum of 5) and per organ (from 5 to 2 per organ), a change in assessment of pathological lymph nodes (measurement of the longest axis has

TABLE 2 Renal cell cancer response evaluation criteria (CT-based)

Criteria	Target Lesions	Maximum Number of Target Lesions	Measurements	Threshold for Change
RECIST (version 1.1) (61,62,72)	CT: tumor size $\geq$ 10 mm			
CXR: tumor size $\geq$ 15 mm	5	Tumor size	20%–30%	
Choi criteria (59)	Tumor size $\geq$ 15 mm	10	Tumor size or tumor attenuation	10%–15%
Modified Choi criteria (67)	Tumor size $\geq$ 15 mm	10	Tumor size and tumor attenuation	10%
SACT criteria (77)	Tumor size $\geq$ 10 mm	10	Tumor size; mean attenuation	10% ($\geq$20 HU)
MASS criteria (78)	Tumor size $\geq$ 10 mm	10	Lesion morphology, attenuation, size, and structure	20% ($\geq$40 HU)

been changed into the shortest; nodes should have a short axis of ≥ 15 mm to be considered as measurable) and the clarification of disease progression in small tumor burden (a 5 mm absolute increase is now required) (76–78).

Many studies have applied RECIST to determine response to targeted therapy in renal carcinoma. Up to 10 months may be required after the start of treatment to determine whether response will be favorable. Use of RECIST at first evaluation in patients with SD is a poor discriminator for long-term patient benefit (79–86).

Some studies suggest that responders (i.e., patients who will benefit from treatment) can be identified earlier with a smaller threshold than with the conventional –30% according to RECIST (87–89).

Contrast-Enhanced Computed Tomography

Tumor attenuation changes during targeted therapy can be detected by contrast-enhanced CT, based on changes in tumor vasculature and angiogenesis. In metastases from renal carcinoma, higher pretreatment values of contrast enhancement are associated with a higher response rate to VEGF pathway-targeted therapy with either sunitinib or sorafenib (Figure 5). Treatment-induced changes in tumor density and the development of necrotic areas are associated with VEGF pathway-directed therapy and may predict for patient benefit. In contrast, the development of a marked central fill-in and new enhancement in homogeneously, hypoattenuating, nonenhancing renal carcinoma lesions are commonly seen at or just before the time of progression late in the course of treatment, suggesting that an increase in contrast enhancement may be associated with disease progression (10).

Tumor response evaluation criteria that incorporate changes in image contrast enhancement have been investigated: the Choi criteria, the modified Choi criteria, the MASS criteria, and the SACT criteria.

Choi Criteria

Using contrast-enhanced CT scans, Choi et al. have developed new evaluation criteria to determine the efficacy of imatinib in patients with gastrointestinal stromal cell tumors (GISTs) (87). In patients with GIST, imatinib is known to induce extensive tumor necrosis that may be accompanied by an increase in tumor size and may even simulate PD. The Choi criteria include changes in tumor attenuation expressed as HU on contrast-enhanced CT. In imatinib-treated patients with GIST, the Choi criteria had a significantly better correlation with disease-specific survival than RECIST (90). However, the Choi criteria were not able to identify renal carcinoma patients with PD and did not change the clinical management of patients treated with sunitinib. The Choi criteria may be more useful to identify renal carcinoma patients with PD during sorafenib treatment, as fewer patients have tumor response to sorafenib as compared to sunitinib (91,92). The modified Choi criteria provided the best segregation of the median time-to-progression (83).

SACT Criteria

As a ≥10% decrease in tumor size or a ≥15% decrease in tumor attenuation is not necessarily associated with a prolonged progression free survival, the SACT criteria have been developed. According to these criteria a favorable response is defined as a decrease in tumor size of ≥20% or a decrease in mean attenuation of ≥40 HU in at least one non-lung target lesion (93).

MASS Criteria

MASS represents further refinement of SACT criteria, which included the detection of central fill-in of formerly necrotic lesions and new enhancement of previously nonenhancing hypoattenuating masses as markers of disease progression. Although SACT criteria were found to improve assessment of tumor response, the 3-D volumetric image analysis required is time-consuming and labor-intensive and hence excluded from MASS criteria (94).

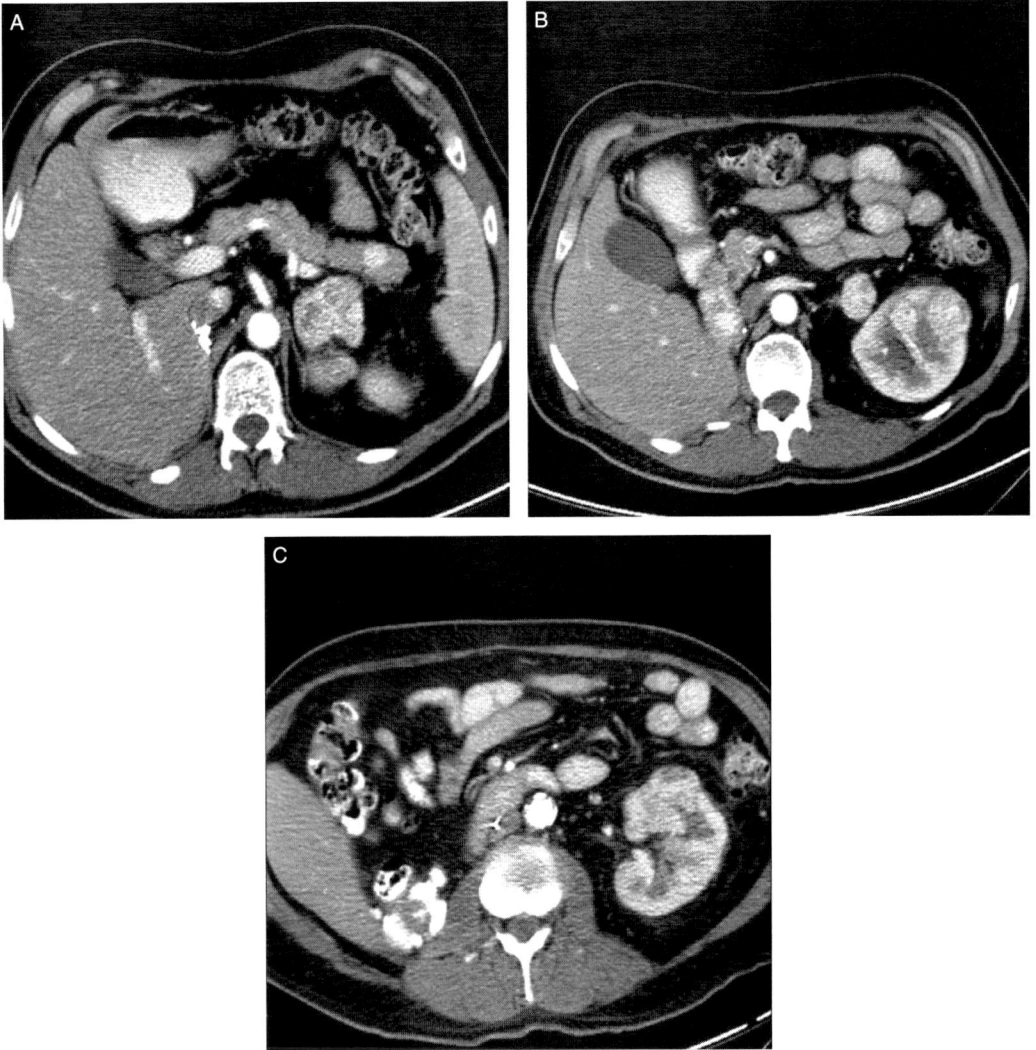

FIGURE 5

CT of a 58-year-old man with metastatic renal cell carcinoma. (A) Lymph node mass in left paraaortic region with focus of enhancement in the pancreas, later shown to be a metastasis. (B) One mass in left kidney and enlarged lymph node medially. (C) Second left kidney mass found at another axial level.

Limitations of Contrast-Enhanced Measurements in Renal Carcinoma

Although incorporation of changes in tumor attenuation appears to be valuable for response assessment, there are limitations. New requirements are imposed, such as consistent scanning protocols and the same timing of IV contrast between the subsequent CT scans, since different phases in IV contrast may dramatically alter lesion attenuation. The targeted agents may also affect the cardiac output and alter the distribution of IV contrast during treatment despite an identical scanning protocol. Contrast-enhanced CT scanning may not be possible in some renal carcinoma patients, since IV contrast may be contraindicated due to impaired renal function.

In sum, incorporation of treatment-induced changes in tumor attenuation on contrast-enhanced CT may have additional value to assess tumor response, but it is not clear whether inclusion of these changes in decision making has significant impact on the current management of metastatic renal carcinoma patients. Functional imaging techniques, including DCE-CT, DCE-MRI, DCE-US, and PET, are thus under investigation. The first reports are promising, but further studies are required to validate the usefulness of these imaging techniques in patients early during targeted therapy.

■ CONCLUSIONS

CT and MR imaging are essential for diagnosis, characterization, and follow-up of renal tumors. US and PET/SPECT have secondary roles. Each imaging modality has strengths and weaknesses but together they provide accurate assessment of most masses. US is safe, widely available, efficient, and avoids radiation exposure, but is user-dependent, has lower spatial resolution than other modalities, and is inadequate for tumor staging. CT is most commonly used, providing sufficient resolution and sensitivity for staging, but causes safety concerns with ionizing radiation and iodinated contrast agents. MRI has superb soft tissue contrast without ionizing radiation, but is expensive, time intensive, and not well-tolerated by some patients. Tumor size and character, local disease extent, and metastasis evaluation are required for renal carcinoma management; combined assessment by CT, MRI, and US can provide this information. Contrast enhancement and vascularity are evaluated to characterize renal tumors. New technologies, including the introduction of MR-PET systems (95–97), low dose whole body CT scanning (42,98,99), dual energy or spectral CT (100,101), targeted diagnostic imaging agents,

functional imaging methods, and numerous other technical innovations, provide the basis of new imaging tests to evaluate renal cell cancer and its treatment. This will likely lead to ever-increasing use of imaging in renal cancer clinical management and the hope for more effective and efficient noninvasive diagnosis and monitoring.

■ REFERENCES

1. Iannicelli P, Rosa A. [Diagnostic imaging of kidney carcinomas. Our experience and review of the literature]. *Minerva Urol Nefrol.* 1992;44(3):177–183.
2. Leveridge MJ, Bostrom PJ, Koulouris G, Finelli A, Lawrentschuk N; Medscape. Imaging renal cell carcinoma with ultrasonography, CT and MRI. *Nat Rev Urol.* 2010;7(6):311–325.
3. Guermazi, A. *Imaging of kidney cancer.* 1st ed. Medical radiology, diagnostic imaging. 2006, Berlin; New York: Springer. xvi, 439 p.
4. Gill IS, Aron M, Gervais DA, Jewett MA. Clinical practice. Small renal mass. *N Engl J Med.* 2010;362(7):624–634.
5. Campbell N, Barrett S, Halpenny D, et al. Imaging patterns of atypical renal cell carcinoma recurrence: a pictorial review. *Can Assoc Radiol J.* 2010. DOI: 10.1016/j.carj.2010.08.001. [Epub ahead of print]
6. Konety BR, Williams RD. Renal parenchymal neoplasms. In: Tanagho EA, McAninch JW, eds. *Smith's General Urology.* McGraw Hill: New York; 2008:328–347.
7. van der Veldt AA, Meijerink MR, van den Eertwegh AJ, Boven E. Targeted therapies in renal cell cancer: recent developments in imaging. *Target Oncol.* 2010;5(2):95–112.
8. Mues AC, Landman J. Small renal masses: current concepts regarding the natural history and reflections on the American Urological Association guidelines. *Curr Opin Urol.* 2010;20(2):105–110.
9. Chen Y, Zhang J, Dai J, Feng X, Lu H, Zhou C. Angiogenesis of renal cell carcinoma: perfusion CT findings. *Abdom Imaging.* 2010;35(5):622–628.
10. Fournier LS, Oudard S, Thiam R, et al. Metastatic renal carcinoma: evaluation of antiangiogenic therapy with dynamic contrast-enhanced CT. *Radiology.* 2010;256(2):511–518.

11. Horton KM. CT urogram. *Crit Rev Comput Tomogr.* 2003;44(4):177–181.

12. Lee SH, Lee JM, Kim KW, et al. Dual-energy computed tomography to assess tumor response to hepatic radiofrequency ablation: potential diagnostic value of virtual noncontrast images and iodine maps. *Invest Radiol* 2011;46(2):77–84.

13. Sommer WH, Graser A, Becker CR, et al. Image quality of virtual noncontrast images derived from dual-energy CT angiography after endovascular aneurysm repair. *J Vasc Interv Radiol.* 2010;21(3):315–321.

14. Maki DD, Birnbaum BA, Chakraborty DP, Jacobs JE, Carvalho BM, Herman GT. Renal cyst pseudoenhancement: beam-hardening effects on CT numbers. *Radiology.* 1999;213(2):468–472.

15. Ho VB, Allen SF, Hood MN, Choyke PL. Renal masses: quantitative assessment of enhancement with dynamic MR imaging. *Radiology.* 2002;224(3):695–700.

16. Abdulla C, Kalra MK, Saini S, et al. Pseudoenhancement of simulated renal cysts in a phantom using different multidetector CT scanners. *AJR Am J Roentgenol.* 2002;179(6):1473–1476.

17. Gokan T, Ohgiya Y, Munechika H, Nobusawa H, Hirose M. Renal cyst pseudoenhancement with beam hardening effect on CT attenuation. *Radiat Med.* 2002;20(4):187–190.

18. Israel GM, Bosniak MA. Pitfalls in renal mass evaluation and how to avoid them. *Radiographics.* 2008;28(5):1325–1338.

19. Wang ZJ, Coakley FV, Fu Y, et al. Renal cyst pseudoenhancement at multidetector CT: what are the effects of number of detectors and peak tube voltage? *Radiology.* 2008;248(3):910–916.

20. Thompson RH, Kurta JM, Kaag M, et al. Tumor size is associated with malignant potential in renal cell carcinoma cases. *J Urol.* 2009;181(5):2033–2036.

21. Frank I, Blute ML, Cheville JC, Lohse CM, Weaver AL, Zincke H. Solid renal tumors: an analysis of pathological features related to tumor size. *J Urol.* 2003;170(6 Pt 1):2217–2220.

22. Smith DR, Tanagho EA, McAninch JW. *Smith's General Urology.* 14th ed. Norwalk, Connecticut: Appleton & Lange; 1995:ix, 823.

23. Herts BR. Imaging for renal tumors. *Curr Opin Urol.* 2003;13(3):181–186.

24. Herts BR. Imaging guided biopsies of renal masses. *Curr Opin Urol.* 2000;10(2):105–109.

25. Silverman SG, Israel GM, Herts BR, Richie JP. Management of the incidental renal mass. *Radiology.* 2008;249(1):16–31.

26. Sheir KZ, El-Azab M, Mosbah A, El-Baz M, Shaaban AA. Differentiation of renal cell carcinoma subtypes by multislice computerized tomography. *J Urol.* 2005;174(2):451–5; discussion 455.

27. Zhang J, Lefkowitz RA, Ishill NM, et al. Solid renal cortical tumors: differentiation with CT. *Radiology.* 2007;244(2):494–504.

28. Kim JK, Park SY, Shon JH, Cho KS. Angiomyolipoma with minimal fat: differentiation from renal cell carcinoma at biphasic helical CT. *Radiology.* 2004;230(3):677–684.

29. Tan YM, Yip SK, Li MK. Clinics in diagnostic imaging (36). Benign renal oncocytoma. *Singapore Med J.* 1999;40(4):314–316.

30. Jinzaki M, Tanimoto A, Mukai M, et al. Double-phase helical CT of small renal parenchymal neoplasms: correlation with pathologic findings and tumor angiogenesis. *J Comput Assist Tomogr.* 2000;24(6):835–842.

31. Hecht EM, Israel GM, Krinsky GA, et al. Renal masses: quantitative analysis of enhancement with signal intensity measurements versus qualitative analysis of enhancement with image subtraction for diagnosing malignancy at MR imaging. *Radiology.* 2004;232(2):373–378.

32. Reuter VE. The pathology of renal epithelial neoplasms. *Semin Oncol.* 2006;33(5):534–543.

33. Siu W, Hafez KS, Johnston WK 3rd, Wolf JS Jr. Growth rates of renal cell carcinoma and oncocytoma under surveillance are similar. *Urol Oncol.* 2007;25(2):115–119.

34. Bosniak MA. The current radiological approach to renal cysts. *Radiology.* 1986;158(1):1–10.

35. Israel GM, Hindman N, Bosniak MA. Evaluation of cystic renal masses: comparison of CT and MR imaging by using the Bosniak classification system. *Radiology.* 2004;231(2):365–371.

36. Israel GM, Bosniak MA. How I do it: evaluating renal masses. *Radiology.* 2005;236(2):441–450.

37. Israel GM, Bosniak MA. An update of the Bosniak renal cyst classification system. *Urology.* 2005;66(3):484–488.

38. Kubo T, Lin PJ, Stiller W, et al. Radiation dose reduction in chest CT: a review. *AJR Am J Roentgenol.* 2008;190(2):335–343.

39. Yu L, Li H, Fletcher JG, McCollough CH. Automatic selection of tube potential for radiation dose reduction in CT: a general strategy. *Med Phys.* 2010;37(1):234–243.

40. Prakash P, Kalra MK, Digumarthy SR, et al. Radiation dose reduction with chest computed

tomography using adaptive statistical iterative reconstruction technique: initial experience. *J Comput Assist Tomogr*. 2010;34(1):40–45.

41. Kalra MK, Francis IR. Personalized dose reduction for computed tomography scanning: size matters, so does prior radiation exposures. *Clin Gastroenterol Hepatol*. 2010;8(3):231–232.

42. Gleeson TG, Byrne B, Kenny P, et al. Image quality in low-dose multidetector computed tomography: a pilot study to assess feasibility and dose optimization in whole-body bone imaging. *Can Assoc Radiol J*. 2010;61(5):258–264.

43. Arana E, Catalá-López F. [Contrast-induced nephropathy in patients at risk of renal failure undergoing computed tomography: systematic review and meta-analysis of randomized controlled trials]. *Med Clin (Barc)*. 2010;135(8):343–350.

44. Garg AX. ACP Journal Club. Review: Evidence on the effectiveness of sodium bicarbonate regimens to prevent contrast-induced nephropathy is unclear. *Ann Intern Med*. 2010;152(10):JC5–J10.

45. Morcos SK, Thomsen HS, Webb JA. Contrast-media-induced nephrotoxicity: a consensus report. Contrast Media Safety Committee, European Society of Urogenital Radiology (ESUR). *Eur Radiol*. 1999;9(8):1602–1613.

46. Goldenberg I, Matetzky S. Nephropathy induced by contrast media: pathogenesis, risk factors and preventive strategies. *CMAJ*. 2005;172(11):1461–1471.

47. Linam LE, Yu X, Calvo-Garcia MA, et al. Contribution of magnetic resonance imaging to prenatal differential diagnosis of renal tumors: report of two cases and review of the literature. *Fetal Diagn Ther*. 2010;28(2):100–108.

48. Wang H, Cheng L, Zhang X, et al. Renal cell carcinoma: diffusion-weighted MR imaging for subtype differentiation at 3.0 T. *Radiology*. 2010;257(1): 135–143.

49. Saremi F, Knoll AN, Bendavid OJ, Schultze-Haakh H, Narula N, Sarlati F. Characterization of genitourinary lesions with diffusion-weighted imaging. *Radiographics*. 2009;29(5):1295–1317.

50. Taouli B, Thakur RK, Mannelli L, et al. Renal lesions: characterization with diffusion-weighted imaging versus contrast-enhanced MR imaging. *Radiology*. 2009;251(2):398–407.

51. Mickisch G, Carballido J, Hellsten S, Schulze H, Mensink H; European Association of Urology. Guidelines on renal cell cancer. *Eur Urol*. 2001; 40(3):252–255.

52. Mainiero MB. Incorporating ACR Practice Guidelines, Technical Standards, and Appropriateness Criteria into resident education. *J Am Coll Radiol*. 2004;1(4):277–279.

53. Berlin L. Commentary: ACR practice guidelines and technical standards. *J Am Coll Radiol*. 2004;1(2):98–99.

54. Ishikawa I, Morita K, Hayama S, et al. Imaging of acquired cystic disease-associated renal cell carcinoma by contrast-enhanced ultrasonography with perflubutane microbubbles and positron emission tomography-computed tomography. *Clin Exp Nephrol*. 2011;15(1):136–140.

55. Xu ZF, Xu HX, Xie XY, Liu GJ, Zheng YL, Lu MD. Renal cell carcinoma and renal angiomyolipoma: differential diagnosis with real-time contrast-enhanced ultrasonography. *J Ultrasound Med*. 2010;29(5):709–717.

56. Lassau N, Koscielny S, Albiges L, et al. Metastatic renal cell carcinoma treated with sunitinib: early evaluation of treatment response using dynamic contrast-enhanced ultrasonography. *Clin Cancer Res*. 2010;16(4):1216–1225.

57. Mazziotti S, Zimbaro F, Pandolfo A, Racchiusa S, Settineri N, Ascenti G. Usefulness of contrast-enhanced ultrasonography in the diagnosis of renal pseudotumors. *Abdom Imaging*. 2010;35(2):241–245.

58. Tamai H, Takiguchi Y, Oka M, et al. Contrast-enhanced ultrasonography in the diagnosis of solid renal tumors. *J Ultrasound Med*. 2005;24(12): 1635–1640.

59. Setola SV, Catalano O, Sandomenico F, Siani A. Contrast-enhanced sonography of the kidney. *Abdom Imaging*. 2007;32(1):21–28.

60. Mariani G, Bruselli L, Kuwert T, et al. A review on the clinical uses of SPECT/CT. *Eur J Nucl Med Mol Imaging*. 2010;37(10):1959–1985.

61. Langer A. A systematic review of PET and PET/CT in oncology: a way to personalize cancer treatment in a cost-effective manner? *BMC Health Serv Res*. 2010;10:283.

62. Shreve P, Chiao PC, Humes HD, Schwaiger M, Gross MD. Carbon-11-acetate PET imaging in renal disease. *J Nucl Med*. 1995;36(9):1595–1601.

63. Oyama N, Okazawa H, Kusukawa N, et al. 11C-Acetate PET imaging for renal cell carcinoma. *Eur J Nucl Med Mol Imaging*. 2009;36(3):422–427.

64. Gambhir SS. Molecular imaging of cancer with positron emission tomography. *Nat Rev Cancer*. 2002;2(9):683–693.

65. de Langen AJ, van den Boogaart VE, Marcus JT, Lubberink M. Use of H2(15)O-PET and DCE-MRI to measure tumor blood flow. *Oncologist*. 2008;13(6):631–644.

66. Middendorp M, Maute L, Sauter B, Vogl TJ, Grünwald F. Initial experience with 18F-fluoroethyl-choline PET/CT in staging and monitoring therapy response of advanced renal cell carcinoma. *Ann Nucl Med*. 2010;24(6):441–446.

67. Shreve PD, Gross MD. Imaging of the pancreas and related diseases with PET carbon-11-acetate. *J Nucl Med* 1997;38(8):1305–1310.

68. Maleddu A, Pantaleo MA, Castellucci P, et al. 11C-acetate PET for early prediction of sunitinib response in metastatic renal cell carcinoma. *Tumori*. 2009;95(3):382–384.

69. Harisankar C, Mittal BR, Bhattacharya A, Singh B. Utility of hybrid SPECT-CT in the detection of unsuspected single lytic vertebral metastases in renal cell carcinoma. *Indian J Nucl Med* 2010;25(1):32–33.

70. Bihl H, Lang O, Schleicher J, Mergenthaler H, Willms K, Eisenberger F. Metastatic renal cell carcinoma (mRCC). Is there a role of F-18-FDG-PET? *Clin Positron Imaging*. 1999;2(6):340.

71. Ramdave S, Thomas GW, Berlangieri SU, et al. Clinical role of F-18 fluorodeoxyglucose positron emission tomography for detection and management of renal cell carcinoma. *J Urol*. 2001;166(3):825–830.

72. Miyakita H, Tokunaga M, Onda H, et al. Significance of 18F-fluorodeoxyglucose positron emission tomography (FDG-PET) for detection of renal cell carcinoma and immunohistochemical glucose transporter 1 (GLUT-1) expression in the cancer. *Int J Urol*. 2002;9(1):15–18.

73. Dilhuydy MS, Durieux A, Pariente A, et al. PET scans for decision-making in metastatic renal cell carcinoma: a single-institution evaluation. *Oncology*. 2006;70(5):339–344.

74. Nakatani K, Nakamoto Y, Saga T, Higashi T, Togashi K. The potential clinical value of FDG-PET for recurrent renal cell carcinoma. *Eur J Radiol*. 2009. DOI:10.1016/j.ejrad.2009.11.019. [Epub ahead of print]

75. Therasse P, Arbuck SG, Eisenhauer EA, et al. New guidelines to evaluate the response to treatment in solid tumors. European Organization for Research and Treatment of Cancer, National Cancer Institute of the United States, National Cancer Institute of Canada. *J Natl Cancer Inst*. 2000;92(3):205–216.

76. Nishino M, Jackman DM, Hatabu H, et al. New Response Evaluation Criteria in Solid Tumors (RECIST) guidelines for advanced non-small cell lung cancer: comparison with original RECIST and impact on assessment of tumor response to targeted therapy. *AJR Am J Roentgenol*. 2010;195(3):W221–W228.

77. Nishino M, Jagannathan JP, Ramaiya NH, Van den Abbeele AD. Revised RECIST guideline version 1.1: What oncologists want to know and what radiologists need to know. *AJR Am J Roentgenol*. 2010;195(2):281–289.

78. van Persijn van Meerten EL, Gelderblom H, Bloem JL. RECIST revised: implications for the radiologist. A review article on the modified RECIST guideline. *Eur Radiol*. 2010;20(6):1456–1467.

79. Baccala A Jr, Hedgepeth R, Kaouk J, Magi-Galluzzi C, Gilligan T, Fergany A. Pathological evidence of necrosis in recurrent renal mass following treatment with sunitinib. *Int J Urol*. 2007;14(12):1095–7; discussion 1097.

80. Bex A, van der Veldt AA, Blank C, et al. Neoadjuvant sunitinib for surgically complex advanced renal cell cancer of doubtful resectability: initial experience with downsizing to reconsider cytoreductive surgery. *World J Urol*. 2009;27(4):533–539.

81. Cowey CL, Fielding JR, Rathmell WK. The loss of radiographic enhancement in primary renal cell carcinoma tumors following multitargeted receptor tyrosine kinase therapy is an additional indicator of response. *Urology*. 2010;75(5):1108–13.e1.

82. Lyrdal D, Boijsen M, Suurküla M, Lundstam S, Stierner U. Evaluation of sorafenib treatment in metastatic renal cell carcinoma with 2-fluoro-2-deoxyglucose positron emission tomography and computed tomography. *Nucl Med Commun*. 2009;30(7):519–524.

83. Nathan PD, Vinayan A, Stott D, Juttla J, Goh V. CT response assessment combining reduction in both size and arterial phase density correlates with time to progression in metastatic renal cancer patients treated with targeted therapies. *Cancer Biol Ther*. 2010;9(1):15–19.

84. Rini BI, Wilding G, Hudes G, et al. Phase II study of axitinib in sorafenib-refractory metastatic renal cell carcinoma. *J Clin Oncol*. 2009;27(27):4462–4468.

85. Rixe O, Bukowski RM, Michaelson MD, et al. Axitinib treatment in patients with cytokine-refractory metastatic renal-cell cancer: a phase II study. *Lancet Oncol*. 2007;8(11):975–984.

86. Thiam R, Fournier LS, Trinquart L, et al. Optimizing the size variation threshold for the CT evaluation of response in metastatic renal cell carcinoma treated with sunitinib. *Ann Oncol.* 2010;21(5):936–941.

87. Benjamin RS, Choi H, Macapinlac HA, et al. We should desist using RECIST, at least in GIST. *J Clin Oncol.* 2007;25(13):1760–1764.

88. Eisenhauer EA, Therasse P, Bogaerts J, et al. New response evaluation criteria in solid tumours: revised RECIST guideline (version 1.1). *Eur J Cancer.* 2009;45(2):228–247.

89. Levine ZH, Borchardt BR, Brandenburg NJ, et al. RECIST versus volume measurement in medical CT using ellipsoids of known size. *Opt Express.* 2010;18(8):8151–8159.

90. van der Veldt AA, Meijerink MR, van den Eertwegh AJ, Haanen JB, Boven E. Choi response criteria for early prediction of clinical outcome in patients with metastatic renal cell cancer treated with sunitinib. *Br J Cancer.* 2010;102(5):803–809.

91. Cowey CL, Amin C, Pruthi RS, et al. Neoadjuvant clinical trial with sorafenib for patients with stage II or higher renal cell carcinoma. *J Clin Oncol.* 2010;28(9):1502–1507.

92. Han KS, Jung DC, Choi HJ, et al. Pretreatment assessment of tumor enhancement on contrast-enhanced computed tomography as a potential predictor of treatment outcome in metastatic renal cell carcinoma patients receiving antiangiogenic therapy. *Cancer.* 2010;116(10):2332–2342.

93. Smith AD, Lieber ML, Shah SN. Assessing tumor response and detecting recurrence in metastatic renal cell carcinoma on targeted therapy: importance of size and attenuation on contrast-enhanced CT. *AJR Am J Roentgenol.* 2010;194(1):157–165.

94. Smith AD, Shah SN, Rini BI, Lieber ML, Remer EM. Morphology, Attenuation, Size, and Structure (MASS) criteria: assessing response and predicting clinical outcome in metastatic renal cell carcinoma on antiangiogenic targeted therapy. *AJR Am J Roentgenol.* 2010;194(6):1470–1478.

95. Catana C, van der Kouwe A, Benner T, et al. Toward implementing an MRI-based PET attenuation-correction method for neurologic studies on the MR-PET brain prototype. *J Nucl Med.* 2010;51(9):1431–1438.

96. Delso G, Martinez-Möller A, Bundschuh RA, Nekolla SG, Ziegler SI. The effect of limited MR field of view in MR/PET attenuation correction. *Med Phys.* 2010;37(6):2804–2812.

97. Herzog H, Pietrzyk U, Shah NJ, Ziemons K. The current state, challenges and perspectives of MR-PET. *Neuroimage.* 2010;49(3):2072–2082.

98. Pontana F, Duhamel A, Pagniez J, et al. Chest computed tomography using iterative reconstruction vs filtered back projection (Part 2): image quality of low-dose CT examinations in 80 patients. *Eur Radiol.* 2011;21(3):636–643.

99. Naidich DP. High-resolution computed tomography of the pulmonary parenchyma: past, present, and future? *J Thorac Imaging.* 2010;25(1):32–33.

100. Eliahou R, Hidas G, Duvdevani M, Sosna J. Determination of renal stone composition with dual-energy computed tomography: an emerging application. *Semin Ultrasound CT MR.* 2010;31(4):315–320.

101. Pan D, Roessl E, Schlomka JP, et al. Computed tomography in color: NanoK-enhanced spectral CT molecular imaging. *Angew Chem Int Ed Engl.* 2010;49(50):9635–9639.

ECAT»»
Emerging Cancer
Therapeutics

demos
MEDICAL

Management of Small Renal Masses: Donating Kidneys to Your Local Pathologist Is Not Advised

Steven C. Campbell* and Byron Lee

Glickman Urological and Kidney Institute, Cleveland Clinic, Cleveland, OH

■ ABSTRACT

Small renal masses (SRMs) are typically discovered incidentally and represent a common and controversial clinical scenario. Biological aggressiveness varies widely—20% are benign and only 20% harbor potentially aggressive features. The results of renal mass sampling have improved and this procedure should be considered more often prior to definitive therapy. Management options range from active surveillance (AS) to radical nephrectomy (RN), also including thermal ablation (TA) and partial nephrectomy (PN). Presuming that adequate oncologic control can be obtained via other approaches, RN should be avoided because it predisposes to chronic kidney disease. In general, nephron-sparing options are preferred, and PN is now the reference standard in the field. Efforts to improve the PN procedure to optimize renal function and minimize morbidity hold great promise for the future. TA has gained considerable traction and represents an attractive alternative for patients with extensive comorbidities, who wish to avoid surgery. However, local recurrence rates are higher with TA, parameters for success during follow up are debated, and surgical salvage can be difficult. AS is ideal for patients with limited life expectancy but entails some oncologic risk otherwise. The elderly with SRMs typically present with competing causes of mortality and declining renal function that must be judiciously considered during counseling and management. American Urologic Association Guidelines provide formal direction with respect to the merits and limitations of these treatment modalities, and their sensible utility for the management of patients with clinical T1 (<7 cm) renal masses. New data and perspectives about SRMs and the guidelines are highlighted reflecting substantial progress in this field in the past few years.

Keywords: renal mass, active surveillance, thermal ablation, partial nephrectomy, radical nephrectomy

* Corresponding author, Glickman Urological and Kidney Institute, Cleveland Clinic, Room Q10–120, Glickman Tower, 9500 Euclid Ave, Q10, Cleveland, OH 44195
   E-mail address: campbes3@ccf.org

Emerging Cancer Therapeutics 2:1 (2011) 57–72.
© 2011 Demos Medical Publishing LLC. All rights reserved.
DOI: 10.5003/2151–4194.2.1.57

■ INTRODUCTION

The generally accepted definition of a small renal mass (SRM) is a solid, enhancing renal mass that is considered suspicious for renal carcinoma based on cross-sectional imaging. These tumors are now being discovered with increased frequency due to the more prevalent use of cross-sectional imaging (1,2). The majority are incidentally discovered, low stage, and relatively small at presentation (3,4). Most studies suggest an increase of SRM incidence of about 3% to 4% per year, although this trend appears to be more substantial in the African American population (5). Overall, clinical T1 renal tumors (< 7.0 cm) are now a common clinical scenario, representing about 40% of all cases of kidney cancer. SRMs also include a fascinating array of benign histologies, most commonly oncocytoma and atypical angiomyolipoma (AML). A reasonable estimate is that there are about 20 to 30,000 new cases of SRMs each year in the United States. Classically managed with radical nephrectomy (RN), which is now recognized as substantial overtreatment, these tumors have engendered much interest over the past decade. Over this time period, we have witnessed substantial progress in our understanding of the tumor biology of SRMs and are beginning to manage them in a more rational manner.

■ TUMOR BIOLOGY

A fundamental principle with respect to SRMs is that they are very heterogeneous from a biological standpoint, with 20% benign, 55% to 60% indolent renal cell cancer (RCC), and only about 20% to 25% presenting with potentially aggressive features (Figure 1) (6–9). As such, oncologic control is potentially obtained through a variety of approaches, and in some patients treatment is not even necessary. A corollary is that cancer-related mortality is somewhat uncommon in this patient population. Nevertheless, hidden among patients with SRMs are subsets with true oncologic risk, which mandate proactive and efficacious management. Numerous lines of evidence support these generalizations.

In our series of 851 patients with clinical T1 renal tumors managed with partial nephrectomy (PN), we reported that 173 (20%) were benign, most commonly oncocytomas or atypical AMLs that were far poor and therefore occult on imaging (8). Benign tumors were more common in young

Clinical T1 Renal Mass: The Future

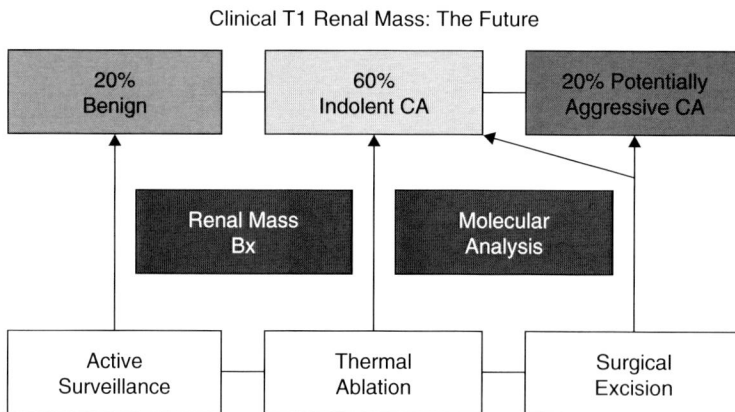

FIGURE 1
Seeing small renal mass (SRM) tumor biology with 20/20 vision. 20% of SRMs are benign and 20% are potentially aggressive. A variety of treatment options are now available ranging from observation to radical nephrectomy. Renal mass sampling and molecular analysis will ultimately facilitate more rational management of patients with SRMs.

women. Our nomogram to predict benign histology for SRMs incorporated gender, tumor size, history of tobacco use, and presence or absence of local symptoms, and yielded a modest c-index of 0.644. This demonstrates that such clinical and preoperative tumor-related factors are inadequate for predicting benign histology. Even for young women, for whom the incidence of benign histology was highest, RCC still predominated and could not be identified *a priori*.

Further analysis of our dataset demonstrated that of the 678 cancers, about 30% were potentially aggressive, that is, either high grade or demonstrating a locally invasive phenotype. Overall, this represented about 24% of the SRMs in our series. This left 56% of all SRMs that appeared to have relatively indolent tumor biology, in that they remained organ confined and were of low to moderate grade. Predictors of potentially aggressive renal cancer in this population included local symptoms, tobacco history, tumor size, and gender; however, the c-index for this analysis was only 0.557, not much better than a coin flip. These data highlight the limited ability of clinical and radiologic features to predict tumor aggressiveness among patients with SRMs.

Other series have confirmed these findings and establish tumor size as the most important indicator of tumor biology. In the series from the Mayo Clinic, benign histology was found in 23.3%, 9.5%, and 6.3% of tumors <4 cm, 4 to 7 cm, and > 7 cm, respectively (6). Similarly, clear cell histology, which tends to be more aggressive, was found in 50.5%, 73.3%, and 83.0% of these same subgroups, respectively. Finally, high tumor grade was found in 12.5%, 29.8%, and 62.1% of these subgroups, respectively. Other studies suggest a potential cut point at 3 cm at which the tumor is more likely to be aggressive, similar to familial kidney cancer, although this remains controversial (10,11). Most data suggest that tumor size is most relevant and powerful as a continuous variable.

Studies of active surveillance (AS) provide a glimpse into the natural history of untreated SRMs, although this literature is notable for strong selection biases and limited follow-up. Nevertheless, primary tumor growth rates and metastatic incidence remain low and most elderly patients on AS appear to die with rather than from their SRM, suggesting a predominance of nonaggressive pathologies.

■ OVERVIEW OF TREATMENT OPTIONS

As illustrated in Figure 1, the treatment options for SRMs vary greatly in their radicality, impact on renal function, and procedural risk. RN was traditionally utilized in the majority of patients with SRMs but predisposes to chronic kidney disease (CKD), a major concern in this patient population that often has preexisting renal dysfunction (12). PN is the reference standard but carries the greatest risk of perioperative complications, although most are readily manageable. Thermal ablation (TA) represents another option for proactive management that is less invasive, and AS is an attractive option for patients with extensive comorbidities or limited life expectancy.

■ RENAL MASS SAMPLING

Renal mass sampling (RMS) can be performed by 18-gauge core biopsy or fine needle aspiration, and by CT or US guidance with each approach presenting potential advantages and limitations (13,14). Perspectives about RMS have evolved substantially from the 1990s when the false-negative rate for this procedure was thought to be too high, namely 18%, to justify its routine incorporation into the evaluation of patients with SRMs (9,15–18). In reality, many of these "false negatives" were actually noninformative biopsies, where the tumor could not be adequately targeted, or the specimen was not sufficient for the pathologist to provide a definitive diagnosis. Prior to 2001, these noninformative biopsies represented 14% of RMS procedures, and the real false-negative rate was only 4% (9).

In the past decade, the false-negative rates for RMS have been consistently below 1% and the overall accuracy has been greater than 95% in most series (14,19,20). These data are much more encouraging, and RMS is now being incorporated into the routine evaluation of SRMs at some centers, particularly for patients that might reasonably be candidates for several treatment options ranging from AS to surgery (14). An example would be a 75-year-old man with modest comorbidities and a 3 cm strongly enhancing renal mass suspicious for RCC. In such a patient, AS, TA, and PN would all be reasonable considerations, and the results of RMS could guide counseling. If TA is performed RMS should be routinely incorporated to guide surveillance on a long-term basis (21). Young, healthy patients with an SRM typically elect proactive management because they are unwilling to accept the low level uncertainty and risk associated with RMS. In this setting, PN represents both diagnosis and cure; it is essentially an excisional biopsy, and presuming negative margins, no further therapy is required.

The risks of RMS include bleeding, pneumothorax, and needle tract seeding, all of which are distinctly uncommon. Symptomatic bleeding requiring transfusion or pneumothorax mandating chest tube placement have both been reported in < 1% of patients (14,20). Needle tract seeding is a very infrequent event presuming that centrally located infiltrative renal masses are precluded from RMS (18). The latter may represent high-grade urothelial cell carcinoma, which is known to be at increased risk for this type of adverse event (18,22,23). Overall, only eight cases of needle tract seeding related to RMS of primary RCC have been reported in the English literature. Importantly, some of these were locally advanced RCC rather than SRMs, and no cases have been reported since 1994 (24). Current technique for RMS uses a cannula, which minimizes the risk of needle tract seeding and allows for placement of sterile, thrombogenic materials directly against the capsule, if substantial bleeding is encountered

(25). Such measures have greatly improved the safety of RMS.

Ongoing challenges with RMS include noninformative biopsies, which represent about 10% of current RMS procedures, and the inherent difficulties differentiating various "oncocytic tumors" on limited pathologic material. Recent studies suggest that noninformative biopsies can undergo repeat RMS with results analogous to initial RMS, that is, repeat sampling will be informative for about 90% of such cases (14). Beyond repeat RMS, other options for the management of noninformative biopsies include surgical excision to provide a definitive diagnosis, or AS if the patient is unwilling or unable to proceed in this direction.

The issue of the oncocytic neoplasm is more challenging, in that it is often difficult to differentiate an oncocytoma from eosinophilic variants of renal carcinoma based on RMS alone. Special stains for cytokeratins and other analyses such as electron microscopy can help, but are not routinely utilized (26–29). Most studies suggest that these oncocytic neoplasms are either oncocytomas or low-grade renal cancers, but definitive data are lacking (14,20). Future molecular profiling may allow for a more accurate definition of tumor histology, grade, and aggressive potential (Figure 1). When available, "enhanced RMS" will facilitate more intelligent counseling and management of patients with SRMs.

■ GUIDELINES FOR MANAGEMENT

Recognizing considerable controversy regarding the management of SRMs and practice patterns that are often discordant with available evidence, the American Urological Association commissioned a panel to provide guidelines for the management of the clinical T1 (≤ 7.0 cm, organ confined) renal mass (12). This document was published in 2009 and presents a detailed algorithm for the management of SRMs (Figure 2). Four index patients were defined based on patient comorbidities, estimated life expectancy, and tumor size, T1a

Key: AS, active surveillance; CKD, chronic kidney disease; CT, computed tomography; FNA, fine needle aspiration; MRI, magnetic resonance imaging; PN, partial nephrectomy; RFA, radiofrequency ablation; RN, radical nephrectomy; TA, thermal ablation

Patient with clinical T1 renal mass

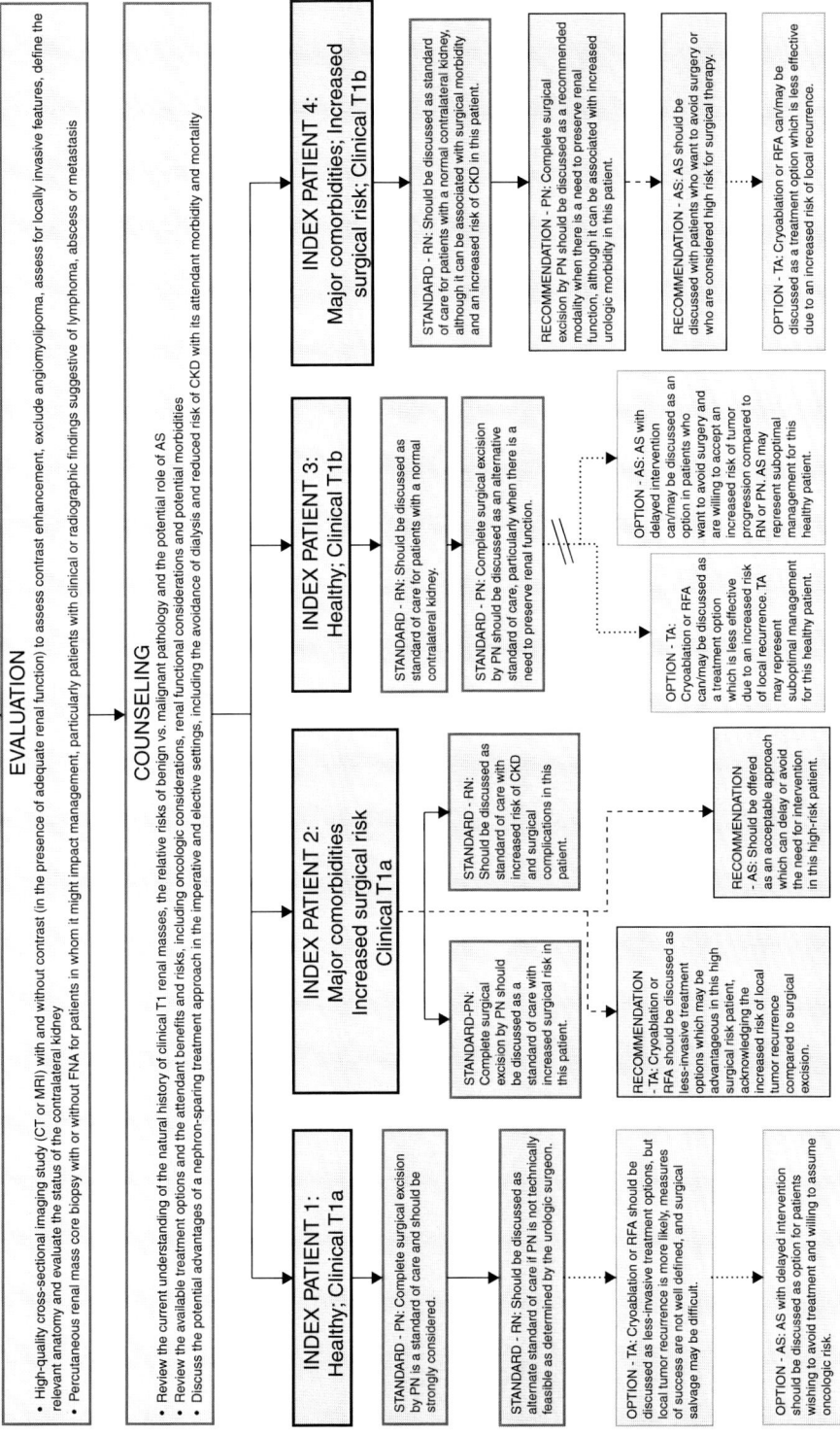

EVALUATION

- High-quality cross-sectional imaging study (CT or MRI) with and without contrast (in the presence of adequate renal function) to assess contrast enhancement, exclude angiomyolipoma, assess for locally invasive features, define the relevant anatomy and evaluate the status of the contralateral kidney
- Percutaneous renal mass core biopsy with or without FNA for patients in whom it might impact management, particularly patients with clinical or radiographic findings suggestive of lymphoma, abscess or metastasis

COUNSELING

- Review the current understanding of the natural history of clinical T1 renal masses, the relative risks of benign vs. malignant pathology and the potential role of AS
- Review the available treatment options and the attendant benefits and risks, including oncologic considerations, renal functional considerations and potential morbidities
- Discuss the potential advantages of a nephron-sparing treatment approach in the imperative and elective settings, including the avoidance of dialysis and reduced risk of CKD with its attendant morbidity and mortality

---

INDEX PATIENT 1: Healthy; Clinical T1a

STANDARD - PN: Complete surgical excision by PN is a standard of care and should be strongly considered.

STANDARD - RN: Should be discussed as alternate standard of care if PN is not technically feasible as determined by the urologic surgeon.

OPTION - TA: Cryoablation or RFA should be discussed as less-invasive treatment options, but local tumor recurrence is more likely, measures of success are not well defined, and surgical salvage may be difficult.

OPTION - AS: AS with delayed intervention should be discussed as option for patients wishing to avoid treatment and willing to assume oncologic risk.

INDEX PATIENT 2: Major comorbidities Increased surgical risk Clinical T1a

STANDARD-PN: Complete surgical excision by PN should be discussed as a standard of care with increased surgical risk in this patient.

STANDARD - RN: Should be discussed as standard of care with increased risk of CKD and surgical complications in this patient.

RECOMMENDATION - TA: Cryoablation or RFA should be discussed as less-invasive treatment options which may be advantageous in this high surgical risk patient, acknowledging the increased risk of local tumor recurrence compared to surgical excision.

RECOMMENDATION - AS: Should be offered as an acceptable approach which can delay or avoid the need for intervention in this high-risk patient.

INDEX PATIENT 3: Healthy; Clinical T1b

STANDARD - RN: Should be discussed as standard of care for patients with a normal contralateral kidney.

STANDARD - PN: Complete surgical excision by PN should be discussed as an alternative standard of care, particularly when there is a need to preserve renal function.

OPTION - TA: Cryoablation or RFA can/may be discussed as a treatment option which is less effective due to an increased risk of local recurrence. TA may represent suboptimal management for this healthy patient.

OPTION - AS: AS with delayed intervention can/may be discussed as an option in patients who want to avoid surgery and are willing to accept an increased risk of tumor progression compared to RN or PN. AS may represent suboptimal management for this healthy patient.

INDEX PATIENT 4: Major comorbidities; Increased surgical risk; Clinical T1b

STANDARD - RN: Should be discussed as standard of care for patients with a normal contralateral kidney, although it can be associated with surgical morbidity and an increased risk of CKD in this patient.

RECOMMENDATION - PN: Complete surgical excision by PN should be discussed as a recommended modality when there is a need to preserve renal function, although it can be associated with increased urologic morbidity in this patient.

RECOMMENDATION - AS: AS should be discussed with patients who want to avoid surgery or who are considered high risk for surgical therapy.

OPTION - TA: Cryoablation or RFA can/may be discussed as a treatment option which is less effective due to an increased risk of local recurrence.

FIGURE 2

Algorithm for the evaluation, counseling, and management of the clinical T1 renal mass. Source: Adapted from Campbell SC, Novick AC, Uzzo RG, et al. *AUA Guidelines for the Management of Clinical T1 Renal Masses.* Available at http://www.auanet.org/content/guidelines-and-quality-care/clinical-guidelines/main-reports/renalmass09.pdf

61

(≤4.0 cm) versus T1b (>4.0 but ≤7.0 cm). Standards, recommendations, and options were defined for each index patient based on a systematic and rigorous meta-analysis of the literature, using strict inclusion and exclusion criteria. Oncologic outcomes such as local recurrence and metastatic rates were prioritized in the analysis, along with renal functional considerations and the risks of various interventions (Table 1). Panel consensus of the various treatment options is summarized in KEY POINTS. Distilled to essentials, the two main statements of this document are as follows:

• Save the kidney whenever possible—donation of functional kidneys to your local pathologist via RN is discouraged and should only be done when necessary.

• The limitations of TA and AS should be recognized and discussed during counseling—these strategies should be used judiciously.

Further progress in the field is beginning to sharpen these perspectives, as highlighted later in this chapter.

Radical Nephrectomy and Chronic Kidney Disease

RN has traditionally been the treatment of choice for SRM, and it is still the most common utilized therapy, even for patients with risk factors for CKD such as hypertension and diabetes (30). Laparoscopic RN has been characterized "The

TABLE 1 Summary of outcomes for patients with a clinical T1 renal mass based on management strategy

	AS	TA	PN	RN
No. studies/No. patients	12/390	35/1389	54/8663	33/7816
Median patient age (years)	68	66–70	60	61–63
Median tumor size (cm)	2.2	2.6–2.7	2.6–3.0	5.1–5.4
Median months follow-up	29	17–19	15–47	18–58
% Urological complication rate	NA	4.9–6.0	6.3–9.0	1.3–3.4
% Local recurrence-free survival rate	20	87.0–90.6	98.0–98.4	98.1–99.2
% Metastatic recurrence-free survival rate	97.7	95.3–97.8	96.7–98.8	89.8–95.7
Reduction in renal function and potential impact on cardiovascular morbidity	None	Minimal	Minimal	High

Gray represents advantageous, black intermediate, and white unfavorable characteristics of the four management types. Data were derived from the meta-analysis reported in AUA Guideline for Management of the Clinical T1 Renal Mass, based on the literature until September of 2007. Data for TA incorporated studies from radiofrequency ablation and cryoablation, PN from studies of open and laparoscopic PN, and RN from open and laparoscopic RN.

AS, active surveillance; TA, thermal ablation; PN, partial nephrectomy; RN, radical nephrectomy.

Median months follow-up for laparoscopic PN was 15 months versus 47 months for open PN. Median months follow-up for laparoscopic RN was 18 months versus 58 for open RN.

Please refer to the guidelines document for a more rigorous analysis and further details. Source: Campbell SC, Novick AC, Uzzo RG, et al. *AUA Guidelines for the Management of Clinical T1 Renal Masses*. Available at http://www.auanet. org/content/guidelines-and-quality-care/clinical-guidelines/main-reports/renalmass09.pdf

Great Seductress" due to its appeal to patients and surgeons alike. Its oncologic radicality, minimal morbidity, and rapid convalescence are all attractive, but it comes at a great price, namely loss of renal function (Figure 3). Interestingly, recognition of the true magnitude of this issue has only been realized within the past 5 to 8 years. A landmark study from Memorial Sloan Kettering evaluated 662 patients with a solitary SRM < 4 cm in size, a normal serum creatinine level and a normal contralateral kidney (31). Such patients were considered for RN or elective PN, although based on the results of this study, PN should no longer be considered elective. The first major finding was that such patients are not analogous to renal transplant donors as was commonly presumed in the past. Renal transplant donors can donate a kidney because they are heavily screened for good renal function and good general health. Patients with SRMs are often older and have comorbidities, and in this study, 26% had preexisting grade 3 CKD (glomerular filtration rate [GFR] < 60 mL/min/1.73 m^2). Of note, 65% of patients treated with RN in this study developed grade 3 CKD postoperatively compared to 20% of patients managed with PN.

The importance of avoiding CKD is supported by an extensive literature that emphasizes the need to optimize renal function, not merely avoid dialysis (32). A landmark study by Go et al. evaluated the relationship between renal function and morbid cardiovascular events and death during longitudinal follow up and is now a cornerstone in this field (33). This population-based study followed over a million subjects for a median of only 2.8 years. The authors reported a strong inverse correlation between baseline renal function and cardiovascular events and mortality, even after controlling for a number of potentially confounding factors, such as hypertension and diabetes. As expected, the risks of cardiovascular events and death were highest for patients requiring dialysis at baseline (GFR < 15 mL/min/1.73 m^2) with adjusted hazard ratios (HR) of 3.4 and 5.9, respectively, compared to patients without CKD. However, increased risks for cardiovascular events and death were also seen for patients with moderate CKD (GFR 30–45 mL/min/1.73 m^2) with adjusted HR of 2.0 and 1.8, respectively, and for severe CKD (GFR 15–30 mL/min/1.73 m^2) with adjusted HR of 2.8 and 3.2, respectively.

A recent study from our institution focused on outcomes for 1,004 patients with pT1b RCC (4–7 cm) managed with either PN (*n* = 524) or RN (*n* = 480) and supports a potential advantage for PN in this population (34). On multivariate analysis that controlled for comorbidities and tumor characteristics, cancer-specific survival was equivalent

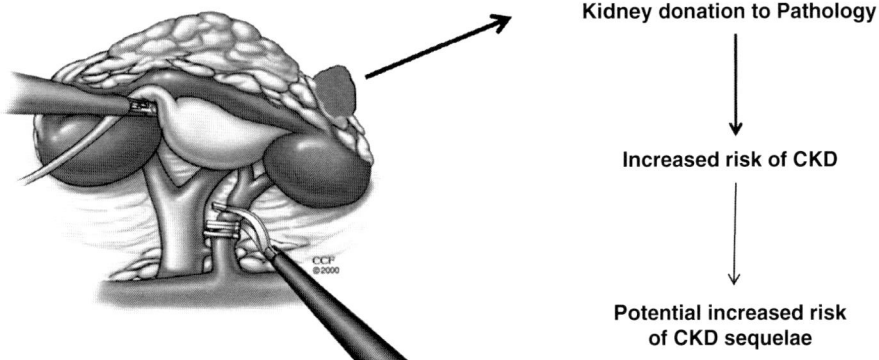

Kidney donation to Pathology

↓

Increased risk of CKD

↓

Potential increased risk of CKD sequelae

FIGURE 3
Laparoscopic RN, The Great Seductress.

for patients treated with PN or RN. As expected, RN was associated with significantly greater loss of renal function than PN. Loss of renal function with RN correlated with a 25% increased risk of cardiac death and a 17% increased risk of death from any cause on multivariate analysis. In summary, postoperative CKD was a significant independent predictor of overall and cardiovascular-specific mortality, and RN was a primary contributor to CKD in this patient population. Several other studies support PN in this population (35,36), suggesting that the guideline statements about Index Patient 3 (Figure 2), a healthy patient with a clinical T1b renal mass, should be reconsidered, with PN being changed from an alternate standard to a reference standard, similar to Index Patient 1.

Partial Nephrectomy

As highlighted earlier, PN is now the reference standard for the management of SRMs, because it provides comparable oncologic outcomes to RN, while also minimizing the risk of developing CKD. This presumes that negative margins can be obtained and multifocality is addressed. In the past, multifocality was considered an indication for RN, but the modern perspective is that such patients are also at high risk to recur in the contralateral kidney and are better served by a nephron-sparing approach up front.

The downside of PN is an increased risk of urologic complications, such as urine leak and postoperative bleed (Table 1). In the guidelines meta-analysis, such complications occurred in 6.3% and 9.0% of patients after open PN (OPN) and laparoscopic PN (LPN), respectively (12). The incidence of complications after LPN was statistically higher than all other modalities, with the exception of OPN. LPN and OPN were used to treat relatively young patients (median age 60) with small tumors, so this was thought to be a real, non-confounded finding. This result is not unexpected, because PN requires a renal reconstruction that must heal, and occasional complications are anticipated. A large study from three centers of excellence provides detailed information about the urologic morbidity associated with LPN (n = 771) and OPN (n = 1,029) (37). Significant selection bias was observed; OPN patients on average were less healthy, had worse performance status, and were more likely to have a symptomatic tumor, solitary kidney, preexisting CKD, larger tumor size, and central tumor location. Nevertheless, urologic complication rates were 5.0% after OPN versus 9.2% after LPN ($P < 0.0001$), perioperative hemorrhage rates were 1.6% for OPN versus 4.2% for LPN ($P < 0.0001$), and the need for subsequent procedures was 3.5% for OPN versus 7.0% for LPN ($P < 0.0001$).

Most complications from PN can be managed conservatively and urologic complications rates for minimally invasive PN appear to be decreasing with further experience (38). Urinary extravasation can be managed with continued drainage to allow for further healing, and a stent should be considered if there is evidence for ureteral obstruction. Open or laparoscopic reoperation for this complication should be a very rare event—almost all urinary leaks will heal with conservative management. Postoperative bleeding can be more problematic and will occasionally require surgical exploration, although the majority can be managed with transfusion and observation or selective angiographic embolization. Loss of the kidney or substantial loss of function is an uncommon event. Further experience and robotic technology are expanding the indications for minimally invasive PN and reducing the morbidity in terms of more rapid convalescence but also reduced urologic complications. Early unclamping allows the surgeon to observe for potential sites of bleeding that can be addressed prior to the final renorrhaphy and can substantially reduce the risk of perioperative bleeding (39).

Other exciting developments include clinical and translational studies to define the determinants of renal function after PN. Until now, the literature has focused on ischemic time and type of ischemia (warm vs. cold) as major determinants of renal function after PN. However, our recent analysis of 660 PN performed in a solitary kidney suggests that factors that are for the most part nonmodifiable, namely the amount of parenchyma that can be spared and the preoperative GFR, are the primary determinants of ultimate renal function ($P < 0.00001$ for both factors on multivariate analysis) (40). When both of these factors were included in the final analysis, ischemia duration and type of ischemia both lost statistical significance as predictors of ultimate renal function. This suggests that within the confines of conventional PN as practiced in this study population, where warm ischemia time was typically < 20 to 30 minutes and hypothermia was liberally utilized, most kidneys will eventually recover from the ischemic insult, leaving the quantity and quality of preserved parenchyma as the primary determinants of ultimate renal function.

Further analysis of a more homogeneous population of 362 patients managed with PN using only warm ischemia is also highly informative. In the initial analysis of this dataset, warm ischemic time was highly predictive of loss of renal function after PN (41). When the percent parenchyma spared and the preoperative GFR were both incorporated into the multivariate analysis, ischemic time retained statistical significance, although the nonmodifiable factors again predominated (*unpublished data*). This suggests that warm ischemic time does matter, particularly if it is extended beyond 20 to 30 minutes, consistent with the recent recommendations of an international consortium that advocated limiting warm ischemic time during PN to 20 minutes or less whenever possible.

Our recent analysis of patients undergoing PN in the presence of a normal contralateral kidney is also consistent with these findings (42). This study included patients managed with no ischemia ($n = 58$), cold ischemia ($n = 265$), or warm ischemia of less than 10 minutes ($n = 63$), 11 to 20 minutes ($n = 389$), or 21 to 30 minutes ($n = 357$). While adverse renal functional outcomes such as de novo CKD were uncommon in this population, they were primarily limited to patients in whom warm ischemia extended beyond 20 minutes.

Moving forward, we will need to reconsider the status of the "nonmodifiable factors" and target these as potential areas for improvement. The amount of parenchyma that can be preserved during PN is primarily determined by tumor size and location, which place constraints on how much vascularized parenchyma can be spared, and baseline functionality is primarily determined by age, comorbidities, body habitus, and history of prior renal disease processes and/or renal surgery. The use of intraoperative ultrasonography and judicious 3D planning both prior to and during intrarenal dissection may optimize the amount of preserved parenchyma, while still achieving negative surgical margins, and careful reconstruction can potentially minimize ischemic areas adjacent to the renorrhaphy. Optimization of renal function prior to and immediately after PN may also be important, and a collaborative approach to the management of these patients involving skilled urologic surgeons and dedicated nephrologists should be strongly considered.

Future studies will use novel biomarkers of renal cellular injury to define the degree of ischemic injury, allowing us to more accurately determine the relative impact of warm versus cold ischemia, and the deleterious effects of prolonged warm ischemia (43). These biomarkers, which are specific to the kidney and analogous to troponins for myocardial injury, will allow us to optimize the PN procedure, allowing it to reach its full potential as a nephron-sparing modality.

Thermal Ablation

TA, including cryoablation (CA) and radiofrequency ablation (RFA), has gained considerable traction in the field due to its relative ease of adoption, favorable economics, minimally invasive characteristics, and inherent appeal to patients (44–49). TA is a reasonable choice for patients with relatively small tumors (< 3.5 cm) and substantial comorbidities, who desire proactive treatment yet are at increased surgical risk. TA also plays an important role for the salvage of patients who recur in the ipsilateral kidney after PN and in patients with multifocal familial disease. However, laparoscopic or percutaneous TA is now supplanting PN at some centers, even for relatively young, healthy patients, and some patients with SRMs are now being managed primarily by interventional radiologists, with no involvement by urologists. It is important to emphasize that the literature does not support these changes in practice pattern (50).

Deficiencies in the TA literature are a major concern, such as limited follow up, lack of pathologic confirmation, and controversies about histologic or radiographic parameters for success (51). In the guidelines meta-analysis, TA had the shortest median follow up, only 17 months for CA and 19 months for RFA (12). Only a minority of studies have included extended follow-up, with all others providing only 1- to 3-year outcomes (44,47,52,53). Many TA studies have not incorporated routine pathologic confirmation prior to treatment, thus including 20% to 25% benign tumors within their efficacy analyses, and thereby inflating the reported success rates (50). Few TA studies have included routine post-ablation biopsies, depending instead on radiographic parameters for determination of success (12,50). We and others have demonstrated that viable cancer can occasionally reside within tumor beds that have lost radiographic enhancement, and false-negative imaging after TA remains a controversial topic in the field (54,55).

The greatest concern with TA relates to its oncologic characteristics, particularly suboptimal local control and difficulty with surgical salvage in the setting of TA failure (Table 1). In the guidelines meta-analysis, 9.4% and 13.0% of patients experienced local recurrence after CA and RFA, respectively, compared to 2% after OPN, although mean tumor size was smaller with TA and median length of follow up was considerably shorter (17–19 months for TA vs. 58 months for OPN) (12). When these confounding factors were taken into account, the local recurrence rates after CA and RFA were estimated to be 7.5- and 18-fold higher than those for PN (56). In one of the few studies

with extended follow up after TA, 5-year cancer-specific and recurrence-free survival rates were 93% and 83%, respectively, substantially lower than what would be expected with surgical excision in a similar patient population (44,53). While most TA failures can be managed with repeat ablation, surgical salvage will be required in about 10% to 20%. However, extensive fibrosis in the perinephric space is typically encountered in this setting that can preclude PN or minimally invasive approaches (57,58). Complication rates for surgical salvage after TA are substantially increased, reflecting challenges related to obliteration of anatomic planes and poor tissue quality adjacent to the tumor bed (57).

Advocates of TA cite better renal functional outcomes and lower morbidity with TA compared with surgical excision, but the literature does not support these presumptions (51,59). In the guidelines meta-analysis, major urologic complication rates after TA (4.9%–6.0%) were similar to those after OPN (6.3%) and major nonurologic complication rates were higher after TA (12). Theoretical advantages related to leaving the renal vasculature unclamped during TA have not correlated with better renal functional outcomes in most studies. In a recent multicenter series new onset CKD was more common after CA than PN (15.6% vs. 9.7%, respectively), and local recurrence (7.8% vs. 1.7%, respectively) and disease-free survival (93% vs. 99%, respectively) were both less favorable for CA (60).

The merits and limitations of TA and its related literature should be acknowledged and conveyed during patient counseling and management, and this modality, which is of great value in select patients, should be utilized in a judicious manner (Figure 2 and KEY POINTS).

Active Surveillance

Meta-analyses of published series of AS from several institutions support this modality as a primary consideration for patients with extensive comorbidities or restricted life expectancy, but the limitations of this literature are still substantial (19). These studies suggest that most SRM grow relatively slow, with a median growth rate of only 0.28 cm per year, and are associated with a low risk of metastasis (1%–2%) during limited follow up (19,61,62). However, substantial selection bias has been practiced, with most AS series consisting of relatively small, well-marginated, and homogeneous tumors. A recent study demonstrated lower RENAL scores associated with tumors on AS, consistent with reduced tumor aggressiveness (63). In some series, the growth rates were calculated backward by obtaining old films for which the lesion of interest was either previously missed or dismissed, introducing further selection bias. In addition, most AS series have not incorporated routine RMS, so a significant proportion of tumors within these meta-analyses are likely benign (56). Another major concern is limited follow-up, which is typically in the 2- to 3-year range in most studies (12).

It is also important to recognize that in many of these series there is a subgroup of patients with rapidly growing tumors that appear to have more aggressive tumor biology. For instance, in the Volpe study, 25% of tumors doubled in volume in 12 months, and one patient developed metastatic disease (64). Clinical T1b tumors in particular are at higher risk for progression with AS, as are tumors with infiltrative appearance. In the study by Sowery and Siemens, T1b tumors demonstrated a growth rate of 1.43 cm per year, and one of nine patients developed metastases (65). Kunkle et al. have shown that the risk of synchronous metastasis goes up 22% with each centimeter increase in tumor size (66). Cure of patients with metastatic renal carcinoma is still extremely uncommon even in the era of targeted molecular agents.

Unfortunately, growth rates of SRMs do not predict malignancy, because even tumors with zero growth rates have proven to be malignant (67). As discussed previously, at present there is no truly reliable way to distinguish benign versus malignant or indolent versus potentially aggressive

tumors based on clinical or radiologic features, which has direct implications with respect to AS.

Taken together, the current literature demonstrates that AS is a viable option for carefully selected patients, who are either unfit for intervention, or do not want to be managed in a proactive manner. Counseling about AS should convey the limitations of the current AS literature and the inherent oncologic risks associated with this pathway, as highlighted in KEY POINTS.

■ SRMs IN THE ELDERLY

The management of SRMs in the elderly is particularly challenging given a high incidence of preexisting CKD and competing causes of mortality (Figure 4). We recently analyzed outcomes with various management strategies in the elderly, defined as those ≥75 years of age (68). Almost a 1,000 patients met the study criteria, which included SRMs (stage T1) and larger or higher stage renal tumors (stage ≥T2), all from our institution between 2000 and 2006. Kaplan-Meier estimates of overall 5-year survival rates for patients with stage T1a, T1b, and T2 cancers were 74%, 66%, and 51%, respectively, with many patients dying of non–cancer-related causes. Cancer-related deaths were infrequent in patients with T1 RCC (7%), yet much more common in patients with stage ≥T2 RCC, with cancer accounting for 51% of deaths in the latter patient population.

We then focused on the subgroup of 537 elderly patients with SRMs, that is, clinical T1 renal tumors. Management was by RN (27%), nephron-sparing approaches (53%) such as PN or TA, or AS in the remaining 20%. The unadjusted Kaplan-Meier estimates of overall survival at 5 years for these patients were 72% with RN, 76% for nephron-sparing approaches, and 58% for AS. Substantial selection bias was observed; the group managed with AS was older and had more comorbidities than the active treatment groups. On multivariate analysis, comorbidity and age were the most powerful predictors of overall survival, as one

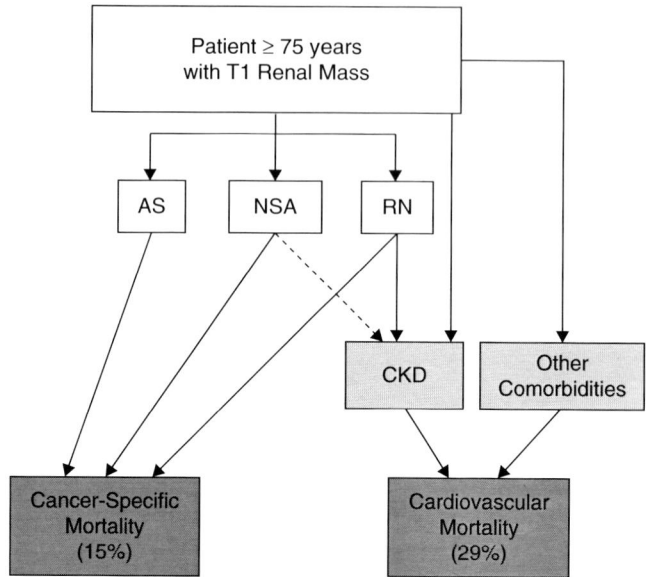

FIGURE 4
T1 renal mass management in the elderly. This special population commonly has comorbidities and pre-existing CKD making cardiovascular mortality more likely than cancer-specific mortality. AS, active surveillance; NSA, nephron sparing approaches; RN, radical nephrectomy; CKD, chronic kidney disease.

would expect in an elderly population. In contrast, management type was not associated with overall survival after adjusting for age, comorbidity, and other relevant variables.

The second main finding of our study was that cardiovascular events, not malignancy, were the leading cause of death, and pretreatment renal dysfunction and comorbidity were significant predictors of cardiovascular death. Pretreatment grade 3 CKD (GFR < 60 mL/min/1.73 m^2) was common in this elderly population and was greatly exacerbated by RN. CKD was present in 45% of patients prior to management of any type, and 86% of patients managed with RN were found to have CKD after surgery, much higher than any other approach. The Kaplan-Meier estimate of cardiovascular death at 5 years was 15% versus 6% for patients with or without CKD, respectively, reflecting the established relationship between CKD and risk of morbid cardiovascular events.

In summary, RN is still necessary in some elderly patients with locally advanced RCC that is potentially life threatening. However, loss of a kidney leaves most elderly patients with CKD and predisposes to cardiovascular morbidity and mortality. The paucity of cancer-related deaths in the elderly with T1 tumors reflects both the limited biological aggressiveness of most SRMs and competing causes of mortality. At our center, nephron-sparing approaches are prioritized, and PN remains an important option for elderly patients with good physiologic status. Treatment should be individualized based on physiologic age and comorbidities, with strong consideration given to AS for those with limited life expectancy.

■ SUMMARY

The elderly represent a unique population that crystallizes all of the basic principles involved in the management of SRMs. Management should be tailored to each individual taking into account oncologic and renal functional concerns, and morbidity should be minimized whenever possible. Physiologic age, comorbidities, and patient preferences all play important roles, and mandate balanced counseling about the merits and limitations of each treatment modality. Prospective, randomized trials are greatly needed to place this field on a more solid foundation. RMS with molecular profiling will likely be the "Holy Grail" that will allow for more rational management of SRMs in the future.

■ KEY POINTS

AUA Guidelines Consensus Statements on Modalities for the Management of the Clinical T1 Renal Mass. Source: Adapted from Campbell SC, Novick AC, Uzzo RG, et al. AUA Guidelines for the Management of Clinical T1 Renal Masses. Available at http://www.auanet.org/content/guide-lines-and-quality-care/clinical-guidelines/main-reports/renalmass09.pdf

Radical Nephrectomy RN, particularly laparoscopic RN, is appealing to patients and physicians but is greatly overutilized. Nephron-sparing approaches should be considered in all patients with a clinical T1 renal mass as an overriding principle, presuming adequate oncologic control can be achieved, based on compelling data demonstrating an increased risk of chronic kidney disease associated with RN, and a direct correlation between CKD and morbid cardiovascular events and mortality on a longitudinal basis. RN is still a viable option when necessary, based on tumor size, location, or radiographic appearance if the surgeon judges that nephron-sparing surgery is not feasible or advisable.

Partial Nephrectomy Surgical excision by PN is a reference standard for the management of clinical T1 renal masses, whether for imperative or elective indications, given the importance of preservation of renal parenchyma and avoidance of CKD. This treatment modality is greatly underutilized. PN has well-established longitudinal oncologic outcomes data comparable to RN. Adequate expertise and careful patient selection are important.

Thermal Ablation TA (cryoablation or RFA), either percutaneous or laparoscopic, is an available treatment option for the patient at high surgical risk who wants active treatment and accepts the need for long-term radiographic surveillance after treatment. Counseling about thermal ablation should include a balanced discussion of the increased risk of local recurrence, a lack of well-proven radiographic parameters for success particularly after RFA, potential for difficult surgical salvage if tumor progression is found and the substantial limitations of the current thermal ablation literature. Larger tumors (> 3.5 cm) and those with infiltrative appearance may be associated with increased risk of recurrence when managed with thermal ablation.

Active Surveillance AS is a reasonable option for the management of localized renal masses that should be discussed with all patients and should be a primary consideration for patients with decreased life expectancy or extensive comorbidities that would make them high risk for intervention. Counseling about AS should include a balanced discussion of the small but real risk of cancer progression, lack of curative salvage therapies if metastases develop, possible loss of window of opportunity for nephron-sparing surgery and substantial limitations of the current AS literature. Larger tumors (> 3 to 4 cm) and those with aggressive appearance, such as infiltrative growth pattern, may be associated with increased risk and should be managed in a proactive manner.

■ REFERENCES

1. Chow WH, Devesa SS, Warren JL, Fraumeni JF Jr. Rising incidence of renal cell cancer in the United States. *JAMA* 1999;281(17):1628–1631.
2. Jayson M, Sanders H. Increased incidence of serendipitously discovered renal cell carcinoma. *Urology* 1998;51(2):203–205.
3. Leslie JA, Prihoda T, Thompson IM. Serendipitous renal cell carcinoma in the post-CT era: continued evidence in improved outcomes. *Urol Oncol* 2003;21(1):39–44.
4. Luciani LG, Cestari R, Tallarigo C. Incidental renal cell carcinoma-age and stage characterization and clinical implications: study of 1092 patients (1982–1997). *Urology* 2000;56(1):58–62.

5. Mathew A, Devesa SS, Fraumeni JF Jr, Chow WH. Global increases in kidney cancer incidence, 1973–1992. *Eur J Cancer Prev* 2002;11(2):171–178.

6. Frank I, Blute ML, Cheville JC, Lohse CM, Weaver AL, Zincke H. Solid renal tumors: an analysis of pathological features related to tumor size. *J Urol* 2003;170(6 Pt 1):2217–2220.

7. Jeldres C, Sun M, Liberman D, et al. Can renal mass biopsy assessment of tumor grade be safely substituted for by a predictive model? *J Urol* 2009; 182(6):2585–2589.

8. Lane BR, Babineau D, Kattan MW, et al. A preoperative prognostic nomogram for solid enhancing renal tumors 7 cm or less amenable to partial nephrectomy. *J Urol* 2007;178(2):429–434.

9. Lane BR, Samplaski MK, Herts BR, Zhou M, Novick AC, Campbell SC. Renal mass biopsy—a renaissance? *J Urol* 2008;179(1):20–27.

10. Pahernik S, Ziegler S, Roos F, Melchior SW, Thüroff JW. Small renal tumors: correlation of clinical and pathological features with tumor size. *J Urol* 2007;178(2):414–417; discussion 416.

11. Remzi M, Ozsoy M, Klingler HC, et al. Are small renal tumors harmless? Analysis of histopathological features according to tumors 4 cm or less in diameter. *J Urol* 2006;176(3):896–899.

12. Campbell SC, Novick AC, Belldegrun A, et al.; Practice Guidelines Committee of the American Urological Association. Guideline for management of the clinical T1 renal mass. *J Urol* 2009;182(4): 1271–1279.

13. Volpe A, Kachura JR, Geddie WR, et al. Techniques, safety and accuracy of sampling of renal tumors by fine needle aspiration and core biopsy. *J Urol* 2007;178(2):379–386.

14. Samplaski MK, Zhou M, Lane BR, Herts B, Campbell SC. Renal mass sampling: an enlightened perspective. *Int J Urol* 2011;18(1):5–19.

15. Brierly RD, Thomas PJ, Harrison NW, Fletcher MS, Nawrocki JD, Ashton-Key M. Evaluation of fine-needle aspiration cytology for renal masses. *BJU Int* 2000;85(1):14–18.

16. Campbell SC, Novick AC, Herts B, et al. Prospective evaluation of fine needle aspiration of small, solid renal masses: accuracy and morbidity. *Urology* 1997;50(1):25–29.

17. Dechet CB, Zincke H, Sebo TJ, et al. Prospective analysis of computerized tomography and needle biopsy with permanent sectioning to determine the nature of solid renal masses in adults. *J Urol* 2003;169(1):71–74.

18. Herts BR, Baker ME. The current role of percutaneous biopsy in the evaluation of renal masses. *Semin Urol Oncol* 1995;13(4):254–261.

19. Chawla SN, Crispen PL, Hanlon AL, Greenberg RE, Chen DY, Uzzo RG. The natural history of observed enhancing renal masses: meta-analysis and review of the world literature. *J Urol* 2006;175(2):425–431.

20. Schmidbauer J, Remzi M, Memarsadeghi M, et al. Diagnostic accuracy of computed tomography-guided percutaneous biopsy of renal masses. *Eur Urol* 2008;53(5):1003–1011.

21. Javadi S, Matin SF, Tamboli P, Ahrar K. Unexpected atypical findings on CT after radiofrequency ablation for small renal-cell carcinoma and the role of percutaneous biopsy. *J Vasc Interv Radiol* 2007;18(9):1186–1191.

22. Slywotzky C, Maya M. Needle tract seeding of transitional cell carcinoma following fine-needle aspiration of a renal mass. *Abdom Imaging* 1994;19(2):174–176.

23. Wehle MJ, Grabstald H. Contraindications to needle aspiration of a solid renal mass: tumor dissemination by renal needle aspiration. *J Urol* 1986;136(2):446–448.

24. Silverman SG, Gan YU, Mortele KJ, Tuncali K, Cibas ES. Renal masses in the adult patient: the role of percutaneous biopsy. *Radiology* 2006;240(1):6–22.

25. Volpe A, Mattar K, Finelli A, et al. Contemporary results of percutaneous biopsy of 100 small renal masses: a single center experience. *J Urol* 2008; 180(6):2333–2337.

26. Leroy X, Moukassa D, Copin MC, Saint F, Mazeman E, Gosselin B. Utility of cytokeratin 7 for distinguishing chromophobe renal cell carcinoma from renal oncocytoma. *Eur Urol* 2000;37(4):484–487.

27. Liu L, Qian J, Singh H, Meiers I, Zhou X, Bostwick DG. Immunohistochemical analysis of chromophobe renal cell carcinoma, renal oncocytoma, and clear cell carcinoma: an optimal and practical panel for differential diagnosis. *Arch Pathol Lab Med* 2007;131(8):1290–1297.

28. Mathers ME, Pollock AM, Marsh C, O'Donnell M. Cytokeratin 7: a useful adjunct in the diagnosis of chromophobe renal cell carcinoma. *Histopathology* 2002;40(6):563–567.

29. Wu SL, Kothari P, Wheeler TM, Reese T, Connelly JH. Cytokeratins 7 and 20 immunoreactivity in chromophobe renal cell carcinomas and renal oncocytomas. *Mod Pathol* 2002;15(7):712–717.

30. Hollenbeck BK, Taub DA, Miller DC, Dunn RL, Wei JT. National utilization trends of partial nephrectomy

for renal cell carcinoma: a case of underutilization? *Urology* 2006;67(2):254–259.

31. Huang WC, Levey AS, Serio AM, et al. Chronic kidney disease after nephrectomy in patients with renal cortical tumours: a retrospective cohort study. *Lancet Oncol* 2006;7(9):735–740.

32. Russo P, Huang W. The medical and oncological rationale for partial nephrectomy for the treatment of T1 renal cortical tumors. *Urol Clin North Am* 2008;35(4):635–43; vii.

33. Go AS, Chertow GM, Fan D, McCulloch CE, Hsu CY. Chronic kidney disease and the risks of death, cardiovascular events, and hospitalization. *N Engl J Med* 2004;351(13):1296–1305.

34. Weight CJ, Larson BT, Fergany AF, et al. Nephrectomy induced chronic renal insufficiency is associated with increased risk of cardiovascular death and death from any cause in patients with localized cT1b renal masses. *J Urol* 2010;183(4):1317–1323.

35. McKiernan J, Simmons R, Katz J, Russo P. Natural history of chronic renal insufficiency after partial and radical nephrectomy. *Urology* 2002;59(6):816–820.

36. Thompson RH, Leibovich BC, Karnes RJ, Bergstralh EJ, Blute ML. Radical retropubic prostatectomy in immunosuppressed transplant recipients. *J Urol* 2008;179(4):1349–52; discussion 1352.

37. Gill IS, Kavoussi LR, Lane BR, et al. Comparison of 1,800 laparoscopic and open partial nephrectomies for single renal tumors. *J Urol* 2007;178:41–46.

38. Stephenson AJ, Hakimi AA, Snyder ME, Russo P. Complications of radical and partial nephrectomy in a large contemporary cohort. *J Urol* 2004;171(1):130–134.

39. Nguyen MM, Gill IS. Halving ischemia time during laparoscopic partial nephrectomy. *J Urol* 2008;179(2):627–32; discussion 632.

40. Lane BR, Russo P, Uzzo RG, et al. Comparison of cold and warm ischemia during partial nephrectomy in 660 solitary kidneys reveals predominant role of nonmodifiable factors in determining ultimate renal function. *J Urol* 2011;185(2):421–427.

41. Thompson RH, Lane BR, Lohse CM, et al. Every minute counts when the renal hilum is clamped during partial nephrectomy. *Eur Urol* 2010;58(3):340–345.

42. Lane BR, Gill IS, Fergany AF, Larson BT, Campbell SC. The use of limited warm ischemia during elective partial nephrectomy has only marginal impact on renal functional outcomes. *J Urol*. in press.

43. Thomas AA, Demirjian S, Lane BR, et al. Acute kidney injury: novel biomarkers and potential utility for patient care in urology. *Urology* 2011;77:5–11.

44. Berger A, Kamoi K, Gill IS, Aron M. Cryoablation for renal tumors: current status. *Curr Opin Urol* 2009;19(2):138–142.

45. Hinshaw JL, Lee FT Jr. Image-guided ablation of renal cell carcinoma. *Magn Reson Imaging Clin N Am* 2004;12(3):429–47, vi.

46. Mabjeesh NJ, Avidor Y, Matzkin H. Emerging nephron sparing treatments for kidney tumors: a continuum of modalities from energy ablation to laparoscopic partial nephrectomy. *J Urol* 2004;171(2 Pt 1):553–560.

47. Matin SF, Ahrar K. Nephron-sparing probe ablative therapy: long-term outcomes. *Curr Opin Urol* 2008;18(2):150–156.

48. Murphy DP, Gill IS. Energy-based renal tumor ablation: a review. *Semin Urol Oncol* 2001;19(2):133–140.

49. Sterrett SP, Nakada SY, Wingo MS, Williams SK, Leveillee RJ. Renal thermal ablative therapy. *Urol Clin North Am* 2008;35(3):397–414, viii.

50. Campbell SC, Palese MA. Laparoscopic cryoablation for a 3 cm nonhilar renal tumor. *J Urol* 2011;185(1):14–16.

51. Kimura M, Baba S, Polascik TJ. Minimally invasive surgery using ablative modalities for the localized renal mass. *Int J Urol* 2010;17(3):215–227.

52. Matin SF, Ahrar K, Cadeddu JA, et al. Residual and recurrent disease following renal energy ablative therapy: a multi-institutional study. *J Urol* 2006;176(5):1973–1977.

53. Aron M, Kamoi K, Remer E, Berger A, Desai M, Gill I. Laparoscopic renal cryoablation: 8-year, single surgeon outcomes. *J Urol* 2010;183(3):889–895.

54. Matin SF. Determining failure after renal ablative therapy for renal cell carcinoma: false-negative and false-positive imaging findings. *Urology* 2010;75(6):1254–1257.

55. Weight CJ, Kaouk JH, Hegarty NJ, et al. Correlation of radiographic imaging and histopathology following cryoablation and radio frequency ablation for renal tumors. *J Urol* 2008;179(4):1277–81; discussion 1281.

56. Kunkle DA, Egleston BL, Uzzo RG. Excise, ablate or observe: the small renal mass dilemma–a meta-analysis and review. *J Urol* 2008;179(4):1227–1233; discussion 1233.

57. Kowalczyk KJ, Hooper HB, Linehan WM, Pinto PA, Wood BJ, Bratslavsky G. Partial nephrectomy after previous radio frequency ablation: the National Cancer Institute experience. *J Urol* 2009;182(5):2158–2163.

58. Nguyen CT, Lane BR, Kaouk JH, et al. Surgical salvage of renal cell carcinoma recurrence after thermal ablative therapy. *J Urol* 2008;180:104–109; discussion 9.

59. Boorjian SA, Uzzo RG. The evolving management of small renal masses. *Curr Oncol Rep* 2009; 11(3):211–217.

60. Stroup S, Choe C, Wong C, et al. 830 Laparoscopic partial nephrectomy versus renal cryoablation: a multicenter comparison of intermediate oncologic outcomes. *J Urol* 2010;183:e324-e5.

61. Crispen PL, Viterbo R, Boorjian SA, Greenberg RE, Chen DY, Uzzo RG. Natural history, growth kinetics, and outcomes of untreated clinically localized renal tumors under active surveillance. *Cancer* 2009;115(13):2844–2852.

62. Jewett MA, Zuniga A. Renal tumor natural history: the rationale and role for active surveillance. *Urol Clin North Am* 2008;35(4):627–34; vii.

63. Kutikov A, Piotrowski ZJ, Manley BJ, et al. 1359 Renal masses under active surveillance are more often radiographically "simple" than those undergoing intermediate intervention. *J Urol* 2010;183:e525-e.

64. Volpe A, Panzarella T, Rendon RA, Haider MA, Kondylis FI, Jewett MA. The natural history of incidentally detected small renal masses. *Cancer* 2004;100(4):738–745.

65. Sowery RD, Siemens DR. Growth characteristics of renal cortical tumors in patients managed by watchful waiting. *Can J Urol* 2004;11(5):2407–2410.

66. Kunkle DA, Crispen PL, Li T, Uzzo RG. Tumor size predicts synchronous metastatic renal cell carcinoma: implications for surveillance of small renal masses. *J Urol* 2007;177(5):1692–1696; discussion 1697.

67. Kunkle DA, Crispen PL, Chen DY, Greenberg RE, Uzzo RG. Enhancing renal masses with zero net growth during active surveillance. *J Urol* 2007; 177:849–853; discussion 53–54.

68. Lane BR, Abouassaly R, Gao T, et al. Active treatment of localized renal tumors may not impact overall survival in patients aged 75 years or older. *Cancer* 2010;116(13):3119–3126.

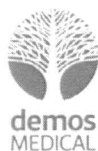

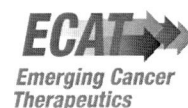

Surgical Management of Renal Cancer

Gautam Jayram and Scott E. Eggener*

University of Chicago Medical Center, Chicago, IL

■ ABSTRACT

Surgery continues to play the predominant role in the treatment of localized renal carcinoma. Appropriate disease staging with cross-sectional imaging and assessment of renal function is critical to determine an appropriate operative plan and approach. Enhancing lesions larger than 3 cm carry a significant risk of malignancy (>75%) and should be given strong consideration for treatment. Nephron-sparing surgery has become the standard of care for T1a lesions (<4 cm) and is encouraged for larger lesions in technically amenable locations. Although associated with greater complications compared to radical nephrectomy, partial nephrectomy (PN) should be offered whenever possible due to lower rates of chronic kidney disease, cardiovascular morbidity, and non-cancer mortality. In experienced hands, laparoscopic and/or robotic approaches to radical and PN have shown comparable outcomes to open surgery. Routine lymphadenectomy does not improve survival but should be selectively considered as it improves staging and disease prognostication. Ipsilateral adrenalectomy should be reserved for patients with large upper pole tumors or radiographic abnormalities in the adrenal gland. Complete removal of a renal cancer-related tumor thrombus in the renal vein or inferior vena cava can lead to long-term durable cure. Cytoreductive nephrectomy should be considered for severe local tumor-related symptoms and for select patients with metastatic disease, but further studies are needed to evaluate its role when combined with modern systemic therapies.

Keywords: renal cell carcinoma, renal surgery, nephrectomy

* Corresponding author, Department of Surgery, University of Chicago Medical Center, 5841 S. Maryland Ave, Mail Code 6038, Chicago, IL 60637
   E-mail address: seggener@surgery.bsd.uchicago.edu

Emerging Cancer Therapeutics 2:1 (2011) 73–88.
© 2011 Demos Medical Publishing LLC. All rights reserved.
DOI: 10.5003/2151–4194.2.1.73

INTRODUCTION

Cancer of the kidney is the sixth most common cause of cancer death worldwide and the incidence appears to be increasing (1). In 2010, it was estimated that approximately 58,000 patients in the United States and 45,000 in Europe would be newly diagnosed for kidney cancer (2). Renal carcinoma, originating in the renal cortex, is the most common type and accounts for more than 85% of all renal tumors. Well-established risk factors include cigarette smoking, obesity, male gender, hypertension, advancing age, acquired cystic disease of the kidney, and several genetic syndromes (3). Due to the relative chemo- and radioresistance of these lesions, surgical excision is the mainstay of management for clinically localized tumors. Contemporary surgical therapy for renal cancer can be traced to Robson's description of radical nephrectomy (RN) 40 years ago (4). Since then, tremendous advances have been made, namely the addition of nephron-sparing and minimally invasive techniques. As such, indications for surgical intervention in renal cancer have expanded and surgery has become an increasingly prominent tool in multimodal therapy for locally advanced and metastatic disease. This chapter addresses all contemporary aspects of the surgical management of renal cancer.

PREOPERATIVE ASSESSMENT

The optimal approach to renal cortical masses includes assessment of the primary lesion, adequate clinical staging, and evaluation of the patient's renal function and overall medical condition. The widespread use of cross-sectional imaging has made the incidental diagnosis of renal cell carcinoma (RCC) much more common (> 80% of all newly diagnosed patients) compared with the classic symptomatic presentation of hematuria, flank pain, or a palpable mass (5). Important features of the primary lesion on imaging include size, location, appearance, and response to intravenous contrast. A renal mass that enhances following the administration of intravenous contrast (increase in Hounsfield units of approximately 10–20 units) represents malignancy over 80% of the time, although this proportion ranges from 54% (less than 1 cm mass) to 94% (>7 cm) depending on tumor size (6,7). Clinical staging of the primary tumor is based on size and relationship with local structures such as the renal capsule, renal vein, inferior vena cava, Gerota's fascia, and adrenal gland (Table 1). Renal biopsy has historically been omitted from the routine evaluation of renal masses due to concerns of tumor seeding, inaccurate sampling, and renal hemorrhage. However, numerous recent series have provided data to counter these claims, demonstrating accurate diagnostic capability in 84% to 100% of small lesions (< 4 cm), with exceedingly rare reports of tumor seeding or bleeding (8–10). The utilization of tissue processing adjuncts, such as fluorescent in-situ hybridization (FISH), can enhance biopsy accuracy, as a recent report demonstrated an accuracy of 86% with FISH compared to 75% with biopsy alone for diagnosis of RCC (11). Although still not widely utilized, renal biopsy is a valuable tool in cases where preoperative knowledge of histopathology would alter management, including imaging or clinical features suggestive of lymphoma or suspicion of a metastasis from another organ, and small lesions in patients with competing health risks.

Contemporary reports suggest a significant correlation between systemic symptoms and tumor stage and prognosis, as more than 70% of patients with stage IV disease have symptoms compared to 24% with stage I disease (12,13). Radiographic assessment also provides information regarding local invasion, vascular involvement, status of regional lymph nodes (LNs), and possible metastases in distant structures. In addition, anatomic detail such as tumor location, multifocality, and presence of renal vascular anomalies should be noted to optimize operative planning. Location of the tumor within the kidney is critical in assessing the likelihood of successfully completing a nephron-sparing procedure. Endophytic and central tumors close to the renal hilum are much more

TABLE 1   Staging of RCC: primary tumor (T)

TX	Primary tumor cannot be assessed.
T0	No evidence of primary tumor.
T1	Tumor ≤7 cm in greatest dimension, limited to the kidney.
T1a	Tumor ≤4 cm in greatest dimension, limited to the kidney.
T1b	Tumor >4 cm but not >7 cm in greatest dimension, limited to the kidney.
T2	Tumor >7 cm in greatest dimension, limited to the kidney.
T2a	Tumor >7 cm but ≤10 cm in greatest dimension, limited to the kidney.
T2b	Tumor >10 cm, limited to the kidney.
T3	Tumor extends into major veins or perinephric tissues but not into the ipsilateral adrenal gland and not beyond Gerota fascia.
T3a	Tumor grossly extends into the renal vein or its segmental (muscle containing) branches, or tumor invades perirenal and/or renal sinus fat but not beyond Gerota fascia.
T3b	Tumor grossly extends into the vena cava below the diaphragm.
T3c	Tumor grossly extends into the vena cava above the diaphragm or invades the wall of the vena cava.
T4	Tumor invades beyond Gerota fascia (including contiguous extension into the ipsilateral adrenal gland).

likely to necessitate RN than peripheral, exophytic lesions. Fortunately, the quality of modern reconstructive computerized tomographic (CT) imaging (e.g., thin slice with 3D reconstruction) nearly always obviates the need for more invasive studies (i.e., arteriography or venacavography) (Figure 1). Magnetic resonance imaging (MRI) is particularly useful in determining the presence and extent of vascular invasion, which is important in determining the need for hepatic mobilization or cardiopulmonary bypass, and when there are concerns regarding invasion into adjacent organs such as the liver, colon, or spleen (14,15). The decision whether to proceed with a metastatic evaluation depends on organ-specific symptoms, laboratory results, and risk for metastases based on kidney tumor features.

Consideration of the patient's overall medical condition is another key component of surgical planning. Patients with significant comorbidity may be better suited for active surveillance or ablative therapy in the setting of a small renal mass, which is discussed elsewhere in this volume. A recent study demonstrated a 5-year non-RCC

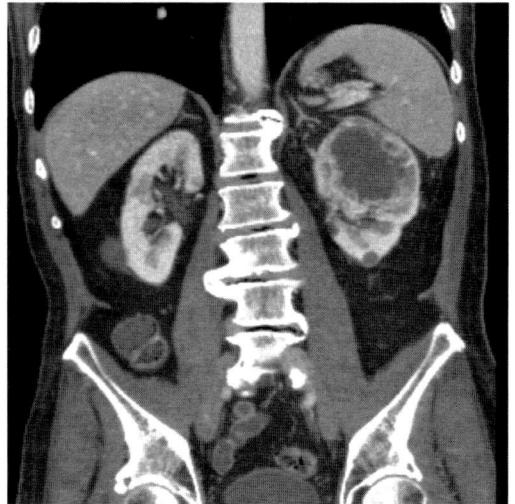

FIGURE 1
Coronal image of large clinically localized left renal mass.

death risk of 18% compared with RCC-specific mortality risk of 4% in more than 30,000 patients with clinically localized RCC (16). The risk of RCC death was directly associated with increasing

TABLE 2 Equations to estimate glomerular filtration rate

CKD-PI:
eGFR = 186*(0.742 if female)*(1.212 if African American)*creatinine$^{-1.153}$*age$^{-0.203}$
MDRD:
eGFR = 141 × min(Scr/k, 1)^a × max(Scr/k, 1)$^{-1.209}$ × 0.993^{Age} × 1.018 [if female] × 1.159 [if African American]

Scr is serum creatinine, k is 0.7 for females and 0.9 for males, a is −0.329 for females and −0.411 for males, min indicates the minimum of Scr/k or 1, and max indicates the maximum of Scr/k or 1.

tumor size. Furthermore, patients with multiple cardiovascular morbidities, including cigarette smoking, obesity, diabetes, and coronary artery disease, are at increased risk of perioperative complications and development or progression of chronic kidney disease. A history of multiple intraabdominal surgeries and/or infections may be more safely managed with a retroperitoneal (RP) compared to a transperitoneal (TP) surgical approach.

Assessment of renal function prior to surgery should be performed with creatinine-based estimations of glomerular filtration rate (GFR), such as Modified Diet in Renal Disease (MDRD) or Chronic Kidney Disease Epidemiology Collaboration (CKD-EPI) (Table 2) (17,18). Radioisotope renal scanning can be helpful in predicting residual renal function following partial or complete removal of a renal unit, and the presence of renal insufficiency can alter surgical approach, which will be discussed later.

■ NEPHRON-SPARING SURGERY

RN consists of removal of the kidney, including Gerota's fascia and the ipsilateral adrenal gland. In 1971, Skinner et al. documented the oncologic efficacy of RN compared with simple nephrectomy (removing the kidney within Gerota's fascia without the adrenal gland) (19). Since then, RN has been considered the gold standard for the surgical treatment of renal cancer. The increased incidental detection of small renal masses, appreciation of the detrimental effects of renal function decline, and advances in surgical techniques have led to the more widespread use of nephron-sparing surgery (NSS), mainly in the form of thermal ablation and partial nephrectomy (PN). The rationale for nephron-sparing techniques is discussed in greater detail later in this volume. PN entails complete resection of a renal tumor while leaving the largest amount of normal functioning parenchyma in the involved kidney. This procedure typically requires clamping of the renal vessels to induce renal ischemia and optimize visualization during tumor resection (20,21). Ischemia and subsequent reperfusion injury to the kidney results in arteriolar vasoconstriction, generation of renotoxic free radicals, which mediate acute kidney injury, and can potentially lead to long-term renal damage. Administration of osmotic diuretic mannitol prior to the ischemic insult has been shown to ameliorate these effects (22). Progressively longer ischemia times are associated with incrementally worse renal outcomes and substantive renal damage can occur as early as 30 to 40 minutes of warm ischemia and 90 minutes of cold ischemia (23,24). The concept of renal ischemia is still controversial in the management of smaller tumors and multiple recent reports have documented the safety of PN without hilar clamping, especially in exophytic lesions with less than 50% penetration into the renal parenchyma (25–28).

Oncologic outcomes following NSS have been closely scrutinized, with major concerns being margin status, tumor multifocality, and subsequent recurrence rates with PN compared to RN. Although occult multifocality has been demonstrated in 5% to 15% of patients with RCC (especially with papillary subtype), the clinical significance of these satellite lesions remain unknown (29,30). Indeed, multiple large, multicenter trials have documented oncologic equivalence between RN and PN for tumors less than 4 cm, with no significant difference in recurrence rates or cancer-specific survival (31). More recent data have also shown similar efficacy of PN for lesions between 4 and 7 cm (T1b), demonstrating 5-year cancer-specific rates of more than 90% following NSS in tumors 4 to 7 cm (32–34). The data regarding PN for tumors more than 7 cm are also encouraging but not as widely accepted (35,36).

The importance of margin status following NSS in RCC remains controversial. Although every effort should be made to ensure a negative margin at the time of surgery, an incidental positive margin does not imply an ominous prognosis and can typically be managed with careful surveillance. In a series of more than 1,300 patients undergoing PN, 6% of patients had a positive margin, and at 5 and 10 years of follow-up, there was no difference in recurrence-free survival compared with patients who had negative margins (31).

Although NSS is surgically more challenging than RN and carries a greater risk of complications, many series have documented its safety in experienced hands (37–40). The complications associated with PN (discussed later in this chapter) and the technical difficulties have adversely impacted the proper utilization of PN. Recent studies have demonstrated the majority of urologists continue to use RN as the predominant treatment for localized (T1) renal masses. Specifically, 7.5% of all renal tumor operations between 1988 and 2002 were PN, and tumor registry data indicate less than 20% of all tumors under 4 cm were treated with PN (41,42). A more updated report suggests that PN use is appropriately increasing, as 35% of a cohort over 18,000 patients received PN between 1999 and 2006 for T1a lesions. Patients over 70 and those in rural communities were identified as being much more likely to undergo RN (43,44). Given the preponderance of data supporting oncologic, safety, and renoprotective outcomes

following NSS, PN (open or laparoscopic) should be given full consideration for patients presenting with renal masses.

■ MINIMALLY INVASIVE APPROACHES

Since the initial report of laparoscopic nephrectomy in 1991 by Clayman and colleagues, the use of minimally invasive techniques for treatment of RCC has steadily increased, with recent reports suggesting more than 70% of all radical nephrectomies are now performed laparoscopically (45,46). Laparoscopic approaches to renal surgery have been shown to have favorable cosmesis, convalescence, hospital stay, and blood loss compared with open procedures. In addition, postoperative pain requirements are significantly less compared with traditional open incisions (46). Early operative times with laparoscopic radical nephrectomy (LRN) were more than 5 hours; however, with improved experience, equipment and techniques, modern operative times are now comparable or less than open radical nephrectomy (ORN) (47). Oncologic data show comparable results between LRN and ORN for both T1 and T2 tumors, with no difference in overall and disease-specific survival at 10 years of follow up (48–51). Furthermore, these reports have demonstrated equivalent complication rates with LRN and ORN at experienced centers. The indications and utilization for LRN have been expanded, and reports of LRN for tumors involving the renal vein, locally advanced disease, and even in a cytoreductive role have been described (52,53). As these situations represent challenging oncologic operations even for experienced surgeons, currently accepted exclusion criteria for LRN include venous involvement and extensive lymphadenopathy.

LRN is performed via either a TP or RP approach. The TP approach is the traditional method to perform LRN and results in small abdominal incisions, giving the urologist ample working space and readily identifiable anatomy.

Violation of the peritoneal cavity makes complications (urine leaks, bleeding, and infection) more morbid and risks injuring vascular and gastrointestinal structures. The RP approach mimics traditional open surgery by developing a working space without entry into the peritoneal cavity. Additional advantages of RP LRN are quicker hilar control and decreased operative time. In the presence of an untoward body habitus or multiple previous abdominal surgeries, an RP approach can be advantageous, and studies have demonstrated comparable results to the TP approach (54,55). Working space and technical facility are more demanding, however, and this approach is still not favored by most urologists.

Minimally invasive techniques have expectedly extended into NSS as the incidence of small, asymptomatic renal masses has increased. Direct vision and real-time incorporation of ultrasonography during laparoscopic and robotic procedures have allowed urologists to reproduce key components of open partial nephrectomy (OPN). In addition, laparoscopic approaches for renal ablative therapies (discussed fully in another chapter) have become more commonly utilized.

Initial experience with laparoscopic partial nephrectomy (LPN) demonstrated a superior recovery profile but was marred by longer ischemia times, inability to provide cold ischemia, and increased postoperative complications compared with OPN (56,57). Following advances in hilar clamping, obtaining adequate cold ischemia, and tumor resection and renorraphy in LPN, outcomes now appear comparable to OPN. In one large multicenter study, patients undergoing LPN had less operative time, estimated blood loss, length of stay, and comparable renal function after 3 months. Cancer-specific survival for patients (all pT1 RCC) was 99.3% for LPN and 99.2% of OPN. LPN patients did have a higher warm ischemia time and more postoperative complications (bleeding and urinary leaks); however, the two cohorts were not matched according to tumor characteristics (58). A more recent, matched study demonstrated improved familiarity with LPN, as complications

and renal function were equivalent between OPN and LPN groups and warm ischemia time was shorter in the LPN group. No difference was seen in 5-year overall cancer-specific or overall survival between the two groups (59). High-volume centers have reported excellent outcomes after LPN for high-risk tumors—those in a solitary kidney, endophytic or with a hilar location, and patients with baseline renal insufficiency (60–62). As the slope of the learning curve appears steeper for this procedure than with LRN, currently accepted criteria for LPN include T1 renal mass, exophytic/peripheral location, and absence of significant renal disease, as warm ischemia times will be longer early in the surgeon's experience.

The technically demanding nature of LPN, specifically concerns for long warm ischemia times, has driven interest in robotic-assisted partial nephrectomy (RALPN). Robotic surgery provides significant advances in ergonomics and visualization with apparently shorter learning curve for complex laparoscopic procedures. Robotic-assisted surgery has already become well established for performing radical prostatectomy and has been used for more diverse indications as experience has grown. Early series have shown equal or shorter operative times in RALPN compared to LPN, with RALPN conferring shorter warm ischemia times and providing greater facility with renorraphy and hemostatic techniques (63–65). Short-term oncologic and renal outcomes appear to be similar as well. Cost of treatment and need for an experienced assistant are limitations of RALPN; however, with refinements in technology, robotic-assisted NSS will likely supersede LPN as the NSS treatment of choice due to a shorter learning curve and familiarity to urologists.

■ LYMPHADENECTOMY

With a downward stage migration of RCC due to a higher proportion of incidentally detected lesions, the incidence of regional LN involvement across all patients with RCC has decreased significantly over the past two decades. This can be most easily inferred from reports of LN metastasis in autopsy series ranging from 14% to 64% compared to recent surgical series reporting LN involvement in 3% to 5% of contemporary patients (66,67). The role of routine lymphadenectomy (LND) in the treatment of RCC still remains a source of debate amongst urologic oncologists. Potential benefits of LND at the time of nephrectomy include more accurate staging and prognostication and the potential for improved survival. Following LND, staging is definitively improved, but the therapeutic benefit and theoretically improved response to systemic therapy are uncertain.

The data are most clear for clinical node-negative patients without metastases. Final results from the only prospective trial comparing RN with and without LND (EORTC 30881) in 772 patients without radiographic evidence of lymphadenopathy demonstrated no survival benefit to LND. Occult incidence of LN positivity was 3.3% amongst all patients (68). This extremely low incidence is not surprising, as this cohort was relatively low-risk group with 69% ≤ T2 and a median tumor size of 5.5 cm. In locally advanced cohorts (≥T3 and/or metastases), LN involvement ranges from 20% to 46% (69,70). The EORTC study thus demonstrates the safety of omitting LND in localized, T1-T2N0 RCC, but the value of an LND for larger or more pathologically advanced tumors is unknown.

The staging value of lymphadenectomy for locally advanced tumors is hampered by the unpredictable and variable metastatic patterns of renal tumors. Clinical experiences demonstrate the frequent presence of distant metastases without regional LN involvement, and autopsy studies have reported this pattern to be as high as 53% (66,67). The hypervascular nature of RCC can distort the normal anatomy, rendering lymphatic drainage unpredictable, and gives these tumors a predilection for early hematogenous dissemination. As such, T3-T4 tumors without visible or radiographic LN abnormalities do not necessarily benefit from LND. However, as CT has been demonstrated to poorly differentiate inflammatory from malignant nodes, LND can serve a valuable staging role in patients in whom borderline lymphadenopathy is identified. Studer et al. demonstrated a 42% incidence of renal cancer within radiographically enlarged LN on pre-operative CT scan (71). As adjuvant therapies continue to improve, the importance of accurately staging patients with locally advanced renal cancer will become more important.

In cases with obvious enlarged nodes on standard cross-sectional imaging preoperatively and no clear evidence of systemic disease, LND does seem to be warranted. Although this situation is rare, retrospective data support a survival benefit in this group as Schafhauser et al. showed 5-year survival rates of 57%, 50%, and 44% in patients undergoing full systematic LND, macroscopic LN excision, and no LND, respectively (72).

The relative value of LND in the setting of regional LN and distant disease is uncertain, a situation more frequently encountered. It was previously noted that interferon-alpha following RN improves survival compared with interferon-alpha alone in the setting of distant disease; however, the more effective VEGF pathway-directed agents have supplanted interferon and the role of aggressive local surgery in the face of widespread metastatic disease treated with such agents is unclear (73–75). Vasselli et al. demonstrated that patients with metastatic disease and detectable preoperative RP lymphadenopathy experienced decreased survival (8 months vs. 14 months) compared to patients without metastatic disease (75). Complete LND following RN in such patients has been further suggested to restore survival to that expected in patients without LN involvement, thus supporting the role of cytoreduction in this situation. Nevertheless, prospective randomized trials evaluating the role of LND have not been performed for patients with preoperative regional lymphadenopathy with or without concomitant distant disease.

Although Robson's early description of LND involved all para-aortic and para-caval LNs from the bifurcation of the aorta to the diaphragmatic crus, in clinical practice most surgeons limit the dissection to the pre-aortic, para-aortic, and hilar nodes on the left and pre-caval, para-caval, and hilar nodes on the right (4). Based on potential understaging because of limited templates, some have argued for more extended lymphadenectomy templates to improve staging. Terrone et al. demonstrated a significantly higher rate of LN positivity with more than 13 nodes resected, suggesting a higher nodal yield, irrespective of template used, would give more accurate staging and prognostic information (76). Furthermore, proponents of LND following RN cite no difference in morbidity between RN only and RN+LND series, even when extended LND templates are used (68,72). In the EORTC prospective trial, the incidence of lymphocele (2.4% vs. 3.9%), significant blood loss (6.5% vs. 9.4%), and bowel injury (1.4% vs. 0.6%) were comparable between the LND and non-LND groups. Although the morbidity of the procedure seems to be low based on this data, LND can be a relatively complex procedure due to the location and nature of the surrounding anatomic structures, and only patients with a reasonable likelihood of clinical benefit should be considered.

■ ADRENALECTOMY

Previously held notions regarding violation of Gerota's fascia and sound oncologic principles dictated routine ipsilateral adrenalectomy at time of RN in patients with renal cancer. The recent demonstration of oncologic efficacy in patients following adrenal-sparing NSS has challenged this notion. This along with downward stage migration of renal cancer has made initial observations and survival data regarding adrenalectomy by Robson et al. 40 years ago inapplicable to a modern cohort. Although adrenalectomy has not been shown to increase morbidity during RN, several contemporary series have questioned routine removal of the adrenal gland (77–80). These studies have demonstrated synchronous, ipsilateral adrenal metastases in 0.7% to 5% of cases. Further studies in patients with higher-grade, higher-stage tumors

have shown a 7% to 8% incidence of adrenal involvement (81,82). A recent meta-analysis suggested patients at high-risk of adrenal involvement sufficient to warrant adrenalectomy include upper pole tumors, tumor multifocality, and increasing tumor size (specifically > T2) (83). Furthermore, adrenal abnormalities on preoperative imaging (CT or MRI) have a poor positive predictive value for malignancy (< 40%) and the decision to proceed with adrenalectomy should not be based on this alone, although most surgeons would favor adrenalectomy in this setting (79,80).

In cases with known or suspected adrenal involvement and no other sites of disease, ipsilateral adrenalectomy can improve survival. In a series of 1,635 RN patients, those with adrenal involvement had an overall 5-year survival of 33%; however, when restricting the analysis to ipsilateral, synchronous lesions, 5-year survival was 61% (84). The potential risk of long-term morbidity following adrenalectomy, especially in renal patients, is the main reason routine adrenalectomy should be discouraged. As 1% to 3% of patients with RCC will have contralateral adrenal metastasis, the goal of preserving functional adrenal tissue is sensible (85). In addition, 20% of patients with metastatic RCC develop some degree of adrenal insufficiency, even in the setting of retained adrenal glands (86).

■ MANAGEMENT OF RCC WITH TUMOR THROMBUS

A unique property of RCC is its ability to invade surrounding venous structures and progress from the renal vein as cranially as the right atrium. This type of presentation is seen in approximately 4% to 10% of all RCC patients, and approximately half of these patients have disease extending past the renal vein at the time of surgery (87). Patients with venous extension are more likely to be symptomatic than patients without venous involvement, presenting commonly with hematuria, flank pain or mass, or lower extremity edema. Adequate preoperative imaging is essential in this setting as the surgical approach relies on defining the cranial most aspect and extent of the tumor thrombus. Complete resection is indicated in these patients as it can lead to symptomatic relief and favorable oncologic outcomes with median survival more than 50 months in T3b disease and more than 25 months in T3c patients (88).

The benefit of preoperative renal embolization (RAE) in bulky cancers with significant feeding vessels is debatable. The theorized advantage is the potential to decrease tumor size, minimize blood loss, and facilitate hilar dissection, particularly the ability to transect the vein prior to dissecting the artery. In addition, embolization-induced tumor necrosis can set off an immunomodulatory effect, which is hypothesized to induce a tumor-specific response (89,90). However, this intervention is not without morbidity, as about 5% of patients will have complications, most frequently "angioinfarction syndrome" consisting of high fevers, leukocytosis, and a systemic inflammatory response (91). Despite the purported benefits, several series have not confirmed any measurable difference in outcomes or operative times following preoperative RAE. A recent comparison of RN alone to RN with preoperative RAE in patients with venous tumor thrombus demonstrated longer operative times, higher transfusion requirement, and greater complication rate in the embolization group (92). Although well-done prospective trials are lacking, the current data do not support routine use of preoperative embolization in RCC, even in the advanced setting.

Surgical strategy should be dictated by the extent of tumor thrombus. Tumors extending above the diaphragm into the cardiac chambers should be managed with cardiopulmonary bypass to provide continuous venous return and arterial output during IVC occlusion. This is typically used in conjunction with a midline sternotomy incision but can also be performed via a thoracoabdominal incision. Tumor thrombus extending into the retrohepatic IVC below the diaphragm are managed best with thoracoabdominal incisions, as often times the coronal, falciform, and

round ligaments of the liver need to be incised to medially mobilize the liver. If the tumor thrombus extends above the liver, a Pringle maneuver is often useful to minimize bleeding during entry into the IVC. A subcostal or flank incision offers adequate exposure to the renal hilum and infrahepatic IVC and is ideal for thrombus extending into this location. A thrombus that appears high in the IVC can often be "milked" caudally, preventing the need for advanced bypass techniques or manipulation above the diaphragm. A subcostal or thoracoabdominal incision provides adequate exposure to the infradiaphragmatic vena cava and renal hilum and is the recommended approach for cases where thrombus is located in this area. In all cases, prior to cavotomy and tumor resection, the IVC should be occluded above and below the thrombus and the contralateral rein vein should be clamped. On rare occasions, tumor thrombus can invade the wall of the IVC. In these situations, the IVC should be resected and caval reconstruction be performed with a patch or graft.

Owing to the nature of the procedure and significant disease burden, patients undergoing RN and tumor thrombectomy are prone to significant intra- and postoperative morbidity. Recent series document an overall complication rate of 12.5% following the procedure, with progressively higher rates according to a more cranial extension of venous tumor (93). Important complications unique to this procedure are venous and tumor embolism, pancreatitis, pneumothorax, acute renal failure, hemorrhage, and vascular bypass-related complications.

■ ROLE OF SURGERY IN METASTATIC DISEASE

In 2001, the results of separate SWOG and EORTC trials documented improved overall survival in patients undergoing cytoreductive nephrectomy (CN) prior to immunotherapy compared to patients undergoing immunotherapy alone (70,73). Immunotherapy in these studies consisted of interferon, which in the modern era has been largely replaced in the front-line setting by tyrosine-kinase inhibitors or interleukin-2. The benefit of CN in the contemporary era of systemic therapies is not as well defined; however, subgroup analyses from comparative data between interferon and TKIs suggest a survival benefit with CN and these newer agents (94,95).

Oncologic and overall outcomes following CN are dependent on multiple clinical and pathological disease features. Although multiple studies have attempted to assign a predictive weight to each of these, consistent data isolating the specific impact of any particular variable is lacking. A consensus panel utilizing all available data indicated that CN was appropriate for patients with good surgical risk, symptoms related to the primary tumor, and limited metastatic burden (96). The main concern with CN is that some patients are unable to receive systemic therapy due to surgery-related morbidity or mortality (97,98). Newer randomized studies describing the efficacy of CN in conjunction with TKIs are needed to update our understanding of the appropriate role of CN.

■ COMPLICATIONS OF SURGICAL MANAGEMENT OF RCC

Complications of renal surgery are dependent on treatment modality, need for renal reconstruction, and experience of the operating surgeon. Minimally invasive approaches to renal masses carry a risk of access injury not encountered in the open approach. Although small, access injuries have been reported in approximately 0.3% of large series, and primarily include injuries to bowel and large vascular structures. Although direct comparison of various access techniques is difficult, the Hasson technique is considered by the majority of urologists to be the safest approach to obtaining pneumoperitoneum, and a large series has confirmed this technique to be associated with the fewest intraabdominal complications (< 0.1%) (99).

Intraoperative bowel injuries are a particular concern during laparoscopic surgery, especially if they are not recognized intraoperatively. A meta-analysis demonstrated the risk of these injuries to be 0.8% with the majority being thermal injuries (100). Management is based on severity and can range from observation, serosal re-approximation, or bowel resection with end-to-end anastamosis in cases of severe injury. If unrecognized, these injuries may lead to peritonitis and need for temporary bowel diversion.

Perioperative complications during RN are relatively rare regardless of surgical approach. Vascular and organ injury rates are similar in laparoscopic approaches (0–4%) and open series (0–9%) (101). Splenic injuries have been reported to be more common in ORN compared to LRN (8% vs. 1.4%) (102,103). This likely is due to larger tumors being managed in an open approach as well as more traction on the splenocolic flexure applied on the upper pole of the kidney during open surgery. Preoperative placement of a nasogastric tube can facilitate the spleen falling medially and minimizing the risk of this complication. Pancreatic injuries are often related to splenic injuries and occur in the setting of a left nephrectomy for large tumors, with a single laparoscopic series reporting a rate of 0.4%(104). Failure to completely mobilize the pancreas and spleen tends to be responsible for this injury. Significant pancreatic dissection should warrant a postoperative drain to assess for pancreatic fistula. Severe pancreatic or splenic injury may necessitate distal pancreatectomy and/or splenectomy. Pleural violation is a complication more commonly seen following open renal surgery, usually occurring in the setting of cranial incisions due to upper pole tumors. A recent study demonstrated a pleural injury incidence of 12%, with 80% of these injuries managed successfully with simple intraoperative evacuation techniques. The remaining 20% required chest tube placement for persistent, symptomatic pneumothorax (105). The presence of rib resection was the only intraoperative factor correlating to the presence of a pleural injury.

Control of the renal hilum is considered the most crucial step during ORN or LRN. Significant bleeding in RN is rare, and transfusion requirements are low in both LRN (0–7%) and ORN (0–2.4%) series (100). Laparoscopically, the renal hilar vessels can be safely secured by an endovascular stapler or locking clips. Although previously thought to be dangerous, en-bloc stapling of the renal hilum is now considered safe. Specifically, no arteriovenous fistula formation was observed in a recent study with 3-year follow-up (106). Stapler and clip malfunction can occur during vascular control and has been reported to be as high as 10% in LRN series (107,108). A recent comprehensive review demonstrated 63% of all hemostatic failures occurred with the endovascular stapler, 33% with titanium clips, and 5% with locking clips. It is recommended at least two clips be placed on the stay side of the artery and vein, and the vessels adequately dissected of lymphatics and perihilar fat in order to maximize clip or staple efficacy. The most common cause of stapler malfunction is thought to be inclusion of metallic clips in the device (108).

Fortunately, long-term complications have proven to be rare following RN. Port-site metastases are extremely uncommon with only six cases reported in the literature (109). The specimen should be isolated in an extraction bag and morcellation should be avoided to minimize risk of tumor spillage. PN is associated with higher complication rates due to the risk of bleeding and the necessity for parenchymal and collecting system reconstruction. Specifically, a prospective randomized trial of OPN versus ORN demonstrated a severe bleeding risk of 3.1% versus 1.2%, a 4.4% urinary fistula rate observed only in OPN patients, and a reoperative rate of 4.4% (OPN) versus 2.4% (ORN) (110). Severe bleeding during OPN is reported to range from 0 to 7.5% and urinary leakage from 0.7% to 17% (38,58,111). These events appear to be decreasing, as Thompson et al. demonstrated decreased morbidity, reduced need for hilar clamping and shorter overall ischemia over the past 10 years (37). Morbidity of PN appears to increase with technical complexity, larger, and more centrally located tumors. Depth of tumor is associated with increased injury to the collecting system and higher risk of urinary fistula. Although equivalent in terms of oncologic and functional outcomes, LPN appears to have a slightly higher risk of postoperative complications. Gill et al. reported a series of 1,800 patients where the risk of postoperative hemorrhage was 4.2% in LPN compared to 1.6% in OPN (58). Furthermore, the rate of urologic complications (urinary leak, infection) was almost twice as high in LPN (9.2% vs. 5.0%). A learning curve appears to be responsible for at least part of this discrepancy, as a recent report demonstrated a complication rate with LPN of 19% in the most recent 200 cases compared to 33% in a previous cohort (112). PN is usually performed with the aid of hemostatic agents or sealants under a bolster to prevent bleeding and urine leakage. These agents may include gelatin matrix thrombin tissue sealant, fibrin glue, and oxidized regenerated cellulose. Postoperative hemorrhage as manifested by decreasing serial hematocrits can be managed conservatively with blood transfusion and bed rest. More serious bleeding as evidenced by orthostatic symptoms can be managed by selective angioembolization or reoperation. A recent report indicated 2% of all LPN patients needed radiologic treatment for refractory bleeding (113). Percutaneous drains should be placed anytime a question of collecting system entry arises. These drains can usually be removed postoperatively if drainage is minimal or proven not to be urine. Prolonged postoperative urine leaks are managed with optimal drainage, usually with ureteral stenting and the occasional addition of bladder catheterization. Leaks not able to be managed in this manner may require percutaneous nephrostomy. When repairing the collecting system, care should be taken not to incorporate interstitial renal tissue in the closure to avoid damaging underlying renal vessels. An arteriovenous fistula or renal pseudoaneurysm typically presents with hematuria and may require angioembolization.

■ REFERENCES

1. http://www.cancer.org/acs/groups/content/@epide-miologysurveilance/documents/document/acspc-026238.pdf

2. http://eu-cancer.iarc.fr/cancer-19-kidney.html,en#block-9–17

3. Lipworth L, Tarone RE, McLaughlin JK. The epidemiology of renal cell carcinoma. *J Urol*. 2006;176(6 Pt 1):2353–2358.

4. Robson CJ, Churchill BM, Anderson W. The results of radical nephrectomy for renal cell carcinoma. *J Urol*. 1969;101(3):297–301.

5. Coll DM, Smith RC. Update on radiological imaging of renal cell carcinoma. *BJU Int*. 2007;99(5 Pt B):1217–1222.

6. Frank I, Blute ML, Cheville JC, Lohse CM, Weaver AL, Zincke H. Solid renal tumors: an analysis of pathological features related to tumor size. *J Urol*. 2003;170(6 Pt 1):2217–2220.

7. Schlomer B, Figenshau RS, Yan Y, Venkatesh R, Bhayani SB. Pathological features of renal neoplasms classified by size and symptomatology. *J Urol*. 2006;176(4 Pt 1):1317–20; discussion 1320.

8. Volpe A, Mattar K, Finelli A, et al. Contemporary results of percutaneous biopsy of 100 small renal masses: a single center experience. *J Urol*. 2008; 180(6):2333–2337.

9. Rybikowski S, Tomatis L, Arroua F, Ragni E, Rossi D, Bastide C. [Value of percutaneous kidney biopsy in the management of solid renal tumours less or equal to 4 cm]. *Prog Urol*. 2008; 18(6):337–343.

10 Thuillier C, Long JA, Lapouge O, et al. Value of percutaneous biopsy for solid renal tumors less than 4 cm in diameter based on a series of 53 cases. *Prog Urol* 2008;18:435–439.

11. Barocas DA, Mathew S, DelPizzo JJ, et al. Renal cell carcinoma sub-typing by histopathology and fluorescence in situ hybridization on a needle-biopsy specimen. *BJU Int*. 2007;99(2):290–295.

12. Lee CT, Katz J, Fearn PA, Russo P. Mode of presentation of renal cell carcinoma provides prognostic information. *Urol Oncol*. 2002;7(4):135–140.

13. Sunela KL, Kataja MJ, Kellokumpu-Lehtinen PL. Changes in symptoms of renal cell carcinoma over four decades. *BJU Int*. 2010;106(5):649–653.

14 Aslam SSA, The J, Nargund VH, et al. Assessment of tumor invasion of the vena caval wall in renal cell carcinoma cases by magnetic resonance imaging. *J Urol* 2002;167:1271–1275.

15. Hallscheidt PJ, Fink C, Haferkamp A, et al. Preoperative staging of renal cell carcinoma with inferior vena cava thrombus using multidetector CT and MRI: prospective study with histopathological correlation. *J Comput Assist Tomogr*. 2005;29(1):64–68.

16. Kutikov A, Egleston BL, Wong YN, Uzzo RG. Evaluating overall survival and competing risks of death in patients with localized renal cell carcinoma using a comprehensive nomogram. *J Clin Oncol*. 2010;28(2):311–317.

17. Soares AA, Eyff TF, Campani RB, Ritter L, Camargo JL, Silveiro SP. Glomerular filtration rate measurement and prediction equations. *Clin Chem Lab Med*. 2009;47(9):1023–1032.

18. Stevens LA, Schmid CH, Greene T, et al. Comparative performance of the CKD Epidemiology Collaboration (CKD-EPI) and the Modification of Diet in Renal Disease (MDRD) Study equations for estimating GFR levels above 60 mL/min/1.73 m2. *Am J Kidney Dis*. 2010;56(3):486–495.

19. Skinner DG, Colvin RB, Vermillion CD, Pfister RC, Leadbetter WF. Diagnosis and management of renal cell carcinoma. A clinical and pathologic study of 309 cases. *Cancer*. 1971;28(5):1165–1177.

20. Kobayashi Y, Saika T, Manabe D, Nasu Y, Kumon H. The benefits of clamping the renal artery in laparoscopic partial nephrectomy. *Acta Med Okayama*. 2008;62(4):269–273.

21. Nadu A, Kitrey N, Mor Y, Golomb J, Ramon J. Laparoscopic partial nephrectomy: is it advantageous and safe to clamp the renal artery? *Urology*. 2005;66(2):279–282.

22. Sheridan AM, Bonventre JV. Cell biology and molecular mechanisms of injury in ischemic acute renal failure. *Curr Opin Nephrol Hypertens*. 2000;9(4):427–434.

23. Thompson RH, Lane BR, Lohse CM, et al. Every minute counts when the renal hilum is clamped during partial nephrectomy. *Eur Urol*. 2010;58(3):340–345.

24. Becker F, Van Poppel H, Hakenberg OW, et al. Assessing the impact of ischaemia time during partial nephrectomy. *Eur Urol*. 2009;56(4):625–634.

25. Finley DS, Lee DI, Eichel L, Uribe CA, McDougall EM, Clayman RV. Fibrin glue-oxidized cellulose sandwich for laparoscopic wedge resection of small renal lesions. *J Urol*. 2005;173(5):1477–1481.

26. Jeon SS, Kim IY. Laparoscopic partial nephrectomy without hilar control. *J Endourol*. 2008;22(9):1937–9; discussion 1941.

27. Weizer AZ, Gilbert SM, Roberts WW, Hollenbeck BK, Wolf JS Jr. Tailoring technique of laparoscopic

partial nephrectomy to tumor characteristics. *J Urol.* 2008;180(4):1273–1278.

28. Koo HJ, Lee DH, Kim IY. Renal hilar control during laparoscopic partial nephrectomy: to clamp or not to clamp. *J Endourol.* 2010;24(8):1283–1287.

29. McKiernan J, Yossepowitch O, Kattan MW, et al. Partial nephrectomy for renal cortical tumors: pathologic findings and impact on outcome. *Urology.* 2002;60(6):1003–1009.

30. Tsivian M, Moreira DM, Caso JR, et al. Predicting occult multifocality of renal cell carcinoma. *Eur Urol* 2010;58(1):118–126

31. Yossepowitch O, Thompson RH, Leibovich BC, et al. Positive surgical margins at partial nephrectomy: predictors and oncological outcomes. *J Urol.* 2008;179(6):2158–2163.

32. Patard JJ, Shvarts O, Lam JS, et al. Safety and efficacy of partial nephrectomy for all T1 tumors based on an international multicenter experience. *J Urol.* 2004;171(6 Pt 1):2181–5, quiz 2435.

33. Crépel M, Jeldres C, Perrotte P, et al. Nephron-sparing surgery is equally effective to radical nephrectomy for T1BN0M0 renal cell carcinoma: a population-based assessment. *Urology.* 2010;75(2):271–275.

34. Thompson RH, Siddiqui S, Lohse CM, Leibovich BC, Russo P, Blute ML. Partial versus radical nephrectomy for 4 to 7 cm renal cortical tumors. *J Urol.* 2009;182(6):2601–2606.

35. Breau RH, Crispen PL, Jimenez RE, Lohse CM, Blute ML, Leibovich BC. Outcome of stage T2 or greater renal cell cancer treated with partial nephrectomy. *J Urol.* 2010;183(3):903–908.

36. Jeldres C, Patard JJ, Capitanio U, et al. Partial versus radical nephrectomy in patients with adverse clinical or pathologic characteristics. *Urology.* 2009; 73(6):1300–1305.

37 http://www.auanet.org/content/media/renalmass09.pdf, 2009 AUA Guidelines

38. Thompson RH, Leibovich BC, Lohse CM, Zincke H, Blute ML. Complications of contemporary open nephron sparing surgery: a single institution experience. *J Urol.* 2005;174(3):855–858.

39 Belldegrun A, Tsui KH, deKernion JB, et al. Efficacy of nephron-sparing surgery for renal cell carcinoma: analysis based on the new 1997 tumor-node-metastasis staging system. *J Clin Oncol* 1999;17:2868–2875.

40. Campbell SC, Novick AC. Surgical technique and morbidity of elective partial nephrectomy. *Semin Urol Oncol.* 1995;13(4):281–287.

41. Hollenbeck BK, Taub DA, Miller DC, Dunn RL, Wei JT. National utilization trends of partial nephrectomy for renal cell carcinoma: a case of underutilization? *Urology.* 2006;67(2):254–259.

42. Miller DC, Hollingsworth JM, Hafez KS, Daignault S, Hollenbeck BK. Partial nephrectomy for small renal masses: an emerging quality of care concern? *J Urol.* 2006;175(3 Pt 1):853–7; discussion 858.

43. Huang WC, Elkin EB, Levey AS, Jang TL, Russo P. Partial nephrectomy versus radical nephrectomy in patients with small renal tumors–is there a difference in mortality and cardiovascular outcomes? *J Urol.* 2009;181(1):55–61; discussion 61.

44. Dulabon LM, Lowrance WT, Russo P, Huang WC. Trends in renal tumor surgery delivery within the United States. *Cancer.* 2010;116(10):2316–2321.

45. Clayman RV, Kavoussi LR, Soper NJ, et al. Laparoscopic nephrectomy: initial case report. *J Urol.* 1991;146(2):278–282.

46. Permpongkosol S, Bagga HS, Romero FR, Solomon SB, Kavoussi LR. Trends in the operative management of renal tumors over a 14-year period. *BJU Int.* 2006;98(4):751–755.

47. Hemal AK, Kumar A, Kumar R, Wadhwa P, Seth A, Gupta NP. Laparoscopic versus open radical nephrectomy for large renal tumors: a long-term prospective comparison. *J Urol.* 2007;177(3):862–866.

48. Colombo JR Jr, Haber GP, Aron M, et al. Oncological outcomes of laparoscopic radical nephrectomy for renal cancer. *Clinics (Sao Paulo).* 2007;62(3):251–256.

49 Cadeddu JA, Ono Y, Clayman RV, et al. Laparoscopic nephrectomy for renal cell cancer: evaluation of efficacy and safety: a multicenter experience. *Urology* 1998;52:773–777.

50. Gill IS, Meraney AM, Schweizer DK, et al. Laparoscopic radical nephrectomy in 100 patients: a single center experience from the United States. *Cancer.* 2001;92(7):1843–1855.

51. Portis AJ, Yan Y, Landman J, et al. Long-term followup after laparoscopic radical nephrectomy. *J Urol.* 2002;167(3):1257–1262.

52. Desai MM, Gill IS, Ramani AP, Matin SF, Kaouk JH, Campero JM. Laparoscopic radical nephrectomy for cancer with level I renal vein involvement. *J Urol.* 2003;169(2):487–491.

53. Rabets JC, Kaouk J, Fergany A, Finelli A, Gill IS, Novick AC. Laparoscopic versus open cytoreductive nephrectomy for metastatic renal cell carcinoma. *Urology.* 2004;64(5):930–934.

54. Desai MM, Strzempkowski B, Matin SF, et al. Prospective randomized comparison of transperitoneal versus retroperitoneal laparoscopic radical nephrectomy. *J Urol.* 2005;173(1):38–41.

55. Berglund RK, Gill IS, Babineau D, Desai M, Kaouk JH. A prospective comparison of transperitoneal and retroperitoneal laparoscopic nephrectomy in the extremely obese patient. *BJU Int.* 2007; 99(4):871–874.

56. Winfield HN, Donovan JF, Godet AS, Clayman RV. Laparoscopic partial nephrectomy: initial case report for benign disease. *J Endourol.* 1993;7(6):521–526.

57. Gill IS, Delworth MG, Munch LC. Laparoscopic retroperitoneal partial nephrectomy. *J Urol.* 1994;152(5 Pt 1):1539–1542.

58. Gill IS, Kavoussi LR, Lane BR, et al. Comparison of 1,800 laparoscopic and open partial nephrectomies for single renal tumors. *J Urol.* 2007;178(1):41–46.

59. Marszalek M, Meixl H, Polajnar M, Rauchenwald M, Jeschke K, Madersbacher S. Laparoscopic and open partial nephrectomy: a matched-pair comparison of 200 patients. *Eur Urol.* 2009;55(5):1171–1178.

60. Gill IS, Colombo JR Jr, Moinzadeh A, et al. Laparoscopic partial nephrectomy in solitary kidney. *J Urol.* 2006;175(2):454–458.

61. Frank I, Colombo JR Jr, Rubinstein M, Desai M, Kaouk J, Gill IS. Laparoscopic partial nephrectomy for centrally located renal tumors. *J Urol.* 2006;175 (3 Pt 1):849–852.

62. Colombo JR Jr, Haber GP, Gill IS. Laparoscopic partial nephrectomy in patients with compromised renal function. *Urology.* 2008;71(6):1043–1048.

63. Scoll BJ, Uzzo RG, Chen DY, et al. Robot-assisted partial nephrectomy: a large single-institutional experience. *Urology.* 2010;75(6):1328–1334.

64. Wang AJ, Bhayani SB. Robotic partial nephrectomy versus laparoscopic partial nephrectomy for renal cell carcinoma: single-surgeon analysis of > 100 consecutive procedures. *Urology.* 2009;73(2):306–310.

65. Jeong W, Park S, Lorenzo E, et al. Laparoscopic partial nephrectomy versus robotic-assisted laparoscopic partial nephrectomy. *J Endourol* 2009;23:1457–1460.

66. Saitoh H, Nakayama M, Nakamura K, Satoh T. Distant metastasis of renal adenocarcinoma in nephrectomized cases. *J Urol.* 1982;127(6):1092–1095.

67. Johnsen JA, Hellsten S. Lymphatogenous spread of renal cell carcinoma: an autopsy study. *J Urol.* 1997;157(2):450–453.

68. Blom JH, van Poppel H, Marechal JM, et al. Radical nephrectomy with and without lymph node dissection: preliminary results of the EORTC randomized phase III protocol 30881. EORTC Genitourinary Group. *Eur Urol.* 1999;36(6):570–575.

69. Blute ML, Leibovich BC, Cheville JC, Lohse CM, Zincke H. A protocol for performing extended lymph node dissection using primary tumor pathological features for patients treated with radical nephrectomy for clear cell renal cell carcinoma. *J Urol.* 2004;172(2):465–469.

70. Tsukamoto T, Kumamoto Y, Miyao N, Yamazaki K, Takahashi A, Satoh M. Regional lymph node metastasis in renal cell carcinoma: incidence, distribution and its relation to other pathological findings. *Eur Urol.* 1990;18(2):88–93.

71. Studer UE, Scherz S, Scheidegger J, et al. Enlargement of regional lymph nodes in renal cell carcinoma is often not due to metastases. *J Urol.* 1990;144(2 Pt 1):243–245.

72. Schafhauser W, Ebert A, Brod J, Petsch S, Schrott KM. Lymph node involvement in renal cell carcinoma and survival chance by systematic lymphadenectomy. *Anticancer Res.* 1999;19(2C):1573–1578.

73. Mickisch GH, Garin A, van Poppel H, de Prijck L, Sylvester R. Radical nephrectomy plus interferon-alfa-based immunotherapy compared with interferon alfa alone in metastatic renal-cell carcinoma: a randomised trial. *Lancet.* 2001;358(9286):966–970.

74. Flanigan RC, Salmon SE, Blumenstein BA, et al. Nephrectomy followed by interferon alfa-2b compared with interferon alfa-2b alone for metastatic renal-cell cancer. *N Engl J Med.* 2001;345(23):1655–1659.

75. Vasselli JR, Yang JC, Linehan WM, White DE, Rosenberg SA, Walther MM. Lack of retroperitoneal lymphadenopathy predicts survival of patients with metastatic renal cell carcinoma. *J Urol.* 2001;166(1):68–72.

76. Terrone C, Guercio S, De Luca S, et al. The number of lymph nodes examined and staging accuracy in renal cell carcinoma. *BJU Int.* 2003;91(1):37–40.

77. Hellström PA, Bloigu R, Ruokonen AO, Vainionpää VA, Nuutinen LS, Kontturi MJ. Is routine ipsilateral adrenalectomy during radical nephrectomy harmful for the patient? *Scand J Urol Nephrol.* 1997;31(1):19–25.

78. Tsui KH, Shvarts O, Barbaric Z, Figlin R, de Kernion JB, Belldegrun A. Is adrenalectomy a necessary component of radical nephrectomy? UCLA experience with 511 radical nephrectomies. *J Urol.* 2000;163(2):437–441.

79. Autorino R, Di Lorenzo G, Damiano R, et al. Adrenal sparing surgery in the treatment of renal cell carcinoma: when is it possible? *World J Urol.* 2003;21(3):153–158.

80. De Sio M, Autorino R, Di Lorenzo G, et al. Adrenalectomy: defining its role in the surgical treatment of renal cell carcinoma. *Urol Int.* 2003;71(4):361–367.

81. Kozak W, Höltl W, Pummer K, Maier U, Jeschke K, Bucher A. Adrenalectomy–still a must in radical renal surgery? *Br J Urol*. 1996;77(1):27–31.

82. Li GR, Soulie M, Escourrou G, Plante P, Pontonnier F. Micrometastatic adrenal invasion by renal carcinoma in patients undergoing nephrectomy. *Br J Urol*. 1996;78(6):826–828.

83. O'Malley RL, Godoy G, Kanofsky JA, Taneja SS. The necessity of adrenalectomy at the time of radical nephrectomy: a systematic review. *J Urol*. 2009; 181(5):2009–2017.

84. Kessler OJ, Mukamel E, Weinstein R, Gayer E, Konichezky M, Servadio C. Metachronous renal cell carcinoma metastasis to the contralateral adrenal gland. *Urology*. 1998;51(4):539–543.

85. Schorr AB. Twenty percent incidence of adrenocortical insufficiency in metastatic hypernephroma. *Clin Res* 1986;34:200A.

86. Siemer S, Lehmann J, Kamradt J, et al. Adrenal metastases in 1635 patients with renal cell carcinoma: outcome and indication for adrenalectomy. *J Urol* 2004;171(6 Pt 1):2155–2159.

87. Kim HL, Zisman A, Han KR, Figlin RA, Belldegrun AS. Prognostic significance of venous thrombus in renal cell carcinoma. Are renal vein and inferior vena cava involvement different? *J Urol*. 2004;171 (2 Pt 1):588–591.

88. Wagner B, Patard JJ, Méjean A, et al. Prognostic value of renal vein and inferior vena cava involvement in renal cell carcinoma. *Eur Urol*. 2009;55(2):452–459.

89. Bakke A, Göthlin JH, Haukaas SA, Kalland T. Augmentation of natural killer cell activity after arterial embolization of renal carcinomas. *Cancer Res*. 1982;42(9):3880–3883.

90. Nakano H, Nihira H, Toge T. Treatment of renal cancer patients by transcatheter embolization and its effects on lymphocyte proliferative responses. *J Urol*. 1983;130(1):24–27.

91. Schwartz MJ, Smith EB, Trost DW, Vaughan ED Jr. Renal artery embolization: clinical indications and experience from over 100 cases. *BJU Int*. 2007;99(4):881–886.

92. Subramanian VS, Stephenson AJ, Goldfarb DA, Fergany AF, Novick AC, Krishnamurthi V. Utility of preoperative renal artery embolization for management of renal tumors with inferior vena caval thrombi. *Urology*. 2009;74(1):154–159.

93. Karnes RJ, Blute ML. Surgery insight: management of renal cell carcinoma with associated inferior vena cava thrombus. *Nat Clin Pract Urol*. 2008;5(6):329–339.

94. Motzer RJ, Figlin RA, Hutson TE, et al. Sunitinib versus interferon-alpha as first-line treatment of metastatic renal cell carcinoma (mRCC): updated results and analysis of prognostic factors. In: 2007 ASCO Annual Meeting Proceedings Part 1 2007, abstract 5024.

95. Rosenberg JE, Motzer RJ, Michaelson MD, et al. Sunitinib therapy for patients with metastatic renal cell carcinoma: updated results of two phase II trials and prognostic factor analysis for survival. In: 2007 ASCO Annual Meeting Proceedings Part 1 2007, abstract 5095.

96. Halbert RJ, Figlin RA, Atkins MB, et al. Treatment of patients with metastatic renal cell cancer: a RAND Appropriateness Panel. *Cancer*. 2006; 107(10):2375–2383.

97. Walther MM, Yang JC, Pass HI, Linehan WM, Rosenberg SA. Cytoreductive surgery before high dose interleukin-2 based therapy in patients with metastatic renal cell carcinoma. *J Urol*. 1997;158(5):1675–1678.

98. Rackley R, Novick A, Klein E, Bukowski R, McLain D, Goldfarb D. The impact of adjuvant nephrectomy on multimodality treatment of metastatic renal cell carcinoma. *J Urol*. 1994;152(5 Pt 1):1399–1403.

99. Catarci M, Carlini M, Gentileschi P, Santoro E. Major and minor injuries during the creation of pneumoperitoneum. A multicenter study on 12,919 cases. *Surg Endosc*. 2001;15(6):566–569.

100. Breda A, Finelli A, Janetschek G, Porpiglia F, Montorsi F. Complications of laparoscopic surgery for renal masses: prevention, management, and comparison with the open experience. *Eur Urol*. 2009;55(4):836–850.

101. Bishoff JT, Allaf ME, Kirkels W, Moore RG, Kavoussi LR, Schroder F. Laparoscopic bowel injury: incidence and clinical presentation. *J Urol*. 1999; 161(3):887–890.

102. Permpongkosol S, Link RE, Su LM, et al. Complications of 2,775 urological laparoscopic procedures: 1993 to 2005. *J Urol*. 2007;177(2):580–585.

103. Cooper CS, Cohen MB, Donovan JF Jr. Splenectomy complicating left nephrectomy. *J Urol*. 1996; 155(1):30–36.

104. Varkarakis IM, Allaf ME, Bhayani SB, et al. Pancreatic injuries during laparoscopic urologic surgery. *Urology*. 2004;64(6):1089–1093.

105. Atmaca AF, Canda AE, Serefoglu EC, Altinova S, Ozdemir AT, Balbay MD. The incidence and management of pleural injuries occurring during open nephrectomy. *Adv Urol*. 2009:948906.

106. Kouba E, Smith AM, Derksen JE, Gunn K, Wallen E, Pruthi RS. Efficacy and safety of en bloc ligation of renal hilum during laparoscopic nephrectomy. *Urology*. 2007;69(2):226–229.

107. Chan D, Bishoff JT, Ratner L, Kavoussi LR, Jarrett TW. Endovascular gastrointestinal stapler device malfunction during laparoscopic nephrectomy: early recognition and management. *J Urol*. 2000;164(2):319–321.

108. His RS, Saint-Elie DT, Zimmerman GJ, et al. Mechanisms of hemostatic failure during laparoscopic nephrectomy. *BJU Int* 2008;101:878–882.

109. Tsivian A, Sidi AA. Port site metastases in urological laparoscopic surgery. *J Urol*. 2003;169(4):1213–1218.

110. Van Poppel H, Da Pozzo L, Albrecht W, et al. A prospective randomized EORTC intergroup phase 3 study comparing the complications of elective nephron-sparing surgery and radical nephrectomy for low-stage renal cell carcinoma. *Eur Urol*. 2007;51(6):1606–1615.

111. Steinbach F, Stöckle M, Müller SC, et al. Conservative surgery of renal cell tumors in 140 patients: 21 years of experience. *J Urol*. 1992;148(1):24–9; discussion 29.

112. Simmons MN, Gill IS. Decreased complications of contemporary laparoscopic partial nephrectomy: use of a standardized reporting system. *J Urol*. 2007;177(6):2067–73; discussion 2073.

113. Montag S, Rais-Bahrami S, Seideman CA, et al. Delayed haemorrhage after laparoscopic partial nephrectomy: frequency and angiographic findings. *BJU Int*. 2010;106(6) [Epub ahead of print].

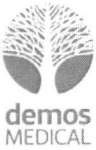

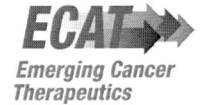

Nonsystemic Approaches to the Management of Metastatic Renal Cell Carcinoma

Brian I. Rini and Lilyana Angelov

Cleveland Clinic Taussig Cancer Center, Cleveland, OH

■ ABSTRACT

Renal cell carcinoma (RCC) is a disease with an inherently variable natural history in which local therapy has been applied to patients with metastatic disease. Traditionally, this has taken the form of surgical removal of metastatic deposits. Inherent challenges of RCC biology, however, have limited surgical removal of brain and bone metastatic sites. More recently, technological advances in radiotherapy have broadened the potential approaches. Focused radiation to tumors (stereotactic radiosurgery) allows conformal delivery of high radiation doses over few treatment sessions. This modality has been applied to both central nervous system and bone metastases, demonstrating excellent local control of tumor growth and palliation of symptoms. Radiofrequency ablation is an alternative local approach, with an electric current causing heating of the tumors with resultant coagulation and cell death. Small case series have emerged of RCC metastasis treatment, with further study required to delineate the risk/benefit ratio of this approach. An observational approach to indolent metastatic RCC has also been adopted before both local and systemic therapy in an attempt to spare patients with low-volume, slow-growing disease from the inherent toxicity of therapy. Further investigation of local approaches in metastatic RCC is ongoing.

Keywords: renal cell carcinoma, radiosurgery, stereotactic, local therapy

*Corresponding author, Cleveland Clinic Taussig Cancer Center, 9500 Euclid Ave, Cleveland, OH 44195
   E-mail address: rinib2@ccf.org

Emerging Cancer Therapeutics 2:1 (2011) 89–100.
DOI: 10.5003/2151–4194.2.1.89

■ INTRODUCTION

Although the emergence of viable systemic therapy has revolutionized the management of metastatic renal cell carcinoma (RCC), there has been simultaneous progress in nonsystemic approaches. These approaches are often applied to patients with a limited volume and number of metastases, and often to organs such as bone and brain where the effect of targeted therapy is uncertain. The use of these approaches has been furthered by advances in technology and is in part driven by the realization of the non-curative and often toxic nature of systemic therapy. Thus, in a subset of patients with limited extent metastatic RCC, an approach of deferred systemic therapy with the use of focal therapy to metastatic sites has been investigated.

Renal carcinoma has always been characterized by an inherently diverse biology. The natural history of metastatic RCC can range from a few months to many years, and this timeline has been further extended by the introduction of targeted therapy. An appreciation of this diverse biology is critical in understanding nonsystemic approaches to this disease. That is, patients with more bulky and/or rapidly growing disease are not good candidates for local approaches, outside those anatomically necessary (e.g., surgery for spinal cord compression or surgery/radiation of brain metastases). However, patients with indolent, low-volume disease, in whom local approaches are most suitable and most likely to be undertaken, are the hardest to prove that treatment of metastatic sites results in clear clinical benefit, such as improved quality of life or increased survival. This review summaries recent advances in this field.

■ ACTIVE SURVEILLANCE

Because of the acute and chronic toxicity and assumed non-curative nature of systemic targeted therapy, a select subset of patients may be better served with initial surveillance. This approach attempts to take advantage of the sometimes indolent RCC biology, applying therapy only

when indicated. Such therapy may include focal approaches, depending on the site and location of metastases, and likely will ultimately involve initiation of systemic therapy. Surveillance is inherently undertaken to some degree in all patients during the period of time where metastatic deposits are below the level of clinical detection.

Although the indolent nature of a small subset of RCC is well-recognized, there is a paucity of data to characterize this approach. A trial was conducted in which 73 patients with metastatic RCC were observed with radiographs monthly until symptoms or WHO-defined disease progression (1). Interferon (IFN) alpha was then started at disease progression. While the median PFS was about 2 months, 10% of patients had not progressed by 12 months. Importantly, the overall response rate to IFN was 15%, identical to a contemporary group treated with IFN without initial observation. These very limited data make some important points. Namely, only a small fraction (likely 5%–10%) of metastatic RCC patients will have indolent enough growth to be candidates for observation. Further, the response to systemic therapy is likely preserved with delayed therapy. More contemporary data involves the randomized discontinuation trial of sorafenib (2). Metastatic RCC patients in this trial were randomized to placebo or sorafenib after a 12-week sorafenib run-in period. Patients who stayed on sorafenib had a median PFS of 24 weeks from the time of randomization. Placebo patients had a median PFS of 7 weeks, but when placebo patients were crossed over to sorafenib, the subsequent PFS was 24 weeks, identical to those patients treated with immediate sorafenib. Although these data are also limited, they generate a hypothesis that treatment benefit is not reduced with deferred treatment and could be a reasonable strategy in a subset of low-volume, indolent metastatic RCC patients. Such patients will have a higher tumor burden upon initiation of therapy, so this approach must be mindful of amount and pace of tumor burden. The critical question of whether or not there is identical clinical benefit to a given agent and overall survival after a period of observation requires prospective study. Currently, a multi-institutional prospective trial of active surveillance in metastatic RCC patients is being undertaken, lead by The Cleveland Clinic. This trial will prospectively follow patients prior to their first systemic treatment for metastatic RCC. Tumor growth characteristics will be measured, and response to subsequent systemic therapy recorded.

■ NONCENTRAL NERVOUS SYSTEM LESIONS

Surgical Removal of Metastatic Sites

RCC has long been a malignancy where surgical removal of limited metastases has been pursued. Several series have documented the feasibility of this approach, with 5-year disease-free survival rates uniformly approximating 30%, encompassing a wide variety of metastatic organ sites. Favorable prognostic factors include a long interval between initial diagnosis and development of metastases, which reflects an indolent course and reinforces the likelihood that the metastasis is truly solitary, and the ability for complete resection (e.g., solitary lung metastasis) (3,4). These series are exclusively retrospective, and thus subject to several inherent biases. Namely, patients who can undergo surgery, usually at a tertiary care referral center, have inherently better performance status and more indolent disease biology. Thus, although all series report long overall survival times that exceed patients who do not undergo surgery, the protoplasm of surgical patients is such that longer survival times are expected, regardless of metastasectomy. It is difficult to prove that the surgical interventions lead to enhanced patient outcomes. It is likely that a subset of patients truly benefit from surgical metastasectomy, whereas the clinical outcome of others is not affected. Evidence from contemporary series demonstrate several consistent factors associated with prolonged survival in this group of patients, such as 1) good performance status, 2) a long disease-free interval from

nephrectomy to metastasectomy, and 3) the ability to completely resect the metastatic lesion. Given the non-curative nature of systemic therapy and associated toxicity, metastasectomy is a reasonable disease control strategy in a highly select subgroup of metastatic RCC patients.

Stereotactic Radiosurgery

Focused radiation to tumors has been termed "stereotactic" radiosurgery (SRS) by many. SRS/stereotactic body radiation therapy represents an evolution in radiation delivery where an accurate and conformal high radiation dose is delivered to the tumor in 1 to 5 sessions. While these treatments are associated with potentially ablative dosing to the tumor, the steep radiation falloff dose gradients associated with the treatment allow for the protection of adjacent normal structures (Figure 1). This technology enables accurate localization of a tumor and provides for delivery of higher radiation doses than possible with standard external beam radiation. Higher radiation doses are thought to overcome somewhat the inherent radioresistance of many RCC tumors. An initial prospective phase II of this approach was reported in 2006 based on a prior retrospective experience report (5) (Table 1). Patients with inoperable RCC and no prior XRT or concurrent systemic therapy were enrolled. Non-bone lesions were treated to a minimum of 8 Gy to the periphery of the tumor volume. Thirty patients were enrolled and a total of 82 lesions treated: 5 patients with inoperable primary RCC tumors, 6 patients with solitary metastases, and 19 patients with multiple metastatic sites. The majority of sites treated (63/82, 77%) were in the lung or mediastinum. Approximately half the patients were MSKCC good risk and half intermediate risk. Local tumor response (% regression) was the primary endpoint and an unspecified number of patients (not 100%) had histologic confirmation of metastatic RCC in the treated lesion(s). Fractionation schema varied from 5 to 15 Gy in 2 to 5 fractions. Fifty-two

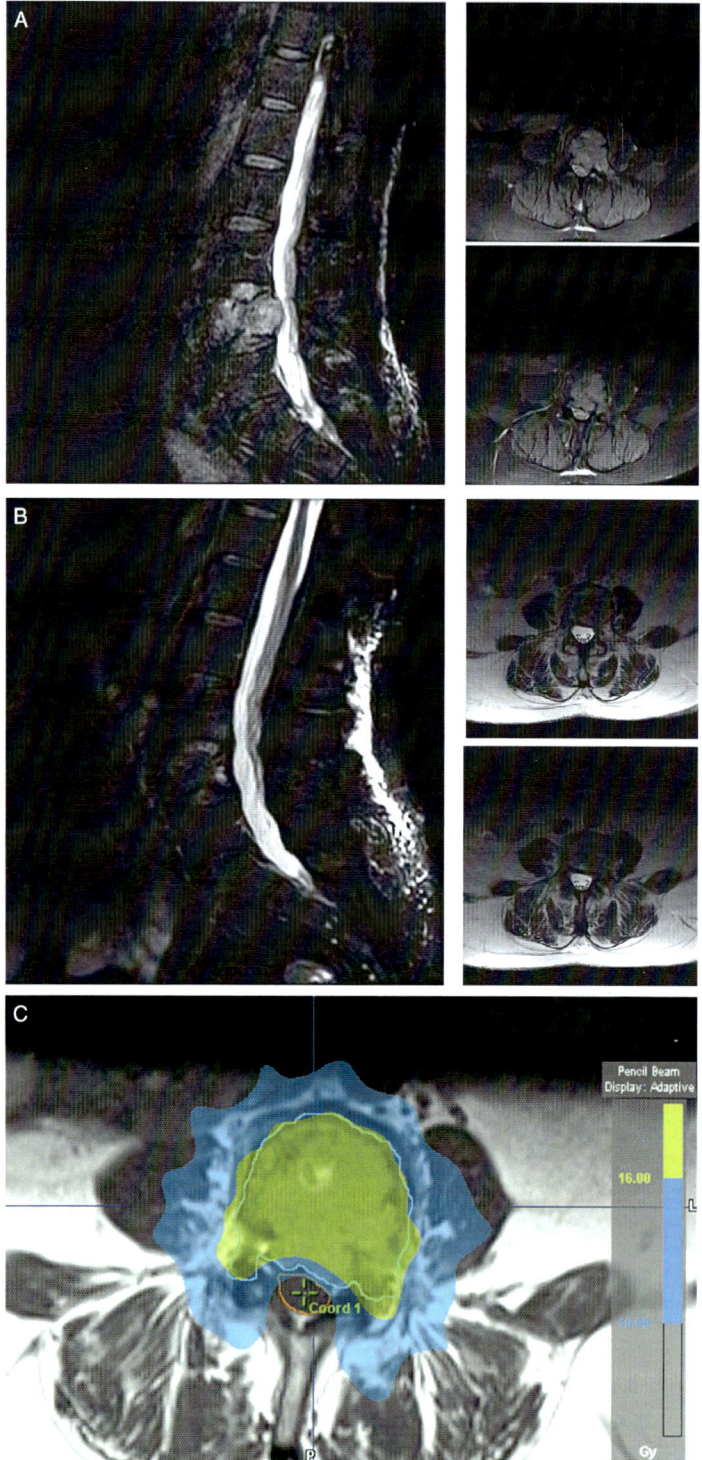

FIGURE 1
(A) MRI of a patient with metastatic renal carcinoma revealing a large heterogeneous expansile mass in the L4 vertebral body with associated moderate epidural disease, anterior thecal sac compression, and left L4/5 nerve root encroachment. The patient had left hip and radicular left leg pain requiring narcotics. (B) The MRI scan demonstrates near-complete resolution of the epidural disease, thecal sac, and nerve root compression. This treatment effect has persisted 20 months post-SRS treatment and the patient reports no pain and does not take any pain medication. (C) SRS plan demonstrating the dose distribution to the tumor and the thecal sac. The desired treatment dose (16 Gy) is conformal to the vertebral body target region. The steep dose falloff results in a lower dose (10 Gy) to the thecal sac.

percent of lesions showed regression, with 21% reported as completely resolved. Interestingly, 6 patients died before 6 months of follow-up (cause not stated), calling into question local therapy in patients with imminent death from systemic disease. Local control rate was 79%, if the early death patients are considered failures.

More commonly, SRS has been applied to bone metastases from RCC. Traditional approaches of treating bone metastases include surgery and radiotherapy but both these alternatives are associated with marked challenges and limitations when applied to the treatment of patients with RCC metastases. These tumors are typically radioresistant, and treatment with conventional radiation is often of modest benefit in terms of either tumor control or pain relief (6,7). Reichel et al. further demonstrated that conventional radiation had no durable impact on pain relief with only a median time to return of pretreatment pain levels and Karnofsky performance score (KPS) decline of only 2 months and 1 month, respectively (8). Specifically, in patients with RCC metastatic epidural spinal cord compression, only 29% of patients showed improvement of motor function after conventional radiation therapy (9). However, renal bone metastases are also considered difficult to treat with open surgery as they are extremely vascular and are associated with a surgical complication rate significantly higher than rates seen with the surgical management of other spinal metastases (7,10–12). Ulmar et al. reported one such surgical series of 37 patients with RCC, where patients experienced significant surgical morbidity (67%) and mortality (10%) in the perioperative period (13). Upon this background of radioresistance and surgical challenges, technological advances through SRS have been applied to RCC metastatic to bone.

One series reported 60 cases of RCC treated with single-fraction SRS (14). Most of the patients (48/60) had progressed through prior conventional radiation therapy. At a median follow-up of 37 months, axial pain had improved in 89% of the patients who initially presented with pain, and

tumor control was achieved in 7 of 8 of patients who presented with tumor progression. Further, no radiation myelopathy or other toxicity was seen in the follow-up period despite the high number of re-irradiated patients in the study. Nguyen et al. demonstrated 82% 1-year progression-free survival in 55 spinal metastases treated with SRS and no grade 3 to 4 neurological treatment-related toxicity was observed in any patient (15). Another series reported 55 consecutive patients with metastatic RCC, who were also receiving antiangiogenic therapy (Table 1). All patients had RCC to bone and were required to have pain, neuroforaminal compromise, or imminent instability (16). The primary endpoint of the trial was local control. Fifty-five patients with 105 lesions were treated with a median of 20 Gy in a single fraction. Local control was 94.1% at 12 months and 90.4% at 24 months. Tumor-associated pain, as measured by a visual analog scale from a median of 5 (range 1–8) pretreatment to 0 (range 0–2) posttherapy ($P < 0.001$). New peritumor enhancement was seen in two patients at 6 months, successfully re-treated with SRS. Our own Cleveland Clinic series reported single-fraction SRS in 29 patients with metastatic RCC (17) (Table 1). This prospective study assessed pain via the Brief Pain Inventory at baseline, 1 week, 1 month, 3 months, and every 3 months thereafter. MRI was done at the same time points as was quality of life assessment via the EORTC QLQ-30 scale. Forty-one percent of patients had mild motor or sensory deficits at baseline, 32% had prior external beam radiation to the treated area and 17% were taking targeted systemic therapy. Pain scores were significantly reduced as early as week 1 posttreatment ($P < 0.01$) and continued to reduce at 12 months posttreatment ($P < 0.05$). This was also associated with an 87.5% local tumor control rate in these patients at last follow up. Last, a recent series, delivered a median of 24 Gy via single-fraction SRS to 50 RCC patients with spine metastases (18) (Table 1). Ninety percent of patients achieved local control and 90% reported symptom palliation. Patients who received <24 Gy had worse local control (including melanoma patients in this series) 77% versus 96%.

Radiofrequency Ablation

Radiofrequency ablation (RFA) is an alternative local approach to metastatic sites that involves insertion of a needle probe into a metastatic site, with an electric current causing heating of the tumors with resultant coagulation and cell death. A retrospective series reported on 39 patients with metastatic RCC in whom lung metastases underwent RFA (19) (Table 1). RFA was performed as an inpatient under moderate sedation using local anesthesia. A single- or multi-timed electrode was placed in the center of lesions 2 cm or less and at multiple sites in larger tumors. Histologic confirmation of metastases was not required. The majority of patients received subsequent immunotherapy and were followed with CT scans every 3 to 4 months to assess response. Sixteen patients had disease outside the lung not addressed by RFA. Local control (absence of tumor growth on CT scan in the ablation zone) was 91% with a mean follow up of 25 months, with significantly more progression (33% vs. 7%) in tumors larger than 3 cm. Seven of 15 patients (47%) with all visible metastatic sites ablated had recurrence, most commonly in nontreated lung sites. These data support the feasibility of this approach, but the benefit to patients of RFA to some but not all metastatic sites is in question. A smaller retrospective series reported RFA on 23 pulmonary lesions in nine metastatic RCC patients (20) (Table 1). Lesion regression was seen in 56% of patients at a median follow up of 19.4 months, with more regression in smaller lesions. Seven patients developed recurrent disease, with five dying from metastatic RCC. An unacceptably high rate of pneumothorax (42%) was seen in this study.

In summary, the experience with SRS to bone metastases in RCC would suggest a high rate of local control and palliation of tumor-related symptoms. Toxicity appears minimal, and this approach seems a useful adjunct to systemic therapy, especially with the observation that patients on targeted therapy can have control of other disease with progression solely in bony sites (21,22). Single-fraction, outpatient delivery offers minimal interference to the patient or the systemic therapy delivery. Prospective investigation is now needed to solidify the retrospective findings, in addition to technique and dose refinement to optimize SRS to bone. In contrast, data regarding SRS and RFA to non-bone sites is limited by the small, highly-selected patient populations and retrospective nature. Significant complications have been reported. Given that RFA has largely been applied to asymptomatic lesions, the risk/benefit balance is not entirely clear. The value of SRS to non-bone sites and RFA in terms of preventing future complications or extending patient survival is not proven. Such interventions should be undertaken with great care in the context of clinical trials to further investigate whether these approaches have merit.

■ CENTRAL NERVOUS SYSTEM LESIONS

Approximately 4% to 17% of metastatic RCC involves the brain, making the estimated incidence of RCC brain metastases 1,200 to 5,100 cases annually in the United States (23). However, the median survival of patients with untreated RCC brain metastases is 3 to 4 months (24). Since effective treatment of brain metastases can improve both quality of life and outcomes in selected patients and can affect eligibility for clinical trials, these patients stand to benefit significantly from early, aggressive control of their CNS disease. However, the early treatment of brain metastases must be weighed against the delays that such interventions may cause for the management of the primary malignancy, and strategies must be designed to maximize the former while minimizing the latter.

A useful tool in the management of patients with brain metastases is the application of validated prognostic indices to estimate a patient's overall survival and potential tailor treatment. Specifically, symptom control and toxicity minimization are typically emphasized in more advanced disease or when comorbidities limit aggressive therapy tolerance while more aggressive measures are favored when they are likely to impact survival. Further, prognostic indices may be used as a benchmark comparison of results in different studies or as inclusion/exclusion criteria in clinical trials. While there are a number of validated prognostic indices for patients with brain metastases (25–31), the Radiation Therapy Oncology Group's 3-tiered prognostic index know as recursive partitioning analysis (RPA) classes are the most widely used and validated indices used to assess the impact of therapy patients with brain metastases and will be referred to in this chapter. The RPA classification system uses the clinical variables of age, KPS, controlled primary, and extent of disease to assign patients with brain metastasis to one of three classes with validated prognostic significance (25,26). Specifically, Class I patients are older than 65 years, have a KPS > 70, controlled primary disease and no extracranial metastases. Class III patients have a KPS < 70 and Class II categorizes all other (i.e., non Class I or III) patients.

Monotherapy with whole brain radiotherapy (WBRT) confers a marginal survival benefit with a median survival of 4 to 6 months and a median survival of 8.5, 3.0, and 0.6 months for RPA Class I, II, and III patients, respectively (6). This modest response to WBXRT is consistent with the "relatively radioresistant" phenotype associated with RCC. This radioresistance is currently believed to be actually a dose-dependent effect where RCC lesions can be effectively treated with higher radiation doses (32,33). The issue however remains the tolerance of the adjacent normal tissue to these higher therapeutic doses and the neurocognitive implications of this. This has lead to the recent trends to treat renal CNS metastases with more conformal strategies such as surgery or radiosurgery with or without the up-front addition of WBRT.

Surgical resection of RCC brain metastases has resulted in reported mean survival times of 12.5 to 27.5 months (34–36). These data however must be viewed with some degree of caution as selection bias toward patients with good performance status, limited systemic disease, surgically accessible tumors, and typically only a single metastasis likely influenced these results. Management with surgery followed by adjuvant WBXRT, a combination known to decrease the recurrence and neurological-associated death in the overall population of patients with metastatic brain lesions (37), confers minimal additional benefit in the subset of patients with metastases from RCC (34–36).

The advent of SRS has provided a new and less invasive local treatment modality that, like surgical resection, has the ability to treat brain metastases while sparing healthy brain tissue. SRS therefore represents an attractive alternative to other therapeutic modalities for patients with RCC brain metastases and has been associated with promising results (38). It confers comparable survival benefits without the risks and side effects inherent in other treatment modalities. The overall survival for patients undergoing monotherapy with SRS is reported to be between 7.5 and 12.5 months (39–44), and stratified by RPA class is reported to be 18 to 24 months for Class I, 8.5 to 9.2 months for Class II, and 5.3 to 7.5 months for Class III patients (45,46). Further, very high local control rates (80%–98%) are reported in patients treated with radiosurgery (32,44,46–48). The concurrent addition of WBXRT to patients treated with SRS does not improve either survival or local or distant recurrences and patients generally die of complications related to their primary malignancy (47,49–51). These findings would suggest that SRS alone is at least as effective as surgery followed by WBXRT in the management of patients with RCC brain metastases.

One particular subgroup that requires special mention is patients presenting with incidentally discovered or asymptomatic brain metastases from RCC primary tumors. In the modern era of CNS surveillance and routine staging evaluation in patients with RCC, up to 86% of patients have brain metastases that are clinically asymptomatic at the time of diagnosis (52). This treatment modality is particularly important to patients who present in this fashion, as they are often eager to minimize

TABLE 1 Select stereotactic radiation and radiofrequency ablation series to non-CNS lesions in metastatic RCC

Study	No. of Patients (No. of Lesions)	Modality (System)/ Organ Site	Median Dose	Local Control	Toxicity	Comments
Svedman (5)	30 (82)	SRS (Elekta System)/ multiple metastatic sites	8 Gy to periphery	79%	16/28 patients with grade 1–2 toxicity including cough, rash, local pain; one treatment-related death	Early deaths reported
Stahler (16)	55 (105)	SRS (Cyber Knife)/ spine metastases	20 Gy	90%	No reported added toxicity to systemic therapy	Significant decrease in tumor-associated pain
Angelov (17)	29 (33)	SRS (Novalis)/spine metastases	14 Gy	87.5%	No neurological/spinal cord toxicity; no additional toxicity with concurrent systemic therapy	Significant improvement at 1 week, 1 month, and 1 year in pain scores
Thiagaragan (18)	50 (NR)	SRS (NR)/spine metastases	24 Gy	90%	Minimal grade 1–2 toxicity; no spinal cord complications	Symptom palliation in 90% as assessed by pain scores
Soga (19)	39 (135)	RFA/lung metastases	n/a	91%	7% pneumothorax rate; no deaths	Retrospective series
Huo (20)	9 (23)	RFA/lung metastases	n/a	NR	43% pneumothorax rate; one bronchopulmonary fistula	Small, retrospective series

NR, not reported; SRS, stereotactic radiosurgery; RFA, radiofrequency ablation.

cognitive side effects, avoid surgery if possible, and expedite treatment of their primary malignancy. SRS is a particularly attractive treatment option for patients with incidentally discovered RCC brain metastases, combining a high local control rate with a favorable side effect profile, a short recovery time, and minimal delay in the treatment of their primary malignancy. A recent study from our center (53) demonstrated that when these patients were treated initially with SRS monotherapy, their mean overall survival was 21.5 months (16.2 months for RPA Class II patients). This treatment was also associated with a 95% local control rate. This is at least comparable to survival after treatment with surgery ± WBRT (53) and is achievable without the risks and side effects inherent in those treatment modalities and should be considered as a key component in the up-front management of these patients.

New preliminary data (largely case reports) are emerging regarding the efficacy of managing patients with known RCC brain metastases with systemic therapy such as multitargeted tyrosine kinase inhibitors (54–56). To date the best available data show that this strategy is associated with only modest clinical efficacy as demonstrated by a 12% objective response rate (54). Given the much higher effectiveness of other therapeutic alternatives, this should not be considered a front-line management option for treating patients with RCC brain metastases.

In summary, focal therapy remains the cornerstone of management of RCC brain metastases. Early detection, minimizing treatment time and hence delay in treating the primary tumor, careful attention to potential treatment-related early and delayed complications, and close patient follow up are all crucial to the successful management of these patients.

■ CONCLUSION

The inherent biology of metastatic RCC results in clinical scenarios in which local therapy may be of benefit. Indolent biology may afford a period of observation before definitive intervention. Similarly, isolated RCC metastases have long been subjected to surgical removal, resulting in significant disease-free intervals in a select subset of patients. Newer modalities such as stereotactic radiation have revolutionized the management of bone and brain metastases in RCC, offering excellent local control and symptom palliation. More experimental are local approaches such as SRS and RFA to non-bone, non-CNS sites. Further prospective investigation is required to fully integrate these modalities into the routine management of metastatic RCC.

■ REFERENCES

1. Oliver RT, Nethersell AB, Bottomley JM. Unexplained spontaneous regression and alpha-interferon as treatment for metastatic renal carcinoma. *Br J Urol* 1989;63(2):128–131.

2. Ratain MJ, Eisen T, Stadler WM, et al. Phase II placebo-controlled randomized discontinuation trial of sorafenib in patients with metastatic renal cell carcinoma. *J Clin Oncol* 2006;24(16):2505–2512.

3. Murthy SC, Kim K, Rice TW, et al. Can we predict long-term survival after pulmonary metastasectomy for renal cell carcinoma? *Ann Thorac Surg* 2005;79(3):996–1003.

4. Pfannschmidt J, Hoffmann H, Muley T, Krysa S, Trainer C, Dienemann H. Prognostic factors for survival after pulmonary resection of metastatic renal cell carcinoma. *Ann Thorac Surg* 2002;74(5):1653–1657.

5. Svedman C, Sandström P, Pisa P, et al. A prospective Phase II trial of using extracranial stereotactic radiotherapy in primary and metastatic renal cell carcinoma. *Acta Oncol* 2006;45(7):870–875.

6. Cannady SB, Cavanaugh KA, Lee SY, et al. Results of whole brain radiotherapy and recursive partitioning analysis in patients with brain metastases from renal cell carcinoma: a retrospective study. *Int J Radiat Oncol Biol Phys* 2004;58(1):253–258.

7. Sundaresan N, Scher H, DiGiacinto GV, Yagoda A, Whitmore W, Choi IS. Surgical treatment of spinal cord compression in kidney cancer. *J Clin Oncol* 1986;4(12):1851–1856.

8. Reichel LM, Pohar S, Heiner J, Buzaianu EM, Damron TA. Radiotherapy to bone has utility in

multifocal metastatic renal carcinoma. *Clin Orthop Relat Res* 2007;459:133–138.

9. Rades D, Freundt K, Meyners T, et al. Dose Escalation for Metastatic Spinal Cord Compression in Patients with Relatively Radioresistant Tumors. *Int J Radiat Oncol Biol Phys.* 2010 Jun 23. [Epub ahead of print]

10. Bowers TA, Murray JA, Charnsangavej C, Soo CS, Chuang VP, Wallace S. Bone metastases from renal carcinoma. The preoperative use of transcatheter arterial occlusion. *J Bone Joint Surg Am* 1982;64(5):749–754.

11. Broaddus WC, Grady MS, Delashaw JB Jr, Ferguson RD, Jane JA. Preoperative superselective arteriolar embolization: a new approach to enhance resectability of spinal tumors. *Neurosurgery* 1990;27(5):755–759.

12. King GJ, Kostuik JP, McBroom RJ, Richardson W. Surgical management of metastatic renal carcinoma of the spine. *Spine* 1991;16(3):265–271.

13. Ulmar B, Catalkaya S, Naumann U, et al. [Surgical treatment and evaluation of prognostic factors in spinal metastases of renal cell carcinoma]. *Z Orthop Ihre Grenzgeb* 2006;144(1):58–67.

14. Gerszten PC, Burton SA, Ozhasoglu C, et al. Stereotactic radiosurgery for spinal metastases from renal cell carcinoma. *J Neurosurg Spine* 2005;3(4):288–295.

15. Nguyen QN, Shiu AS, Rhines LD, et al. Management of spinal metastases from renal cell carcinoma using stereotactic body radiotherapy. *Int J Radiat Oncol Biol Phys* 2010;76(4):1185–1192.

16. Staehler M, Haseke N, Nuhn P, et al. Simultaneous antiangiogenic therapy and single fraction radiotherapy in RCC. *J Clin Oncol* 2010;28:15s.

17. Angelov L. Stereotactic spine radiosurgery (SRS) for pain and tumor control in patients with spinal metastases from renal cell carcinoma: a prospective study. *Int J Radiat Oncol Biol Phys* 2009;75(3):s112–s113.

18. Thiagaragan A, Yamada Y, Lovelock D, et al. Stereotactic radiosurgery: a new paradigm for melanoma and RCC metastases. *J Clin Oncol* 2010; 28:15s.

19. Soga N, Yamakado K, Gohara H, et al. Percutaneous radiofrequency ablation for unresectable pulmonary metastases from renal cell carcinoma. *BJU Int.* 2009;104(6):790–794.

20. Shu Yan Huo A, Lawson Morris D, King J, Glenn D. Use of percutaneous radiofrequency ablation in pulmonary metastases from renal cell carcinoma. *Ann Surg Oncol.* 2009;16(11):3169–3175.

21. Plimack ER, Tannir N, Lin E, Bekele BN, Jonasch E. Patterns of disease progression in metastatic renal cell carcinoma patients treated with antivascular agents and interferon: impact of therapy on recurrence patterns and outcome measures. *Cancer.* 2009;115(9):1859–1866.

22. Basappa NS, Elson P, Golshayan AR, et al. The impact of tumor burden characteristics in patients with metastatic renal cell carcinoma treated with sunitinib. *Cancer.* 2010 Oct 19. [Epub ahead of print]

23. Sheehan JP, Sun MH, Kondziolka D, Flickinger J, Lunsford LD. Radiosurgery in patients with renal cell carcinoma metastasis to the brain: long-term outcomes and prognostic factors influencing survival and local tumor control. *J Neurosurg.* 2003;98(2):342–349.

24. Decker DA, Decker VL, Herskovic A, Cummings GD. Brain metastases in patients with renal cell carcinoma: prognosis and treatment. *J Clin Oncol.* 1984;2(3):169–173.

25. Gaspar L, Scott C, Rotman M, et al. Recursive partitioning analysis (RPA) of prognostic factors in three Radiation Therapy Oncology Group (RTOG) brain metastases trials. *Int J Radiat Oncol Biol Phys.* 1997;37(4):745–751.

26. Gaspar LE, Scott C, Murray K, Curran W. Validation of the RTOG recursive partitioning analysis (RPA) classification for brain metastases. *Int J Radiat Oncol Biol Phys.* 2000;47(4):1001–1006.

27. Lagerwaard FJ, Levendag PC, Nowak PJ, Eijkenboom WM, Hanssens PE, Schmitz PI. Identification of prognostic factors in patients with brain metastases: a review of 1292 patients. *Int J Radiat Oncol Biol Phys.* 1999;43(4):795–803.

28. Lorenzoni J, Devriendt D, Massager N, et al. Radiosurgery for treatment of brain metastases: estimation of patient eligibility using three stratification systems. *Int J Radiat Oncol Biol Phys.* 2004;60(1):218–224.

29. Rades D, Dunst J, Schild SE. A new scoring system to predicting the survival of patients treated with whole-brain radiotherapy for brain metastases. *Strahlenther Onkol.* 2008;184(5):251–255.

30. Sperduto PW, Berkey B, Gaspar LE, Mehta M, Curran W. A new prognostic index and comparison to three other indices for patients with brain metastases: an analysis of 1,960 patients in the RTOG database. *Int J Radiat Oncol Biol Phys.* 2008;70(2):510–514.

31. Weltman E, Salvajoli JV, Brandt RA, et al. Radiosurgery for brain metastases: a score index for predicting prognosis. *Int J Radiat Oncol Biol Phys.* 2000;46(5):1155–1161.

32. Beitler JJ, Makara D, Silverman P, Lederman G. Definitive, high-dose-per-fraction, conformal,

stereotactic external radiation for renal cell carcinoma. *Am J Clin Oncol*. 2004;27(6):646–648.

33. Epstein BE, Scott CB, Sause WT, et al. Improved survival duration in patients with unresected solitary brain metastasis using accelerated hyperfractionated radiation therapy at total doses of 54.4 gray and greater. Results of Radiation Therapy Oncology Group 85–28. *Cancer*. 1993;71(4):1362–1367.

34. O'dea MJ, Zincke H, Utz DC, Bernatz PE. The treatment of renal cell carcinoma with solitary metastasis. *J Urol*. 1978;120(5):540–542.

35. Salvati M, Scarpinati M, Orlando ER, Celli P, Gagliardi FM. Single brain metastases from kidney tumors. Clinico-pathologic considerations on a series of 29 cases. *Tumori*. 1992;78(6):392–394.

36. Wronski M, Arbit E, Russo P, Galicich JH. Surgical resection of brain metastases from renal cell carcinoma in 50 patients. *Urology*. 1996;47(2):187–193.

37. Patchell RA, Tibbs PA, Regine WF, et al. Postoperative radiotherapy in the treatment of single metastases to the brain: a randomized trial. *JAMA*. 1998;280(17):1485–1489.

38. Doh LS, Amato RJ, Paulino AC, Teh BS. Radiation therapy in the management of brain metastases from renal cell carcinoma. *Oncology (Williston Park, NY)*. 2006;20(6):603–13; discussion 613, 616, 619.

39. Chang EL, Selek U, Hassenbusch SJ 3rd, et al. Outcome variation among "radioresistant" brain metastases treated with stereotactic radiosurgery. *Neurosurgery*. 2005;56(5):936–45; discussion 936.

40. Hoshi S, Jokura H, Nakamura H, et al. Gamma-knife radiosurgery for brain metastasis of renal cell carcinoma: results in 42 patients. *Int J Urol*. 2002;9(11):618–25; discussion 626; author reply 627.

41. Manon R, O'Neill A, Knisely J, et al.; Eastern Cooperative Oncology Group. Phase II trial of radiosurgery for one to three newly diagnosed brain metastases from renal cell carcinoma, melanoma, and sarcoma: an Eastern Cooperative Oncology Group study (E 6397). *J Clin Oncol*. 2005;23(34):8870–8876.

42. Petrovich Z, Yu C, Giannotta SL, O'Day S, Apuzzo ML. Survival and pattern of failure in brain metastasis treated with stereotactic gamma knife radiosurgery. *J Neurosurg*. 2002;97(5 Suppl):499–506.

43. Schöggl A, Kitz K, Ertl A, Dieckmann K, Saringer W, Koos WT. Gamma-knife radiosurgery for brain metastases of renal cell carcinoma: results in 23 patients. *Acta Neurochir (Wien)*. 1998;140(6):549–555.

44. Shuto T, Inomori S, Fujino H, Nagano H. Gamma knife surgery for metastatic brain tumors from renal cell carcinoma. *J Neurosurg*. 2006;105(4):555–560.

45. Hernandez L, Zamorano L, Sloan A, et al. Gamma knife radiosurgery for renal cell carcinoma brain metastases. *J Neurosurg*. 2002;97(5 Suppl):489–493.

46. Muacevic A, Kreth FW, Mack A, Tonn JC, Wowra B. Stereotactic radiosurgery without radiation therapy providing high local tumor control of multiple brain metastases from renal cell carcinoma. *Minim Invasive Neurosurg*. 2004;47(4):203–208.

47. Mori Y, Kondziolka D, Flickinger JC, Logan T, Lunsford LD. Stereotactic radiosurgery for brain metastasis from renal cell carcinoma. *Cancer*. 1998; 83(2):344–353.

48. Noel G, Valery CA, Boisserie G, et al. LINAC radiosurgery for brain metastasis of renal cell carcinoma. *Urol Oncol*. 2004;22(1):25–31.

49. Flickinger JC. Radiosurgery of brain metastases from renal cell carcinoma: how can you improve on results like this? *Cancer J*. 2000;6(6):360–361.

50. Goyal LK, Suh JH, Reddy CA, Barnett GH. The role of whole brain radiotherapy and stereotactic radiosurgery on brain metastases from renal cell carcinoma. *Int J Radiat Oncol Biol Phys*. 2000;47(4):1007–1012.

51. Kondziolka D, Patel A, Lunsford LD, Kassam A, Flickinger JC. Stereotactic radiosurgery plus whole brain radiotherapy versus radiotherapy alone for patients with multiple brain metastases. *Int J Radiat Oncol Biol Phys*. 1999;45(2):427–434.

52. Seaman EK, Ross S, Sawczuk IS. High incidence of asymptomatic brain lesions in metastatic renal cell carcinoma. *J Neurooncol*. 1995;23(3):253–256.

53. Marko NF, Angelov L, Toms SA, et al. Stereotactic radiosurgery as single-modality treatment of incidentally identified renal cell carcinoma brain metastases. *World Neurosurg*. 2010;73(3):186–93; discussion e29.

54. Gore ME, Hariharan S, Porta C, et al. Sunitinib in metastatic renal cell carcinoma patients with brain metastases. *Cancer*. 2011;117(3):501–509

55. Zeng H, Li X, Yao J, et al. Multifocal brain metastases in clear cell renal cell carcinoma with complete response to sunitinib. *Urol Int*. 2009;83(4):482–485.

56. Valcamonico F, Ferrari V, Amoroso V, et al. Long-lasting successful cerebral response with sorafenib in advanced renal cell carcinoma. *J Neurooncol*. 2009;91(1):47–50.

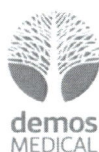

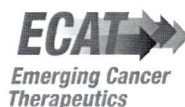

IL-2 and Other Immunotherapy in Renal Cancer

Jacalyn Rosenblatt and David F. McDermott

*Beth Israel Deaconess Medical Center, Harvard Medical School,
Dana-Farber/Harvard Cancer Center, Boston, MA*

■ ABSTRACT

The ability of some renal tumors to evoke an immune response and the lack of benefit seen with standard chemotherapy and radiation led to the application of immunotherapy for patients with metastatic renal carcinoma (1,2). In an attempt to reproduce or accentuate this response, various immunotherapeutic strategies have been used, including adoptive immunotherapy, the induction of a graft-versus-tumor response via allogeneic hematopoietic stem cell transplantation, and the administration of partially purified or recombinant cytokines (3–7). Although a number of cytokines have shown antitumor activity in renal carcinoma, the most consistent results have been reported with interleukin-2 (IL-2). In contrast to the results seen with molecularly targeted therapies (e.g., sunitinib), the administration of high-dose bolus IL-2 (HD IL-2) has consistently produced durable responses, including complete responses, in a small percentage of patients with advanced renal cell cancer (8). However, the substantial toxicity and limited efficacy that is associated with HD IL-2 limits its application to highly selected patients treated at specialized centers (9). HD IL-2's use, though once the standard of care, has decreased with the advent of novel therapies that target angiogenesis and signal transduction pathways, producing significant clinical benefits; this development prompted a reassessment of the role of immunotherapy for metastatic renal carcinoma (10–13). Recent insights into how the immune response to a tumor is regulated may allow patients to obtain a durable response to immunotherapy without the significant toxicity associated with conventional approaches. This review describes how improvements in patient

*Corresponding author, Beth Israel Deaconess Medical Center, 375 Longwood Ave, MS-428, Boston, MA 02215
E-mail address: dmcdermo@bidmc.harvard.edu

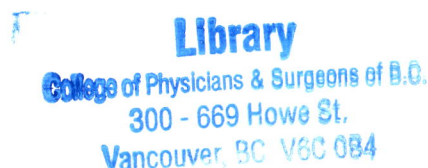

Emerging Cancer Therapeutics 2:1 (2011) 101–114.
© 2011 Demos Medical Publishing LLC. All rights reserved.
DOI: 10.5003/2151-4194.2.1.101

demosmedpub.com/ecat

selection, combination therapy, and investigational agents might expand and better define the role of IL-2 in metastatic renal carcinoma.

Keywords: renal cell carcinoma, PD-1 blockade, immunotherapy

■ CYTOKINE THERAPY

Although a number of cytokines have shown antitumor activity in renal carcinoma, the most consistent results have been reported with interleukin-2 (IL-2) and interferon alpha (IFN-α). In contrast to the results seen with molecularly targeted therapies (e.g., sorafenib, sunitinib), which lead to tumor shrinkage in most treated patients but do not produce remissions of cancer when therapy is discontinued, the administration of high-dose bolus IL-2 has consistently produced durable and even complete responses in a small percentage of patients with advanced renal carcinoma (8,14,15). However, the substantial toxicity and limited efficacy that are associated with IL-2 have narrowed its application to highly selected patients treated at specialized centers (9,16). Although IFN-α has produced modest benefits in unselected patients, randomized clinical trials have revealed a small survival benefit with manageable toxic effects when compared with non–IFN-α control arms (17–23). As it became the de facto standard of care worldwide, regulatory agencies have supported the use of IFN-α as the control arm for randomized trials with targeted therapies that are described elsewhere in this issue (10–13). The results of these investigations have, in general, established the superiority of targeted agents in previously untreated patients, thereby narrowing the future use of IFN-α as a single agent in this setting.

In recent years, the relative merits of these low- and high-dose cytokine regimens have been clarified by the results of four randomized trials (Table 1) (24–27). In the most consequential trial, the French Immunotherapy Group randomized patients with an intermediate likelihood of response to IL-2 and IFN-α to receive medroxyprogesterone (control group), subcutaneous IFN-α, subcutaneous IL-2, or the combination of IFN-α and IL-2 (27). Although significant toxicity

was more common in the IL-2 and IFN-α arm, median overall survival did not differ between the arms. The investigators concluded that subcutaneous IFN-α and IL-2 should no longer be recommended in patients with metastatic renal cell carcinoma and intermediate prognosis.

Taken together, these studies suggest that high-dose intravenous (IV) bolus IL-2 is superior in terms of response rate and possibly response quality to regimens that involve low-dose IL-2 and IFN-α, intermediate- or low-dose IL-2 alone, or low-dose IFN-α alone. Consequently, although low-dose single cytokine therapy has a limited role in patients with metastatic renal carcinoma, high-dose IV IL-2 remains a reasonable option for appropriately selected patients with access to such therapy. More significantly, correlative biomarker investigations associated with these trials suggest that the potential exists for identifying predictors of response (or resistance) and limiting IL-2 therapy to those most likely to benefit.

■ PATHOLOGIC AND MOLECULAR PREDICTORS OF RESPONSE TO IL-2

Influence of Histologic Subtype

Responses to immunotherapy are most frequently seen in patients with clear cell renal carcinoma (28–30). This observation was detailed in a retrospective analysis of pathology specimens obtained from 231 patients (163 primary and 68 metastatic tumor specimens), who had received IL-2 therapy in Cytokine Working Group (CWG) clinical trials (30). For patients with primary tumor specimens available for review, the response rate to IL-2 was 21% (30 of 146 patients) in the case of clear cell histologic primary tumors, compared to the 6% response rate in the case of non–clear cell histologic tumors (1 responder in 17 patients). Among the patients with clear cell carcinoma, response to IL-2

TABLE 1 Select randomized trials of cytokine therapy in metastatic renal cell cancer

Trial	Treatment Regimens	N	Response Rate (%)	Durable Complete Response (%)	Overall Survival (months)[a]
French Immunotherapy Group (32)	CIV IL-2	138	6.5	1	12
	LD SC IFN-α	147	7.5	2	13
	CIV IL-2 + IFN-α	140	18.6	5	17
	MPA	123	2.5	1	14.9
French Immunotherapy Group (35)	LD SC IFN-α	122	4.4	3	15.2
	LD SC IL-2	125	4.1	0	15.3
	SC IL-2 + IFN	122	10.9	0	16.8
National Cancer Institute Surgery Branch (33)	HD IV IL-2	156	21	8	NR
	LD IV IL-2	150	13	3	NR
	HD IV IL-2	95	23	7	17.5
Cytokine Working Group (34)	LD SC IL-2/IFN-α	91	10	0	13
	HD IV IL-2	95	23	7	17.5

CIV, continuous IV infusion; CR, complete response; HD, high dose; IFN-α, interferon alpha; IL-2, interleukin 2; IV, intravenous; LD, low dose; MPA, medroxyprogesterone acetate; NR, not reported; RR, response rate; SC, subcutaneous.

[a]The overall survival difference was not statistically significant in all cases.

was also associated with the presence of good predictive features (e.g., more than 50% alveolar and no granular or papillary features) and the absence of poor predictive features (e.g., more than 50% granular or any papillary features). As a result of these data, it may be appropriate for patients whose primary tumor is of non–clear cell histologic type or of clear cell histologic type but with poor predictive features to forgo IL-2–based treatment altogether.

Immunohistochemical Markers

Carbonic anhydrase IX (CAIX) has been identified as an immunohistochemical marker that might predict the outcomes of patients with renal carcinoma. In an analysis by Bui et al., CAIX expression in more than 85% of tumor cells (high CAIX expression) has been associated with improved survival and a higher objective response rate in IL-2–treated patients (31). Building on this work, Atkins et al. developed a two-component model that combined pathology analysis and immunohistochemical staining for CAIX (32). In a retrospective analysis, this model was able to identify a good-risk group that contained 26 (96%) of 27 responders to IL-2 compared with only 18 (46%) of 39 nonresponders (odds ratio, 30; $P < 0.01$). A significant survival benefit was also seen for this group ($P < 0.01$).

Molecular Markers

Through gene expression profiling of tumor specimens, Pantuck et al. were able to identify a set of 73 genes whose expression distinguished complete responders from nonresponders after IL-2 therapy (33). In their hands, complete responders to IL-2 have a signature gene and protein expression pattern that includes CAIX, PTEN, and CXCR4. A similar analysis identified loss of chromosome 4, 9, and 17p as possible predictors of IL-2 nonresponse (34). Further investigation into these regions may improve our understanding of the molecular basis of an effective immune response in renal carcinoma. Although this approach requires prospective validation, it may become a powerful aid for clinicians in selecting appropriate treatment options.

CURRENT INVESTIGATION IN PATIENT SELECTION

The CWG conducted the high-dose IL-2 "Select" trial to determine, in a prospective fashion, if the predictive model proposed by Atkins et al. can identify a group of patients with advanced renal carcinoma who are significantly more likely to respond to high-dose IL-2–based therapy (good risk) than a historical, unselected patient population (32). The preliminary clinical results of this trial revealed a response rate (28%) that was significantly higher than the historical experience with high-dose IL-2 (35). Analysis of tumor (central pathology review and staining for CAIX) and blood-based predictive markers is going to further improve the selection criteria for IL-2 and limit its application to those patients most likely to benefit. As the list of effective therapies for metastatic renal carcinoma grows, improvements in patient selection will be necessary to ensure that patients who might attain a durable remission with IL-2 will not miss this opportunity.

IL-2 THERAPY AFTER VEGF PATHWAY–DIRECTED THERAPY

The emergence of molecularly targeted therapies has offered hope for improved clinical outcome for patients with renal carcinoma. Vascular endothelial growth factor (VEGF) pathway–directed therapy

has been recommended for frontline use with other treatments reserved for time of disease progression. However, a retrospective analysis suggests that the toxicity of IL-2 therapy may be higher in patients who have received prior VEGF-targeted therapy, particularly sunitinib, and antitumor activity may be diminished (36). Although the mechanism for the observed increased incidence of cardiovascular complications remains speculative, the assumption that IL-2 can be given safely after VEGF pathway–targeted therapy may not be valid.

COMBINATION OF IMMUNOTHERAPY AND TARGETED/ ANTIANGIOGENIC THERAPY

Although the role of low-dose single-agent cytokines is limited, combinations of cytokines with targeted therapy may have merit. Bevacizumab and IL-2 have been combined in a CWG trial. Preliminary results suggest that these two agents can be given safely in combination and produce efficacy improvements that are additive but not synergistic (37). Two recently completed large phase 3 trials of interferon plus bevacizumab versus interferon alone have demonstrated superior efficacy with the combination regimen compared with cytokine monotherapy and suggest the potential of an additive effect (13,38). Confirmation of the benefit of combination therapy will require a randomized trial comparing the combination to bevacizumab alone.

INVESTIGATIONAL IMMUNOTHERAPY

Metastatic renal carcinoma has long been a testing ground for novel immunotherapies. Several such approaches, including vaccination and allogeneic bone marrow transplant, have been tested over the past two decades. Allogeneic bone marrow transplant attempts to induce a graft-versus-tumor effect in the patient through transfer of sibling bone marrow stem cells. The initial reports of applying allogeneic bone marrow transplantation in renal carcinoma were encouraging, but further clinical trials have highlighted the potential toxicity and limited applicability of this approach (6,39,40).

An improved understanding of the molecular mechanisms that govern the interaction between a tumor and host immune response has provided insight into why immunotherapies too often fail to achieve satisfactory results. In renal carcinoma, obstacles to effective immunotherapy likely include the physiological down-modulation of the immune response through the increased expression of molecules such as *cytotoxic T-lymphocyte antigen 4* (CTLA4) on the surface of activated T cells and proliferation of regulatory (CD4+ CD25+) T cells (T-regs) in response to nonspecific cytokine administration (41–45). These insights have encouraged investigators to pursue agents that block T-cell regulation (e.g., programmed death 1 [PD-1] and CTLA-4 antibodies), inhibit tumor-induced immunosuppression (e.g., transforming growth factor beta [TGF-β] antibody, programmed death ligand 1 [PD-L1] antibody), and more specifically activate T-cells (e.g., CD137

antibody, IL-21) and dendritic cells (e.g., toll-like receptor agonists) (Table 2) (46–51). Several of these agents have shown encouraging efficacy in early trials. These targeted immunotherapies may allow patients to obtain a durable response to immunotherapy without the significant toxicity associated with HD IL-2.

In a single-institution phase 2 trial, the CTLA-4 antibody ipilimumab produced major tumor regressions but also significant toxicities in patients with metastatic renal carcinoma who had failed prior immunotherapy (47). Toxicities associated with CTLA-4 antibodies, including enteritis, skin rash, and hypophysitis, have occasionally been life threatening and have also been associated with tumor response. Combination of cytokines and agents that block immune down-regulation may prove particularly effective in select patients. A recent report of high-dose IL-2 and ipilimumab (CTLA4 antibody) in patients with metastatic melanoma revealed manageable toxicity with a complete response rate of 17% suggesting a potential role for this combination in renal carcinoma patients (52). However, the development

TABLE 2 Investigational immunotherapeutic approaches to the treatment of renal carcinoma

Target	Drug	Class	Development Phase
Blockade of T-cell regulation			
PD-1 antibody (46)	MDX-1106	Fully human mAb	Phase 1
CTLA-4 antibody (47)	Ipilimumab	Fully human IgG1 mAb	Phase 3 (melanoma)
Inhibition of tumor-induced T-cell function			
TGF-β (48)	GC1008	Fully human mAb	Phase 1
TGF-β2	AP12009	Fully human mAb	Phase 1
T-cell activation			
CD137 (49)	BMS-663513	mAb	Phase 1
Cytokines (50)	Interleukin-21	Recombinant molecule	Phase 2 (melanoma)
Dendritic cell activation			
Toll-like receptor (51)	HYB2055	TLR9 agonist	Phase 2

Mrenal carcinoma, metastatic renal cell carcinoma; PD-1, programmed death-1; mAb, monoclonal antibodies; IgG1, immunoglobulin 1; TGF-β, tumor growth factor beta; TLR9, toll-like receptor 9.

of targeted immunotherapy for renal carcinoma is complicated by the increasing array of other treatment options and their potential impact on the immune system.

One of the most critical pathways responsible for tumor-induced immune suppression in renal carcinoma is the interaction between B7–1, otherwise known as PD-1, and its ligand B7-H1 (PD-L1) interaction, which serves to restrict the cytolytic function of tumor-infiltrating T lymphocytes. Renal tumors that express B7-H1 have been shown to behave more aggressively, which leads to a shorter survival (Figure 1) (53). Blocking the receptor (PD-1)/ligand (PD-L1) interaction with monoclonal antibodies (e.g., PD-1 antibody MDX-1106, PD-L1 antibody MDX–1105), may facilitate immunotherapy and represents one of the most promising therapeutic strategies being studied in patients with renal carcinoma. These agents have recently completed phase 1 testing (46).

■ PD-1/PD-L1 BIOLOGY

The PD-1/PD-L1 pathway is an important inhibitory pathway that regulates T-cell activation and mediates T-cell tolerance (Figure 2) (54). The PD-1 receptor is expressed on T cells, B cells, monocytes, and natural killer T cells, following activation. PD-L1 (B7-H1) and PD-L2 (B7-dendritic cell), the two ligands for PD-1, are expressed on antigen presenting cells, including dendritic cells and macrophages. In addition, PD-L1 is expressed on nonhematopoietic cells, including pancreatic islet cells, endothelial cells, and epithelial cells, and they play a role in protecting tissue from immune mediated injury (55). Binding of PD-1 to PD-L1 or PD-L2 inhibits T-cell proliferation, decreases secretion of Th1 cytokines, and results in T-cell apoptosis (55,56).

The critical role that PD-1 plays in blunting activated T-cell responses was first demonstrated by the autoimmune phenotypes that develop in

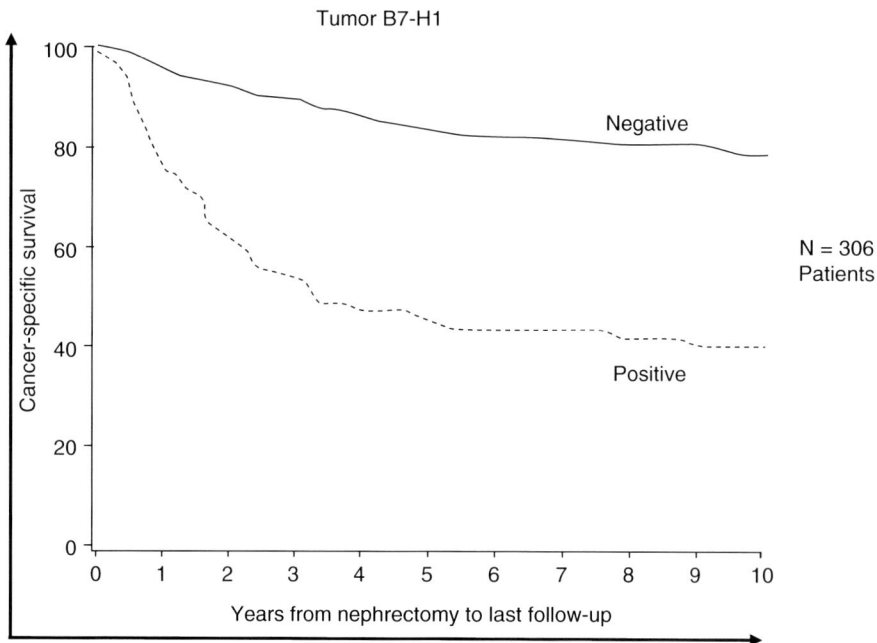

FIGURE 1
Increased PD-L1 (B7-H1) expression in renal cell carcinoma diminishes survival.

PD-1 knockout mice, including cardiomyopathy, diabetes, glomerulonephritis, and arthritis (54,57–60). In a non-obese diabetic mouse model, it has been shown that pancreatic islet cells express PD-L1 and that PD-1 blockade results in exacerbation of diabetes (55,61,62). Similarly, it has been shown in models of experimental autoimmune encephalitis that PD-1 blockade exacerbates disease and increases inflammatory infiltrates in the central nervous system (63,64). In addition, PD-L1 expression on nonhematopoeitic cells, including renal tubular epithelial cells, inhibits immune-mediated tissue damage, which indicates that the PD-1/PD-L1 pathway is a critical mediator of tissue tolerance (55,61,65,66).

The PD-1/PD-L1 pathway plays an important role in modulating immune response to infection.

T-cell expression of PD-1 is upregulated during chronic viral infection, which results in an "exhausted" T-cell phenotype. The lymphocytic choriomeningitis virus (LCMV) model was the first to demonstrate the impact of the PD-1/PD-L1 pathway in limiting clearance of virally infected cells (55,67). Barber et al. (67) demonstrate that PD-1 expression is upregulated in mice chronically infected with LCMV, and that PD-1 blockade enhanced the clearance of virus. Similarly, it has been shown in models of chronic HIV, hepatitis C, and hepatitis B that T cells upregulate expression of PD-1 and that PD-1 blockade restores T-cell proliferative capacity and effector function (55,68–72). In patients with hepatitis C, it has been shown that PD-1 is upregulated on T cells during acute infection, remains high in patients who

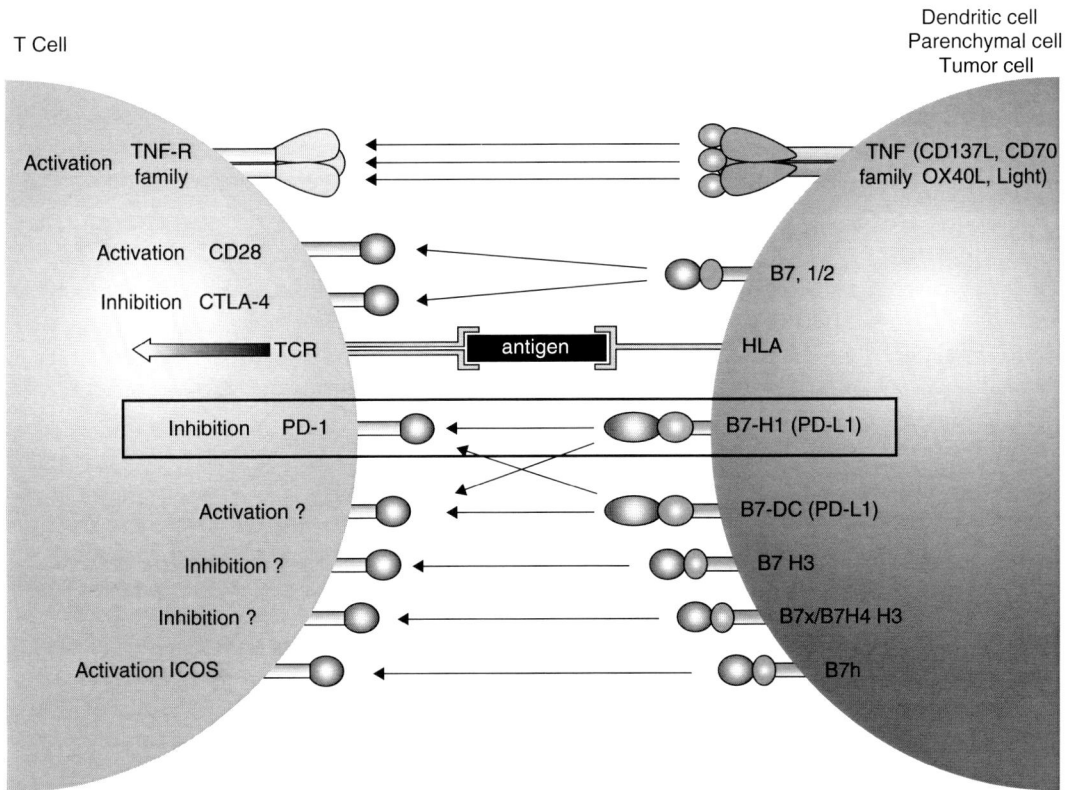

FIGURE 2
T-cell regulatory pathways.

develop chronic infection, and declines in patients who effectively clear the virus (70). Similarly, in HIV patients, PD-1 expression on CD8+ T cells correlates with viral load and declines following antiretroviral therapy (68).

■ PD-1 AND TUMOR IMMUNITY

There has been increasing interest in exploring the contribution of the PD-1/PD-L1 pathway to tumor evasion of host immunity. Tumor cells secrete inhibitory cytokines, including TGF-β and IL-10, which creates an immunosuppressive milieu and limits effective anti-tumor immunity.

Recent studies suggest that tumor expression of PD-L1 may play an important role in contributing to tumor-mediated immunosuppression. A variety of tumors have been shown to express PD-L1, including renal, melanoma, stomach, breast, and lung carcinoma (53,73–83). In addition, PD-LI expression on tumor cells has been shown to correlate with a poor prognosis not only in renal carcinoma but also in breast, pancreatic, stomach, and ovarian cancer (53,77,79–83).

In a murine model, it was shown that transgenic expression of PD-L1 rendered a mastocytoma cell line less susceptible to cytotoxic T-lymphocytes–mediated killing and enhanced their tumorigenicity in vivo. These effects were reversed in the presence of PD-1 blockade (84). Likewise, Dong et al (76) showed that tumor expression of PD-L1 enhanced T-cell apoptosis both in vitro and in vivo. Recently, Ahmadzadeh and colleagues (85) demonstrated in a melanoma model that PD-1 expression on tumor-infiltrating lymphocytes (TIL) is significantly higher than on a T cell isolated from the peripheral blood or normal tissue of the same individuals. In this study, PD-1+ TIL were shown to have impaired effector function, as measured by interferon γ secretion, which suggests that PD-1 expression on TILs limits their capacity to mount an effective immune response. Blank et al. (60) also showed higher levels of PD-1 expression on TIL than on peripheral blood lymphocytes

isolated from melanoma patients. In addition, PD-1 blockade increased interferon γ secretion by T-cell populations in response to stimulation by antigen-loaded dendritic cells. In a murine model of chronic myelogenous leukemia (CML), leukemia-specific cytotoxic T lymphocytes were shown to express high levels of PD-1 and were functionally exhausted. PD-L1 blockade was shown to restore the function of CML-specific cytotoxic T lymphocytes and prolong survival (86). The effect of PD-1 blockade on enhancing activated antitumor T-cell responses makes it an ideal therapeutic target to study in the setting of malignancy.

PD-L1 expression on renal cell carcinoma may play a significant role in promoting T-cell tolerance by binding PD-1 on activated T cells and suppressing their capacity to secrete stimulatory cytokines. Inhibition of this pathway may significantly augment the capacity of tumor-reactive T cells to eliminate tumor cells. Monoclonal antibodies that target the PD-1/PD-L1 interaction are being evaluated in clinical studies and hold promise as an important immunotherapeutic approach in renal carcinoma.

■ MDX-1106 IN PHASE 1 TRIALS

Brahmer et al. (46) reported the first in human phase 1/2 trial of MDX-1106 (ONO-4538), a fully human IgG4 anti-PD-1 blocking antibody, in patients with selected refractory or relapsed malignancies. This single-dose trial established the maximum tolerance of MDX-1106 at 10 mg/kg without evidence of serious toxicity (arthritic symptoms: 2 patients; thyroid-stimulating hormone elevation: 1 patient). Flow cytometric analysis showed sustained occupancy of the majority of PD-1 molecules on patient T cells for at least 3 months following a single dose. In a dose-expansion cohort at the MTD, patients with stable disease or better were able to receive repeat doses of MDX-1106. Tumor responses were seen in melanoma and renal carcinoma without increased toxicity. One patient with renal carcinoma, who had received several prior therapies, achieved a partial remission that has lasted more than 18 months despite having received only three MDX-1106 infusions. This small efficacy signal prompted investigators to include a larger cohort of renal carcinoma patients in a subsequent biweekly MDX-1106 trial that reported results at the American Society of Clinical Oncology meeting in June 2010 (87). In the cohort of patients with renal carcinoma, 5 of 16 patients experienced major tumor responses that have remained durable for 8 to 17+ months.

■ VACCINATION + IMMUNE CHECKPOINT BLOCKADE

Metastatic renal carcinoma has long been a testing ground for novel immunotherapies. Vaccination therapy has demonstrated potentially relevant immune responses, although clinical benefit and objective responses have not been consistently observed (88–90). Avigan et al. (88) conducted a series of clinical trials with a dendritic cell/tumor fusion vaccine approach that have shown encouraging clinical responses in patients with a variety of malignancies including renal carcinoma. To realize the full potential of a vaccine approach in renal carcinoma, combinations with immune stimulants (e.g., granulocyte macrophage colony-stimulating factor) and inhibitors of natural T-cell regulation pathways (e.g., CTLA4 blockade, T reg depletion) may be necessary.

The PD-1/PD-L1 pathway may play an important role in blunting immune response to tumor vaccines. PD-1 is upregulated on T-cell populations in response to antigenic and nonantigenic stimulation. Study findings suggest that stimulation with DC/tumor fusion cells results in increased T-cell expression of PD-1, which potentially blunts response to vaccination (91). In preclinical studies, stimulation of T cells with a dendritic cell/tumor fusion vaccine in the presence of PD-1 blockade results in an increase in Th1 cytokines, a decrease in regulatory T cells, and enhanced tumor killing (91). As such, combining

dendritic cell-based tumor vaccines with PD-1 blockade may be an effective means of enhancing immunological and clinical response to vaccination. A clinical trial is planned in which patients with metastatic renal carcinoma will be treated with dendritic cell/tumor fusion vaccination in conjunction with PD-1 blockade following debulking nephrectomy.

■ CONCLUSIONS

Renal carcinoma has long been considered an immunologically influenced malignancy and thus served as a platform for the clinical testing of anticancer immunotherapy. The nonspecific cytokines, IL-2 and IFN-α, have undergone the most testing and produced only modest benefits for unselected patients. High-dose IL-2 remains the only approach to produce durable responses in patients with metastatic renal carcinoma and can thus be considered in appropriately selected patients. For patients unlikely to benefit from, unable to receive, or who progress after IL-2, the emergence of molecularly targeted therapies offers hope for improved clinical outcome (15–18). Additional molecular and pathologic selection opportunities exist for cytokines but considerable validation work is needed before these selection features can be used clinically. Cytokine therapy optimally should be given in the context of a clinical trial investigating combination therapy and/or patient selection to maximize the benefit of this approach. Targeted immunotherapeutic strategies have been tested in metastatic renal carcinoma but definitive evidence of clinical benefit is only emerging.

In recent years, the list of effective therapies (e.g., angiogenesis inhibition, signal transduction inhibition, and immunotherapy) for metastatic renal carcinoma has increased substantially. The advent of targeted therapy in renal carcinoma does not eliminate the potential utility of immunotherapy in renal carcinoma but rather requires a rational refinement of this therapy through patient selection, combination regimens, and novel agents that together may extend overall survival and increase the cure rate for patients with this disease.

■ ACKNOWLEDGMENT

This study was supported in part by the DF/HCC Renal Cancer SPORE: P50 CA101942–01.

■ REFERENCES

1. Gleave ME, Elhilali M, Fradet Y, et al. Interferon gamma-1b compared with placebo in metastatic renal-cell carcinoma. Canadian Urologic Oncology Group. *N Engl J Med* 1998;338(18):1265–1271.
2. Vogelzang NJ, Priest ER, Borden L. Spontaneous regression of histologically proved pulmonary metastases from renal cell carcinoma: a case with 5-year follow up. *J Urol* 1992;148(4):1247–1248.
3. Chang AE, Li Q, Jiang G, Sayre DM, Braun TM, Redman BG. Phase II trial of autologous tumor vaccination, anti-CD3-activated vaccine-primed lymphocytes, and interleukin-2 in stage IV renal cell cancer. *J Clin Oncol* 2003;21(5):884–890.
4. Lesimple T, Moisan A, Guillé F, et al. Treatment of metastatic renal cell carcinoma with activated autologous macrophages and granulocyte–macrophage colony-stimulating factor. *J Immunother* 2000;23(6):675–679.
5. Schwaab T, Heaney JA, Schned AR, et al. A randomized phase II trial comparing two different sequence combinations of autologous vaccine and human recombinant interferon gamma and human recombinant interferon alpha2B therapy in patients with metastatic renal cell carcinoma: clinical outcome and analysis of immunological parameters. *J Urol* 2000;163(4):1322–1327.
6. Childs R, Chernoff A, Contentin N, et al. Regression of metastatic renal-cell carcinoma after nonmyeloablative allogeneic peripheral-blood stem-cell transplantation. *N Engl J Med* 2000;343(11):750–758.
7. Rosenberg SA, Mulé JJ, Spiess PJ, Reichert CM, Schwarz SL. Regression of established pulmonary metastases and subcutaneous tumor mediated by the systemic administration of high-dose recombinant interleukin 2. *J Exp Med* 1985;161(5):1169–1188.
8. Fisher RI, Rosenberg SA, Fyfe G. Long-term survival update for high-dose recombinant interleukin-2 in patients with renal cell carcinoma. *Cancer J Sci Am* 2000;6(suppl 1):S55–S57.
9. Margolin KA, Rayner AA, Hawkins MJ, et al. Interleukin-2 and lymphokine-activated killer cell therapy of solid tumors: analysis of toxicity and management guidelines. *J Clin Oncol* 1989;7(4):486–498.
10. Escudier B, Eisen T, Stadler WM, et al. Sorafenib in advanced clear-cell renal-cell carcinoma. *N Engl J Med* 2007;356(2):125–134.
11. Motzer RJ, Hutson TE, Tomczak P, et al. Sunitinib versus interferon alfa in metastatic renal-cell carcinoma. *N Engl J Med* 2007;356(2):115–124.
12. Hudes G, Carducci M, Tomczak P, et al. Temsirolimus, interferon alfa, or both for advanced renal-cell carcinoma. *N Engl J Med* 2007;356(22):2271–2281.
13. Escudier B, Pluzanska A, Koralewski P, et al. Bevacizumab plus interferon alfa-2a for treatment of metastatic renal cell carcinoma: a randomised, double-blind phase III trial. *Lancet* 2007;370(9605):2103–2111.
14. Fyfe G, Fisher RI, Rosenberg SA, Sznol M, Parkinson DR, Louie AC. Results of treatment of 255 patients with metastatic renal cell carcinoma who received high-dose recombinant interleukin-2 therapy. *J Clin Oncol* 1995;13(3):688–696.
15. Rosenberg SA, Yang JC, White DE, Steinberg SM. Durability of complete responses in patients with metastatic cancer treated with high-dose interleukin-2: identification of the antigens mediating response. *Ann Surg* 1998;228(3):307–319.
16. Belldegrun A, Webb DE, Austin HA 3rd, Steinberg SM, Linehan WM, Rosenberg SA. Renal toxicity of interleukin-2 administration in patients with metastatic renal cell cancer: effect of pre-therapy nephrectomy. *J Urol* 1989;141(3):499–503.
17. Neidhart JA. Interferon therapy for the treatment of renal cancer. *Cancer* 1986;57(8 suppl):1696–1699.
18. Muss HB. Interferon therapy for renal cell carcinoma. *Semin Oncol* 1987;14(2 suppl 2):36–42.
19. Muss HB, Costanzi JJ, Leavitt R, et al. Recombinant alfa interferon in renal cell carcinoma: a randomized trial of two routes of administration. *J Clin Oncol* 1987;5(2):286–291.
20. Négrier S, Caty A, Lesimple T, et al. Treatment of patients with metastatic renal carcinoma with a combination of subcutaneous interleukin-2 and interferon alfa with or without fluorouracil. Groupe Français d'Immunothérapie, Fédération Nationale

des Centres de Lutte Contre le Cancer. *J Clin Oncol* 2000;18(24):4009–4015.

21. Interferon-alpha and survival in metastatic renal carcinoma: early results of a randomised controlled trial. Medical Research Council Renal Cancer Collaborators. *Lancet* 1999;353:14–17

22. Pyrhönen S, Salminen E, Ruutu M, et al. Prospective randomized trial of interferon alfa-2a plus vinblastine versus vinblastine alone in patients with advanced renal cell cancer. *J Clin Oncol* 1999;17(9):2859–2867.

23. Coppin C, Porzsolt F, Awa A, Kumpf J, Coldman A, Wilt T. Immunotherapy for advanced renal cell cancer. *Cochrane Database Syst Rev* 2005:CD001425

24. Negrier S, Escudier B, Lasset C, et al. Recombinant human interleukin-2, recombinant human interferon alfa-2a, or both in metastatic renal-cell carcinoma. Groupe Français d'Immunothérapie. *N Engl J Med* 1998;338(18):1272–1278.

25. Yang JC, Sherry RM, Steinberg SM, et al. Randomized study of high-dose and low-dose interleukin-2 in patients with metastatic renal cancer. *J Clin Oncol* 2003;21(16):3127–3132.

26. McDermott DF, Regan MM, Clark JI, et al. Randomized phase III trial of high-dose interleukin-2 versus subcutaneous interleukin-2 and interferon in patients with metastatic renal cell carcinoma. *J Clin Oncol* 2005;23(1):133–141.

27. Negrier S, Perol D, Ravaud A, et al. Medroxyprogesterone, interferon alfa-2a, interleukin 2, or combination of both cytokines in patients with metastatic renal carcinoma of intermediate prognosis: results of a randomized controlled trial. *Cancer* 2007;110(11):2468–2477.

28. Cangiano T, Liao J, Naitoh J, Dorey F, Figlin R, Belldegrun A. Sarcomatoid renal cell carcinoma: biologic behavior, prognosis, and response to combined surgical resection and immunotherapy. *J Clin Oncol* 1999;17(2):523–528.

29. Motzer RJ, Bacik J, Mariani T, Russo P, Mazumdar M, Reuter V. Treatment outcome and survival associated with metastatic renal cell carcinoma of non-clear-cell histology. *J Clin Oncol* 2002;20(9):2376–2381.

30. Upton MP, Parker RA, Youmans A, McDermott DF, Atkins MB. Histologic predictors of renal cell carcinoma response to interleukin-2-based therapy. *J Immunother* 2005;28(5):488–495.

31. Bui MH, Seligson D, Han KR, et al. Carbonic anhydrase IX is an independent predictor of survival in advanced renal clear cell carcinoma: implications for prognosis and therapy. *Clin Cancer Res* 2003;9(2):802–811.

32. Atkins M, Regan M, McDermott D, et al. Carbonic anhydrase IX expression predicts outcome of interleukin 2 therapy for renal cancer. *Clin Cancer Res* 2005;11(10):3714–3721.

33. Pantuck AJ, Fang Z, Liu X, et al. Gene expression and tissue microarray analysis of interleukin-2 complete responders in patients with metastatic renal cell carcinoma. *J Clin Oncol* 2005;23(16S, pt 1): abstract 4535.

34. Jones J, Otu HH, Grall F, et al. Proteomic identification of interleukin-2 therapy response in metastatic renal cell cancer. *J Urol* 2008;179(2):730–736.

35. McDermott DF, Ghebremichael MS, Signoretti S, et al. The high-dose Aldesleukin (HD IL-2) "SELECT" trial in patients with metastatic renal cell carcinoma (mRCC). *J Clin Oncol* 2010;28:15s:abstr 4514.

36. Cho DC, Puzanov I, Regan MM, et al. Retrospective analysis of the safety and efficacy of interleukin-2 after prior VEGF-targeted therapy in patients with advanced renal cell carcinoma. *J Immunother* 2009;32(2):181–185.

37. Dandamudi UB, Ghebremichael MS, Sosman JA, et al. A phase II study of bevacizumab and high dose bolus aldesleukin (IL-2) in metastatic renal cell carcinoma patients: A Cytokine Working Group Study. *J Clin Oncol* 2010;28:15s:abstr 5044.

38. Rini BI, Halabi S, Rosenberg JE, et al. Phase III trial of bevacizumab plus interferon alfa versus interferon alfa monotherapy in patients with metastatic renal cell carcinoma: final results of CALGB 90206. *J Clin Oncol* 2010;28(13):2137–2143.

39. Childs R, Srinivasan R. Advances in allogeneic stem cell transplantation: directing graft-versus-leukemia at solid tumors. *Cancer J* 2002;8(1):2–11.

40. Rini BI, Zimmerman T, Stadler WM, Gajewski TF, Vogelzang NJ. Allogeneic stem-cell transplantation of renal cell cancer after nonmyeloablative chemotherapy: feasibility, engraftment, and clinical results. *J Clin Oncol* 2002;20(8):2017–2024.

41. Thompson CB, Allison JP. The emerging role of CTLA-4 as an immune attenuator. *Immunity* 1997;7(4):445–450.

42. Walunas TL, Lenschow DJ, Bakker CY, et al. CTLA-4 can function as a negative regulator of T cell activation. *Immunity* 1994;1(5):405–413.

43. Krummel MF, Allison JP. CD28 and CTLA-4 have opposing effects on the response of T cells to stimulation. *J Exp Med* 1995;182(2):459–465.

44. Chambers CA, Sullivan TJ, Allison JP. Lymphoproliferation in CTLA-4-deficient mice is mediated by costimulation-dependent activation of CD4+ T cells. *Immunity* 1997;7(6):885–895.

45. Cesana GC, DeRaffele G, Cohen S, et al. Characterization of CD4+CD25+ regulatory T cells in patients treated with high-dose interleukin-2 for metastatic melanoma or renal cell carcinoma. *J Clin Oncol* 2006;24(7):1169–1177.

46. Brahmer JR, Topalian S, Wollner I, et al. Safety and activity of MDX-1106 (ONO-4538), an anti-PD-1 monoclonal antibody, in patients with selected refractory or relapsed malignancies. *J Clin Oncol* 2008;26 (May 20 suppl; abstr 3006).

47. Yang JC, Hughes M, Kammula U, et al. Ipilimumab (anti-CTLA4 antibody) causes regression of metastatic renal cell cancer associated with enteritis and hypophysitis. *J Immunother* 2007;30(8):825–830.

48. Morris J, Shapiro G, Tan A, et al. Phase I/II study of GC1008: A human anti-transforming growth factor-beta (TGFβ) monoclonal antibody (MAb) in patients with advanced malignant melanoma (MM) or renal cell carcinoma (RCC). *J Clin Oncol* 2008;26 (May 20 suppl; abstr 9028).

49. Sznol M, Hodi F, Margolin K, et al. Phase I study of BMS-663513, a fully human anti-CD137 agonist monoclonal antibody, in patients (pts) with advanced cancer (CA). *J Clin Oncol* 2008;26 (May 20 suppl: abstr 3007).

50. Schmidt H, Selby P, Mouritzen U, et al. Subcutaneous (SC) dosing of recombinant human interleukin-21 (rIL-21) is safe and has clinical activity: Results from a dose-escalation study in stage 4 melanoma (MM) or renal cell cancer (RCC). *J Clin Oncol* 2008;26 (May 20 suppl: abstr 3041).

51. Moore DJ, Hwang J, McGreivy J, et al. Phase I trial of escalating doses of the TLR9 agonist HYB2055 in patients with advanced solid tumors. *J Clin Oncol,* 2005 ASCO Annual Meeting Proceedings. Vol 23, No. 16S, Part I of II (June 1 Supplement), 2005: 2503.

52. Prieto PA, Yang JC, Sherry RM, et al. Cytotoxic T lymphocyte-associated antigen 4 blockade with ipilimumab: Long-term follow-up of 179 patients with metastatic melanoma. *J Clin Oncol* 2010;28:15s:abstr 8544.

53. Thompson RH, Gillett MD, Cheville JC, et al. Costimulatory B7-H1 in renal cell carcinoma patients: Indicator of tumor aggressiveness and potential therapeutic target. *Proc Natl Acad Sci USA* 2004;101(49):17174–17179.

54. Keir ME, Francisco LM, Sharpe AH. PD-1 and its ligands in T-cell immunity. *Curr Opin Immunol* 2007;19(3):309–314.

55. Keir ME, Butte MJ, Freeman GJ, Sharpe AH. PD-1 and its ligands in tolerance and immunity. *Annu Rev Immunol* 2008;26:677–704.

56. Carter L, Fouser LA, Jussif J, et al. PD-1:PD-L inhibitory pathway affects both CD4(+) and CD8(+) T cells and is overcome by IL-2. *Eur J Immunol* 2002;32(3):634–643.

57. Okazaki T, Honjo T. The PD-1-PD-L pathway in immunological tolerance. *Trends Immunol* 2006;27(4):195–201.

58. Nishimura H, Nose M, Hiai H, Minato N, Honjo T. Development of lupus-like autoimmune diseases by disruption of the PD-1 gene encoding an ITIM motif-carrying immunoreceptor. *Immunity* 1999;11(2):141–151.

59. Nishimura H, Okazaki T, Tanaka Y, et al. Autoimmune dilated cardiomyopathy in PD-1 receptor-deficient mice. *Science* 2001;291(5502):319–322.

60. Blank C, Kuball J, Voelkl S, et al. Blockade of PD-L1 (B7-H1) augments human tumor-specific T cell responses in vitro. *Int J Cancer* 2006;119(2):317–327.

61. Keir ME, Liang SC, Guleria I, et al. Tissue expression of PD-L1 mediates peripheral T cell tolerance. *J Exp Med* 2006;203(4):883–895.

62. Ansari MJ, Salama AD, Chitnis T, et al. The programmed death-1 (PD-1) pathway regulates autoimmune diabetes in nonobese diabetic (NOD) mice. *J Exp Med* 2003;198(1):63–69.

63. Salama AD, Chitnis T, Imitola J, et al. Critical role of the programmed death-1 (PD-1) pathway in regulation of experimental autoimmune encephalomyelitis. *J Exp Med* 2003;198(1):71–78.

64. Magnus T, Schreiner B, Korn T, et al. Microglial expression of the B7 family member B7 homolog 1 confers strong immune inhibition: implications for immune responses and autoimmunity in the CNS. *J Neurosci* 2005;25(10):2537–2546.

65. Grabie N, Gotsman I, DaCosta R, et al. Endothelial programmed death-1 ligand 1 (PD-L1) regulates CD8+ T-cell mediated injury in the heart. *Circulation* 2007;116(18):2062–2071.

66. Keir ME, Freeman GJ, Sharpe AH. PD-1 regulates self-reactive CD8+ T cell responses to antigen in lymph nodes and tissues. *J Immunol* 2007;179(8):5064–5070.

67. Barber DL, Wherry EJ, Masopust D, et al. Restoring function in exhausted CD8 T cells during chronic viral infection. *Nature* 2006;439(7077):682–687.

68. Trautmann L, Janbazian L, Chomont N, et al. Upregulation of PD-1 expression on HIV-specific CD8+ T cells leads to reversible immune dysfunction. *Nat Med* 2006;12(10):1198–1202.

69. Day CL, Kaufmann DE, Kiepiela P, et al. PD-1 expression on HIV-specific T cells is associated with T-cell exhaustion and disease progression. *Nature* 2006;443(7109):350–354.

70. Urbani S, Amadei B, Tola D, et al. PD-1 expression in acute hepatitis C virus (HCV) infection is associated with HCV-specific CD8 exhaustion. *J Virol* 2006;80(22):11398–11403.

71. Boni C, Fisicaro P, Valdatta C, et al. Characterization of hepatitis B virus (HBV)-specific T-cell dysfunction in chronic HBV infection. *J Virol* 2007; 81(8):4215–4225.

72. Boettler T, Panther E, Bengsch B, et al. Expression of the interleukin-7 receptor alpha chain (CD127) on virus-specific CD8+ T cells identifies functionally and phenotypically defined memory T cells during acute resolving hepatitis B virus infection. *J Virol* 2006;80(7):3532–3540.

73. Brown JA, Dorfman DM, Ma FR, et al. Blockade of programmed death-1 ligands on dendritic cells enhances T cell activation and cytokine production. *J Immunol* 2003;170(3):1257–1266.

74. Oflazoglu E, Swart DA, Anders-Bartholo P, et al. Paradoxical role of programmed death-1 ligand 2 in Th2 immune responses *in vitro* and in a mouse asthma model in vivo. *Eur J Immunol* 2004; 34(12):3326–3336.

75. Fukushima A, Yamaguchi T, Azuma M, Yagita H, Ueno H. Involvement of programmed death-ligand 2 (PD-L2) in the development of experimental allergic conjunctivitis in mice. *Br J Ophthalmol* 2006;90(8):1040–1045.

76. Dong H, Strome SE, Salomao DR, et al. Tumor-associated B7-H1 promotes T-cell apoptosis: a potential mechanism of immune evasion. *Nat Med* 2002;8(8):793–800.

77. Hamanishi J, Mandai M, Iwasaki M, et al. Programmed cell death 1 ligand 1 and tumor-infiltrating CD8+ T lymphocytes are prognostic factors of human ovarian cancer. *Proc Natl Acad Sci USA* 2007;104(9):3360–3365.

78. Strome SE, Dong H, Tamura H, et al. B7-H1 blockade augments adoptive T-cell immunotherapy for squamous cell carcinoma. *Cancer Res* 2003; 63(19):6501–6505.

79. Inman BA, Sebo TJ, Frigola X, et al. PD-L1 (B7-H1) expression by urothelial carcinoma of the bladder and BCG-induced granulomata: associations with localized stage progression. *Cancer* 2007;109(8):1499–1505.

80. Konishi J, Yamazaki K, Azuma M, Kinoshita I, Dosaka-Akita H, Nishimura M. B7-H1 expression on non-small cell lung cancer cells and its relationship with tumor-infiltrating lymphocytes and their PD-1 expression. *Clin Cancer Res* 2004;10(15):5094–5100.

81. Nakanishi J, Wada Y, Matsumoto K, Azuma M, Kikuchi K, Ueda S. Overexpression of B7-H1 (PD-L1) significantly associates with tumor grade and postoperative prognosis in human urothelial cancers. *Cancer Immunol Immunother* 2007;56(8):1173–1182.

82. Nomi T, Sho M, Akahori T, et al. Clinical significance and therapeutic potential of the programmed death-1 ligand/programmed death-1 pathway in human pancreatic cancer. *Clin Cancer Res* 2007;13(7):2151–2157.

83. Wu C, Zhu Y, Jiang J, Zhao J, Zhang XG, Xu N. Immunohistochemical localization of programmed death-1 ligand-1 (PD-L1) in gastric carcinoma and its clinical significance. *Acta Histochem* 2006;108(1):19–24.

84. Iwai Y, Ishida M, Tanaka Y, Okazaki T, Honjo T, Minato N. Involvement of PD-L1 on tumor cells in the escape from host immune system and tumor immunotherapy by PD-L1 blockade. *Proc Natl Acad Sci USA* 2002;99(19):12293–12297.

85. Ahmadzadeh M, Johnson LA, Heemskerk B, et al. Tumor antigen-specific CD8 T cells infiltrating the tumor express high levels of PD-1 and are functionally impaired. *Blood* 2009;114:1537–1544.

86. Mumprecht S, Schürch C, Schwaller J, Solenthaler M, Ochsenbein AF. Programmed death 1 signaling on chronic myeloid leukemia-specific T cells results in T-cell exhaustion and disease progression. *Blood* 2009;114(8):1528–1536.

87. Sznol M, Powderly JD, Smith DC, et al. Safety and antitumor activity of bi-weekly MDX1106 in patients with advanced or refractory malignancies. *J Clin Oncol* 2010;28:15s, 2010 (suppl; abstr 2506).

88. Avigan DE, Vasir B, George DJ, et al. Phase I/II study of vaccination with electrofused allogeneic dendritic cells/autologous tumor-derived cells in patients with stage IV renal cell carcinoma. *J Immunother* 2007;30(7):749–761.

89. Oosterwijk-Wakka JC, Tiemessen DM, Bleumer I, et al. Vaccination of patients with metastatic renal cell carcinoma with autologous dendritic cells pulsed with autologous tumor antigens in combination with interleukin-2: a phase 1 study. *J Immunother* 2002;25(6):500–508.

90. Wierecky J, Müller MR, Wirths S, et al. Immunologic and clinical responses after vaccinations with peptide-pulsed dendritic cells in metastatic renal cancer patients. *Cancer Res* 2006;66(11):5910–5918.

91. Rosenblatt J, Glotzbecker B, Mills H, et al. CT-011, Anti-PD-1 antibody, enhances ex-vivo T cell responses to autologous dendritic/myeloma fusion vaccine developed for the treatment of multiple myeloma. *Blood* (ASH Annual Meeting Abstracts) 2009;114:781.

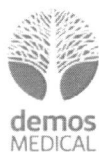

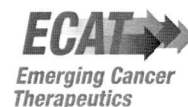

VEGF Pathway–Directed Therapies in Renal Carcinoma

C. Lance Cowey* and Thomas E. Hutson

Genitourinary Oncology Program, Baylor Sammons Cancer Center, Texas Oncology, Dallas, TX

■ ABSTRACT

Tumor angiogenesis has long been recognized as a hallmark of cancer, and antiangiogenic drugs have recently become an important part of cancer therapy. In the last several years, the management of metastatic renal carcinoma has become dominated by the use of angiogenesis-targeted therapeutics, particularly those affecting the vascular endothelial growth factor (VEGF) pathway. Currently, there are four VEGF pathway inhibitors that have gained FDA approval for the treatment of renal carcinoma, with more similar agents in development. Efforts to improve on outcomes with these agents are ongoing and include evaluation of potential drug resistance mechanisms, discovery and incorporation of predictive biomarkers, and evaluation of optimal combinations and sequencing approaches to renal carcinoma management.

Keywords: VEGF, targeted therapy, clear cell renal cell cancer, sequential therapy, combination therapy, biomarkers

■ INTRODUCTION

Renal cell carcinoma is a common malignancy with an estimated 58,240 new cases diagnosed in 2009 and 13,040 deaths (1). Renal carcinoma is potentially curable with surgical resection; however, the recurrence risk increases with greater stage (2) and metastatic disease is incurable. Several different histologic subtypes of renal carcinoma occur, including clear cell (~75% of cases), papillary (~15%, types 1 and 2), chromophobe (~5%), and oncocytoma (~5%). Metastatic renal carcinoma is notoriously resistant to cytotoxic chemotherapeutics (3) and, until recently, the mainstay of therapy has been cytokine-based treatments such as interferon (IFN) and interleukin-2 (IL-2). During this era of immune-based therapies, clinical prognostic methods were developed (4), which have been

*Corresponding author, 3535 Worth Street, Dallas, TX 75246

E-mail address: Lance.Cowey@USOncology.com

Emerging Cancer Therapeutics 2:1 (2011) 115–136.
DOI: 10.5003/2151–4194.2.1.115

utilized in stratification of patients in clinical trials evaluating new therapies. The clinical features of poor performance status (Karnofsky performance status, KPS < 80%), elevated serum LDH, elevated serum calcium, low hemoglobin, and initiation of systemic therapy of less than 1 year from nephrectomy remain poor risk indicators in patients treated with vascular endothelial growth factor (VEGF)– and mTOR-directed agents as well.

Currently, VEGF pathway–directed agents have had the highest rate of clinical responses and form the mainstay of renal carcinoma therapy. Approved VEGF pathway inhibitors include sunitinib (Sutent), sorafenib (Nexavar), bevacizumab (Avastin), and pazopanib (Votrient). This review will focus on a summary of the available VEGF inhibitor agents for use in metastatic renal carcinoma and upcoming novel VEGF inhibitors. Although VEGF-directed therapy has resulted in a paradigm shift in treatment, multiple clinical questions remain to be answered: What is the mechanism of resistance to these new therapies? What is the optimal combination or proper sequencing with these agents? What prognostic or predictive biomarkers can be identified and incorporated into the modern management of renal carcinoma? Can these therapies be incorporated into earlier stages of renal carcinoma management to improve outcomes? Most importantly, VEGF pathway–directed agents are not curative in metastatic renal carcinoma, and thus addressing these questions will hopefully improve outcomes in these patients.

■ VEGF AND RENAL CELL CARCINOMA MOLECULAR BIOLOGY

The development of VEGF pathway targeted therapeutics for renal carcinoma stemmed from scientific discoveries in the molecular pathogenesis of the disease (5). As reviewed in Chapter 1, the landmark finding of von Hippel Lindau (VHL) mutation as the sentinel genetic event responsible for both hereditary and sporadic forms of renal carcinoma was a critical step (6–8). As discussed, the *VHL* gene encodes a tumor-suppressor protein that functions as part of an E3 ubiquitin ligase complex, targeting various proteins, including a family of transcription factors known as hypoxia inducible factors (HIF) (9,10) for destruction by the cellular proteosome (Figure 1) (11,12).

HIF-1 and HIF-2 play considerable roles promoting cell survival under hypoxic conditions (13). Their overexpression in renal cancer initiates transcription of a variety of different "hypoxia-inducible" genes that stimulate tumor cell survival, proliferation, and invasiveness (14). Among the HIF-targeted genes are those that help to promote angiogenesis, such as platelet-derived growth factor (PDGF), fibroblast growth factor (FGF), angiopoietin-1 (Ang-1), and VEGF.

In a landmark angiogenesis study from 1948, Michaelson et al. described a factor that could induce the growth and expansion of vessels in the retina (15). He termed this factor as "angiogenic factor X," which is now known as VEGF. Although VEGF can be secreted by fibroblasts and stromal support cells (16), renal carcinoma tumors are capable of producing large amounts of VEGF (17). There are several different gene loci that make up the VEGF family and each have several isoforms possible through genetic splicing (18); however, the VEGF-A isoforms that bind to VEGF receptor-1 (VEGFR-1, also called Flt-1) and VEGFR-2 (Flk-1 or FDR) are likely the most important in promoting tumor angiogenesis. VEGFR-1 and -2 function as transmembrane receptor tyrosine kinases, located on the cellular surface of vascular endothelial cells. Activation of the VEGF receptor through ligand binding results in receptor dimerization and subsequent intracellular growth pathway activation with an end-result of new blood vessel formation. Given the strong relationship between the VEGF pathway and renal carcinoma carcinogenesis via VHL-HIF dysregulation, the development of VEGF-inhibiting agents for the management of renal carcinoma has been particularly rewarding and unlike other cancer types, monotherapy with VEGF inhibitors has become the standard of care.

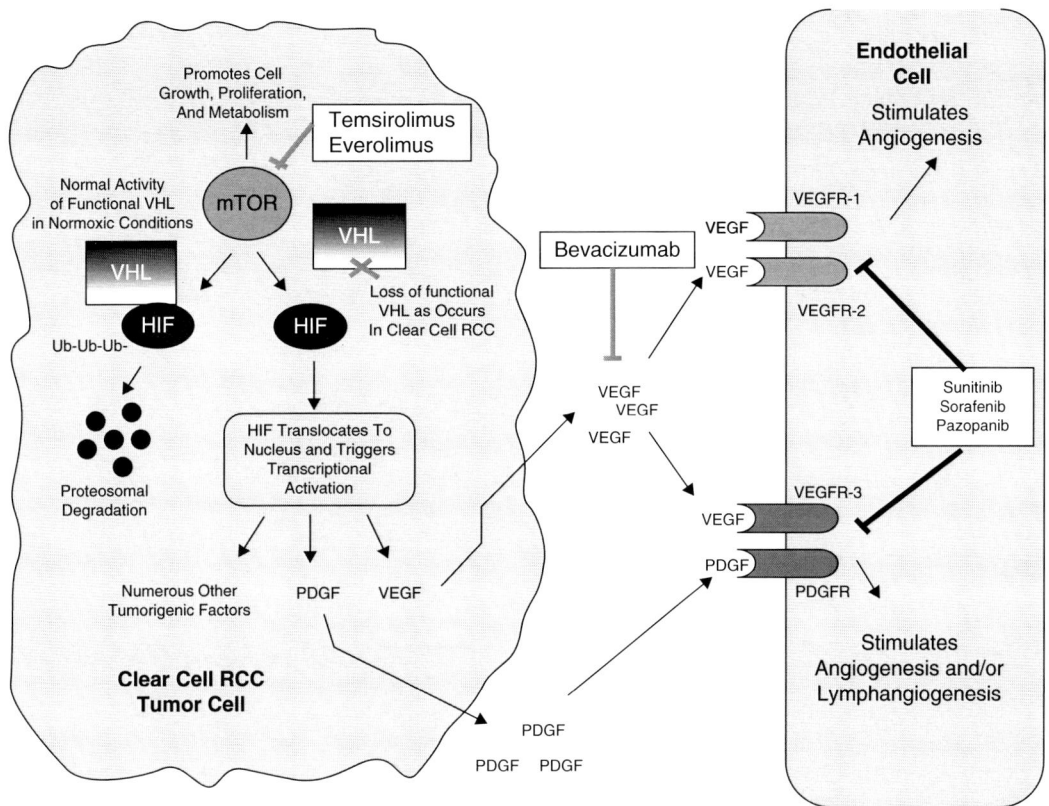

FIGURE 1

Pathogenesis of VHL-deficient clear cell renal cell carcinoma (renal carcinoma) and drug targets. In normal oxygen conditions, the von Hippel Lindau protein (VHL) recognizes prolyl hydroxylated hypoxia-inducible factor (HIF) and marks it for degradation by the cellular proteosome by adding a polyubiquitin tail (Ub). However, in hypoxia or in absence of functional VHL, as seen in clear cell renal carcinoma tumors, HIF is stabilized and translocates to the nucleus where it results in transcriptional activation of multiple pro-tumorigenic factors. Among these factors are vascular endothelial growth factor (VEGF) and platelet-derived growth factor (PDGF) and which are able to bind to their respective receptors (VEGFR, PDGFR) on the cell surface of stromal endothelial cells and promote tumor angiogenesis and lymphogenesis. The currently FDA-approved VEGF-inhibitors are shown in white boxes with their respective molecular targets.

■ CURRENTLY APPROVED VEGF PATHWAY INHIBITORS IN RENAL CARCINOMA

Sunitinib

This orally bioavailable compound inhibits a broad range of tyrosine kinases, including VEGFR-1, -2, -3, PDGF-α, -β, ckit, and Flt-3 (19). The inhibitory profile of sunitinib compared with other VEGF TKIs is shown in Table 1. After displaying adequate tolerability and efficacy profiles in phase I and II clinical trials (20–23), an international multicenter randomized controlled phase III study was performed in patients with advanced/metastatic renal carcinoma (24,25). In this trial, 750 patients with previously untreated clear cell renal carcinoma were randomized 1:1 to receive either sunitinib or IFN. The primary endpoint of

TABLE 1 Inhibition profiles of select TKIs

VEGF TKI	Tyrosine Kinase Receptor, IC$_{50}$ (nM)							
	VEGFR-1	VEGFR-2	VEGFR-3	PDGFR-α	PDGFR-β	c-kit	Flt-3	Raf
Sunitinib	21	34	3	143	75	40	4	–
Sorafenib	–	90	20	–	57	68	58	6
Pazopanib	10	30	47	71	84	74	>2000	–
Axitininb[†]	0.1	0.2	0.1–0.3	5	1.6	1.7	>1000	–
Tivozanib[†]	0.21	0.16	0.24	–	1.72	1.63	–	–

TKI, tyrosine kinase inhibitor; VEGFR, vascular endothelial growth factor receptor; PDGF, platelet-derived growth factor receptor.

[†]Of note, axitinib and tivozanib have not gained FDA approval; however, are shown to demonstrate their respective potency for the VEGFR-2 TKI in comparison to the others.

this trial was progression-free survival (PFS) with additional secondary endpoints of safety, overall survival (OS) and overall response rate (ORR). The results showed a significantly improved PFS of 11 months in the sunitinib treated cohort compared to 5 months for those in the IFN cohort (HR 0.42, 95% CI 0.32–0.54, P < 0.001). In addition, the ORR for sunitinib was 47% versus 12% for IFN. Survival data were potentially impacted by the fact that a significant proportion of patients in the IFN group went on to receive sunitinib or other VEGF TKIs. Nevertheless, the intent-to-treat final OS analysis showed a survival of 26.4 months for the sunitinib group compared to 21.8 months for the IFN group (HR 0.821, 95%CI 0.673–1.001, P = 0.051 unstratified log-rank test; P = 0.013 unstratified Wilcoxin test). In the phase III study, the most common adverse events included diarrhea, fatigue, nausea, hypertension, hand-foot syndrome and rash, whereas the most common laboratory abnormalities included neutropenia, anemia, lymphopenia, thrombocytopenia, elevated creatinine, elevated liver transaminases, and elevated lipase. Postmarketing experience indicates that liver dysfunction can be severe and occasionally fatal. Most of these symptoms have been noted as VEGF TKI class-associated side effects as will be seen with the discussions of trials with

similar agents below. Sunitinib gained approval for use in advanced or metastatic renal carcinoma in early 2006.

Sorafenib

The development of the agent called sorafenib began based on its potential as an RAF inhibitor, but it was additionally found to be a potent inhibitor of VEGFR 2–3, PDGFR-β, RAF, FLT-3, and c-kit (26–29). Promising activity in a phase II randomized discontinuation study (30) led to its evaluation in a large multicenter placebo-controlled trial in patients with metastatic clear cell renal carcinoma who had received prior cytokine therapy (31). In this trial, 903 patients were randomized to either sorafenib or placebo with a primary endpoint of OS and secondary endpoints of PFS and ORR. The final results of the OS analysis did not demonstrate significance (17.8 months for sorafenib vs. 15.2 months for placebo, HR = 0.88, P = 0.146); although when patients who crossed over from placebo to sorafenib were excluded, the analysis did suggest a survival improvement (17.8 months for sorafenib vs. 14.3 months for placebo, HR = 0.78, P = 0.029) (32). The ORR for sorafenib was 10% compared to 2% in the placebo group.

PFS was significantly extended in the sorafenib group compared to placebo (5.5 vs. 2.8 months, respectively, HR = 0.44 95%CI 0.35–0.55, $P < 0.000001$). Adverse effects seen in the phase III trial included diarrhea, fatigue, hypertension, HFS, and rash.

Bevacizumab

Unlike sunitinib and sorafenib, which are VEGF receptor inhibitors, bevacizumab is an intravenously administered recombinant monoclonal antibody (IgG1) that binds the VEGF TKI ligand, effectively neutralizing all soluble VEGF-A isoforms (33). Bevacizumab has been evaluated in combination with IFN in treatment-naïve metastatic renal carcinoma patients in two large randomized controlled trials. The phase III AVOREN study compared the combination of bevacizumab and IFN with IFN alone (34). In this study, 649 patients with clear cell metastatic renal carcinoma were randomized and the primary endpoint of PFS was found to be 10.2 months in the bevacizumab/IFN arm compared to 5.4 months in the IFN alone arm (HR 0.63, 95% CI 0.52–0.75, $P = 0.0001$). A subsequent report of the OS data showed no significant difference between bevacizumab/IFN and IFN alone (unstratified HR 0.91, 95% CI, 0.76–1.10; $P = 0.3360$) (35), likely secondary to the high rate of subsequent effective therapy in patients randomized to the IFN alone arm. In a similarly designed phase III study performed by the CALGB, patents with treatment-naïve clear cell renal carcinoma ($n = 732$) were randomized to receive the combination of bevacizumab and IFN or IFN alone (36). In this study, the PFS of bevacizumab/IFN was 8.5 months, whereas the PFS of IFN alone was 5.2 months (HR 0.71 95% CI 0.61–0.83, $P < 0.0001$). Similar to the AVOREN trial, this CALGB comparison did not result in a statistically significant OS benefit (37). The common side effects seen in the bevacizumab and IFN arms of these two trials included fatigue, hypertension, proteinuria, and anorexia.

Pazopanib

Pazopanib, which is the most recently approved agent for metastatic renal carcinoma, shares similarities with sunitinib and sorafenib where it is also an orally bioavailable multitargeted VEGF TKI. Pazopanib potently targets the tyrosine kinase receptors VEGF 1–3, PDGF-α, -β, and c-kit (38,39). Because of promising results from a phase II randomized discontinuation trial, an international, multicenter randomized controlled phase III trial with pazopanib was initiated (40). Similar to the phase II trial, this study included patients with metastatic clear cell renal carcinoma who had progressed on one prior cytokine or were treatment naïve. A total of 435 patients were randomized (2:1) to receive pazopanib or placebo with a primary endpoint of PFS and secondary endpoints of RR, OS, DOR, and safety. The median PFS for those in the pazopanib arm was 9.2 months compared with 4.2 months for the placebo control arm (HR 0.46, 95% CI 0.34–0.62, $P < 0.0001$). The ORR of pazopanib in this trial was 30% with a median duration of response of 58.7 weeks. When patients were stratified based on prior therapy or not, the difference in PFS for pazopanib compared to placebo was more prominent in the treatment naïve patients (11.1 months for pazopanib vs. 2.8 months for placebo, HR 0.40 95% CI 0.27–0.60, $P < 0.0001$). Final OS data for this trial remains to be reported. In terms of safety, pazopanib was felt to be well tolerated with common adverse events including diarrhea, nausea, hypertension, hair depigmentation, and liver transaminase elevation. The most common grade 3/4 toxicity was liver transaminase elevation (grade 3/4 increased ALT in 12% and AST in 8%) which led the FDA to place a black box warning regarding this particular adverse event (hepatotoxicity) on the drug's label. A head-to-head noninferiority study comparing pazopanib to sunitinib for front-line therapy has recently completed accrual (National Cancer Institute/www.clinicaltrials.gov Identification Number: NCT00720941).

■ PLACEMENT OF APPROVED VEGF PATHWAY INHIBITORS IN PRACTICAL CARE OF PATIENTS

The evidence-based approach to management of patients diagnosed with metastatic renal carcinoma is based upon the aforementioned phase 3 trials and is summarized in Table 2. For patients with good or intermediate risk clear cell renal carcinoma, front-line VEGF pathway inhibitor options with level 1 evidence include sunitinib, bevacizumab plus IFN and pazopanib.

TABLE 2   Summary of phase III data involving FDA-approved VEGF pathway inhibitors

VEGF Pathway Inhibitor	Phase III Setting	Comparator Arm	Outcomes	References
Sunitinib	Treatment-naïve	Interferon ORR: 47% vs. 12% OS: unstratified analysis insignificant ($P = 0.051$); stratified analysis significant ($P = 0.013$)	PFS: 11 vs. 5 months ($P < 0.001$)	24,25
Sorafenib	Cytokine-refractory	Placebo ORR: 10% vs. 2% OS: intent-to-treat analysis insignificant ($P = 0.146$); when cross-over excluded, significant ($P = 0.029$)	PFS: 5.5 vs. 2.8 ($P < 0.000001$)	31,32
Bevacizumab (plus interferon)	Treatment-naïve	Interferon ORR: AVOREN trial 31% vs.13%; CALGB 25.5% vs. 13.1% OS intent-to-treat analysis insignificant in both studies	PFS: AVOREN trial: 10.2 vs. 5.4 months ($P = 0.0001$);CALGB trial: 8.5 vs. 5.2 months ($P < 0.0001$)	34–37
Pazopanib	Treatment-naïve or cytokine-refractory	Placebo	*Treatment-naïve:* PFS: 11.1 vs. 2.8 months ($P < 0.001$) ORR: 32% OS: NA *Cytokine-refractory:* PFS: 7.4 vs. 4.2 months ($P < 0.001$) ORR: 29% OS: NA	40

VEGF, vascular endothelial growth factor; PFS, progression-free survival; ORR, overall response rate; OS, overall survival.

Although none of these trials have data with head-to-head comparison, they all have PFS outcomes in a similar 9 to 11 month range. However, in patients with poor risk clear cell renal carcinoma or non–clear cell renal carcinoma, there is level 1 evidence to support the use of temsirolimus, an mTOR inhibitor (see Chapter 9) (41). In addition, appropriate patients should be considered for high dose IL-2 (see Chapter 7) (42). In the second-line setting, both sorafenib and pazopanib have a high level of evidence supporting its use following front-line cytokine-based therapy. In the post-VEGF TKI setting, phase III evidence for the mTOR inhibitor, everolimus, exists (see Chapter 9) (43,44). The optimal therapy for renal carcinoma variants, such as Xp11 translocation-associated carcinoma and papillary cancers, are unknown due to a dearth of prospective data; however, retrospective studies have shown that these subtypes can also respond to VEGF-targeted therapies (45,46).

■ VEGF PATHWAY INHIBITORS IN DEVELOPMENT

Currently, four VEGF pathway inhibitors have been approved for the management of renal carcinoma and to add to this panoply are several other VEGF-targeted drugs, which have distinguished themselves in early testing. The experimental agents, axitinib and tivozanib, inhibit the VEGF receptors much more potently than their predecessors (Table 1). This may give them a potential tactical advantage over the currently approved ones, which still needs to be clinically demonstrated. In addition, dovitinib is a potent inhibitor of FGF in addition to VEGF, which may provide value by targeting a potential escape mechanism simultaneously. VEGF TRAP is a monoclonal peptibody that binds all VEGF ligands as compared to bevacizumab, which binds the isoforms of VEGF A alone. These agents are currently in clinical testing and their early phase clinical experience will be described as follows (Table 3).

TABLE 3 VEGF pathway inhibitors currently in development for renal carcinoma

VEGF Pathway Inhibitor	Type	Status of Development	Published Data	References
Axitinib	VEGFR TKI	First- and second-line phase III trials ongoing	*Phase II Cytokine-refractory (single arm):* ORR 44.2%; mPFS 15.7 months	47–49
			Phase II Sorafenib-refractory (single arm): ORR 22.6%; mPFS 7.4 months	
Tivozanib	VEGFR TKI	First-line phase III trial ongoing	*Phase II Treatment-naïve or cytokine-refractory (RDT with placebo):* ORR 25.4%; mPFS 11.8 months	50,51
Dovitinib	FGFR/VEGFR TKI	Refractory phase III trial ongoing	*Phase I:* Safety and tolerability demonstrated	52
ABT-869	VEGFR TKI	Second-line phase II trial complete	*Phase II Sunitinib-refractory (single arm):* ORR 6.8%; mPFS 4.9 months	53,54
Aflibercept (VEGF Trap)	Peptibody Against VEGF	Second-line trial ongoing	*Phase I:* Safety and tolerability demonstrated	55

VEGF TKI, vascular endothelial growth factor receptor tyrosine kinase inhibitor; FGFR, fibroblast growth factor receptor; ORR, overall response rate; mPFS, median progression-free survival; OS, overall survival.

Axitinib

Axitinib is a orally bioavailable TKI with potent inhibition of VEGFR1–3, PDGF, and c-kit (47). Renal carcinoma-specific trials that have been reported include phase II studies evaluating the drug's efficacy in the second-line setting. A single-arm phase II study in 52 metastatic renal carcinoma patients refractory to IFN, IL-2 or both (48) revealed a 44% response rate (complete response, $n = 2$; partial response, $n = 21$), a median time to progression of 15.7 months and a median survival of 29.9 months. The most common grade 3/4 adverse events were hypertension, fatigue, and diarrhea.

In a separate single-arm phase II study of metastatic renal carcinoma patients who were sorafenib-refractory, a total of 62 patients were enrolled (49). Dose-escalation of axitinib was allowed in patients who tolerated the drug with less than grade 2 toxicity and in the absence of hypertension. In more than half of the patients (53.2%), the dose was able to be titrated above the initial 5 mg twice daily dosing, while 35.5% of patients required dose reduction that was less than the starting dose. Although prior sorafenib therapy was required, other previous treatments were allowed with 61.3% having had received prior cytokines and 22.6% prior sunitinib. The ORR was 22.6% with a median PFS of 7.4 months (95% CI, 6.7–11.0 months). The OS was 13.6 months (95% CI, 8.4–18.8 months). The common adverse events on this trial included fatigue, diarrhea, hypertension, nausea, anemia, and lymphopenia.

On the basis of these data, two large randomized phase III trials have been initiated. In the second-line setting (post-VEGF TKI), axitinib is being compared to sorafenib with primary endpoint of OS (NCT00678392). This study has completed accrual and preliminary results are anticipated soon. In addition, a phase III trial comparing the efficacy of axitinib to sorafenib in a treatment-naïve population is currently accruing patients with a anticipated completion date in 2011(NCT00920816).

Tivozanib

Tivozanib is a more potent VEGF receptor inhibitor than its predecessors similar to axitinib. Tivozanib (AV-951) is an oral multitargeted VEGF TKI which potently targets VEGFR 1–3 at picomolar concentrations. It has been tested in the phase I setting in solid tumors and demonstrated good tolerability (50). Tivozanib was subsequently evaluated in a phase II randomized discontinuation trial in patients with metastatic renal carcinoma (51). In this study, 272 patients with no prior VEGF-targeted therapy were treated. In the intent-to-treat analysis, the ORR for tivozanib was 25.4% and the median PFS was 11.8 months (95% CI 253–450 days). Hypertension, diarrhea, fatigue, and dysphonia were reported as the most common adverse events.

Recently a subset analysis showed that patients with clear cell type histology ($n = 225$) and prior nephrectomy ($n = 199$) had better PFS results than their counterparts. A phase III randomized trial of tivozanib versus sorafenib in the front-line setting has recently completed accrual and results are expected in 2011 (NCT01030783).

Dovitinib

Dovitinib (TKI258), a multitargeted TKI, possesses potent inhibitory properties against VEGF and FGF receptors, as well as PDGFR-b, Flt3, and ckit. In a phase I clinical study involving 20 patients with metastatic renal carcinoma refractory to standard therapy, the agent was found to be tolerable with common adverse events including nausea, diarrhea, vomiting, hypertension, and rash (52). Dovitinib is currently being evaluated in a phase II study in refractory renal carcinoma patients (NCT00715182).

ABT-869

Another orally bioavailable TKI, ABT-869, inhibits VEGFR 1–3, PDGFR, Flt3, and CSF1R.

ABT-869 has undergone phase I testing showing tolerable side effects (53). Tannir et al. presented a phase II study of 53 patients with metastatic clear cell renal carcinoma who were sunitinib refractory (54). The ORR for ABT-869 was 6.8% (with an additional 54% obtaining stable disease) and the median PFS was 4.9 months. Common adverse effects were fatigue, diarrhea, nausea, and hand-foot syndrome.

Aflibercept

Aflibercept, also known as VEGF Trap (aflibercept, Regeneron Pharmaceuticals, Inc.), is a peptibody that is composed of the Fc portion of human IgG antibody and part of the extracellular domains of VEGFR-1 and-2. This molecule is thus able to bind and clear all isoforms of VEGFA and PDGF. Tolerability of aflibercept was demonstrated in a phase I trial in patients with solid tumors (55). Currently, the efficacy of aflibercept in metastatic renal carcinoma is being evaluated in a randomized phase II study by the Eastern Cooperative Oncology Group (NCT00357760).

■ VEGF PATHWAY TOXICITY AND MANAGEMENT

Toxicities from inhibitors of the VEGF pathway have been well described and are typically easily managed. Several class-related toxicities have been demonstrated with these drugs and the most notable overlapping toxicities common to all include hypertension and proteinuria. Other side effects such as skin, hepatic, thyroid and hematopoietic toxicities appear to be associated with specific VEGF tyrosine kinase inhibitors. Fortunately, most toxicities are reversible following cessation of the agent, and some patients require dose reduction to avoid intolerable side effects.

Hypertension is considered an on-target side effect of VEGF pathway inhibition. The mechanism behind the development of hypertension with VEGF pathway inhibitors is not fully understood

but available data support that decreased nitrous oxide availability plays a role (56). Management of hypertension in the setting of VEGF pathway inhibitor agents depends on the severity. The treating clinician should make every effort to keep the blood pressure below 140/90 during the course of VEGF therapy treatment, and commonly used blood pressure medications such as calcium channel blockers, β-blockers, angiotensin-receptor blockers, and diuretics are all reasonable options. It should be noted that severe hypertension (> 200/110) can occur and management includes holding the VEGF agent until blood pressure can be controlled. Posterior reversible encephalopathy syndrome can occur, and neurologic symptoms (e.g., altered mental status, seizure) should trigger brain imaging to rule out this serious complication (57). In addition, in the sequential use of VEGF pathway agents, it should be noted that the half life of bevacizumab is long (~21 days), and therefore, a wash out period should occur prior to initiating another VEGF pathway agent as the concomitant use of these medications can lead to increased potential for overlapping side effects such as hypertension. Although less common than hypertension, congestive heart failure has also been associated with both VEGF tyrosine kinase inhibitors and VEGF ligand inhibitors. In patients with pre-existing cardiac issues, evaluation of cardiac function prior to VEGF inhibitor administration is reasonable and subsequent development of cardiac dysfunction warrants discontinuation of this class of agents.

Treatment with VEGF tyrosine kinase inhibitors can produce a variety of adverse effects involving the skin, including rash, hand-foot syndrome, and skin or hair depigmentation. While hair or skin depigmentation can have cosmetic impacts for patients, hand-foot syndrome can impair functionality, and aggressive management is required to keep this side effect to a minimum. It is thought that hand-foot syndrome from VEGF tyrosine kinase inhibitors occurs secondary to the impairment of wound healing and microtrauma to the palms and soles with repetitive activity. The symptoms of hand-foot syndrome include the development of increased sensitivity, erythema, paresthesias, callous over the palms or surfaces of the feet, and in some cases skin breakdown. The management depends on the severity of the symptoms; however, frequent use of good quality emollient lotions, protective cotton gloves, and thick soled shoes are important preventative measures. In severe cases, temporary discontinuation of the drug is required and use of steroid or urea-based creams may be helpful. With the proactive management of side effects, the treating physician has a better opportunity to maintain dose intensity, which is important for anti-cancer effects with these agents.

■ MECHANISMS OF RESISTANCE TO VEGF PATHWAY INHIBITORS

Although the introduction of VEGF pathway inhibitors has dramatically impacted patient outcomes in the treatment of metastatic renal carcinoma, this disease remains incurable. Most patients experience tumor shrinkage with initial VEGF inhibitor treatment; however, further growth is typically inevitable. Such acquired drug resistance differs from drug refractoriness in which certain patient's tumors are never sensitive to VEGF-targeted therapies, which likely occurs through different mechanism(s). One potential mechanism for acquired resistance in initial VEGF therapy responsive patients is that tumoral response to VEGF pathway–directed therapy results in a hypoxic insult via disruption of intratumoral blood supply. This hypoxic environment would theoretically further increase HIF levels in tumor and stromal support cells, and thus create a vicious cycle of pro-tumorigenic hypoxia-inducible gene transactivation. Although specific molecular mechanisms of acquired VEGF inhibitor resistance continue to be explored, this phenomenon likely occurs due to an angiogenic escape mechanism, which is multifactorial.

Several molecular pathways have been implicated, including upregulation of other pro-angiogenic molecules such as ang-2, IL-8, FGF, and PlGF (58). For instance IL-8 production was recently evaluated in a sunitinib-resistant xenograft model of renal carcinoma by Teh et al (59). In this experiment, renal carcinoma xenografts were created that mimicked sunitinib resistance and re-vascularization (angiogenic escape) coincided with increased IL-8 production by the tumors. Subsequent blockade of IL-8 via an antibody resulted in subsequent re-response to sunitinib therapy. Although the mechanisms of VEGF inhibitor resistance are likely complex and may be different for the various VEGF inhibitors, a better understanding of these pathways will help guide treatment selection for patients and hopefully identify novel druggable molecular targets.

■ SEQUENCING AND COMBINATIONS OF VEGF INHIBITORS

Sequencing

Because of the inability of any single agent to commonly produce complete, durable responses, efforts have been made to improve upon clinical outcomes by exploration of optimal sequencing or combination strategies with the available agents. Substantial retrospective evidence exists supporting the lack of cross-resistance to sequential VEGF-targeted therapies (60–63). For example, Sablin et al. reported a retrospective study of 90 consecutive patients with metastatic renal carcinoma who were treated with sorafenib followed by sunitinib (*n* = 68) or sunitinib followed by sorafenib (*n* = 22) (60). In the patients that received sorafenib first, the partial response rate was 16% for sorafenib followed by a response rate of 15% with subsequent sunitinib. For patients that received sunitinib first, the partial response rate was 23% with sunitinib and then 9% with subsequent sorafenib treatment.

Although the reasons why patients who develop acquired resistance to one VEGF agent can go on to receive benefit from another VEGF agent are not completely understood; it is perceivable that the differences involve VEGF inhibition potency, drug metabolism (pharmacogenomic variation), and drug tolerance (which often correlates with being able to maintain drug intensity) all play a role. Interestingly, a retrospective analysis of renal carcinoma patients who have been re-challenged with sunitinib has recently been reported (Rini et al., ASCO Genitourinary Cancers Symposium 2010, abstract 319). In this review, 23 patients were identified who underwent a rechallenge of sunitinib after being off of the drug for a median of 6.7 months. Between the sunitinib treatment periods, patients received a variety of agents, including other VEGF TKIs, bevacizumab, and mTOR inhibitors. In these patients sunitinib retreatment resulted in a 22% ORR and a median PFS of 7.2 months (range, 1.2–28.5⁺). Patients who were off of sunitinib for longer than 6 months did better than those retreated with a shorter interval (median PFS 16.5 vs. 6.0 months, respectively; $P = 0.03$). This study supports the concept of a VEGF-dominant angiogenesis physiology that can be "reset."

Multiple prospective studies have been performed, which have provided further evidence for the sequential use of VEGF inhibitors and these are outlined in Table 4. Rini et al. evaluated 61 patients in a single-arm phase II study of bevacizumab-refractory metastatic renal carcinoma patients who were treated with sunitinib (64). The median PFS for patients treated with sunitinib in this study was 30.4 weeks with a PR rate of 23% and SD rate of 59%. Adverse toxicities for sunitinib were similar to that seen in front-line use. In a separate prospective phase II study, Di Lorenzo et al. evaluated the efficacy of sorafenib in 52 sunitinib refractory patients (65). Of note, 42% of these patients had a response with prior sunitinib therapy. The ORR after two cycles of sorafenib was 9.6% and median time-to-progression was 16 weeks (range 8–40).

Ongoing phase III studies will provide a higher level of evidence on the sequential VEGF inhibitor to VEGF inhibitor treatment approach, including the phase III AXIS trial, which has recently completed accrual (NCT00678392).

In this study, 650 patients were randomized to receive either axitinib or sorafenib following failure of sunitinib, bevacizumab, temsirolimus, or cytokine. The primary outcome of this study is PFS with secondary outcome measures, including ORR, OS, and safety. Another phase III trial will randomize patients to receive the sequence of sorafenib followed by sunitinib or the sequence of sunitinib followed by sorafenib (Switch study, NCT00732914). The primary endpoint of this study is to compare the additive PFS of each sequence with other endpoints including OS and the development of cardiotoxicity.

Combination Therapy

There are two main approaches to combination molecular targeted therapy—horizontal blockade and vertical blockade. Horizontal blockade uses two or more agents to block separate molecular pathways, for example, the VEGF pathway and the mTOR pathway. The vertical blockade approach blocks two different points in the same pathway (e.g., VEGF ligand and VEGF receptor). While serial use of targeted agents allows for exposure to single agents, with the efficacy and toxicity limited to the individual agent employed, the use of combination targeted therapy provides a platform for additive or synergistic response (as well as additive or synergistic toxicity). Since the field of renal carcinoma therapeutics has been dominated by two classes of agents, the VEGF inhibitors and mTOR inhibitors, attempts have been made to study the combination of these agents. The results of these studies are summarized in Table 4.

In an example of vertical pathway inhibition, the combination of bevacizumab and sunitinib was evaluated in a phase I clinical study by Feldman et al. (66). In this trial, 26 patients were enrolled and treated with fixed dose bevacizumab with escalating sunitinib, in a dose-escalation cohort fashion. The ORR was 52% (including 1 complete response) and 36% had SD. Unfortunately, the adverse events seen in this study were notable.

TABLE 4 Prospective studies of sequential targeted therapies and combination-based therapies involving VEGF pathway inhibitors

Sequencing or Combination	Trial Type	Comparator Arm	Results	Reference
A. Sequencing Trials				
VEGF TKI → everolimus	Phase III	Placebo	PFS 4.9 vs. 1.9 months	43,44
Sorafenib → Axitinib	Phase II	Single arm	ORR 22.6%, PFS 7.4 months, OS 13.6 months	49
Bevacizumab → sunitinib	Phase II	Single arm	ORR 23%, PFS 7 months	64
Sunitinib → ABT869 (VEGF TKI)	Phase II	Single arm	ORR 18.1%, PFS 4.9 months	54
Sunitinib → Sorafenib	Phase II	Single arm	ORR 9.6%, TTP 16 weeks, OS 32 weeks	65
VEGF inhibitor ± mTOR i → perifosine	Phase II	Single arm	ORR 9%, PFS 15 weeks	116
Bevacizumab or sunitinib → sorafenib	Phase II	Single arm	ORR 0%, PFS 3.8 months	117
Sorafenib → Sunitinib	Phase II	Single arm	ORR 18%, PFS 4.8 months	118
B. Combination Trials				
VEGF + VEGF				
Bevacizumab + sorafenib	Phase I	Single arm	ORR 46%, TTP 11.2 months; increased toxicity	70
Bevacizumab + sunitinib	Phase I	Single arm	ORR 52%; increased toxicity	119
VEGF + mTOR				
Bevacizumab + temsirolimus	Phase I/II	Single arm	ORR 16%	71
Bevacizumab + everolimus	Phase II	Single arm	ORR 28%, PFS 8.1 months	72
Bevacizumab + temsirolimus (BT)	Phase II	Sunitinib (S)	NPR@48 weeks: 30.7% (BT), 40.5%(S), 65.9%(BI).	35
		Bevacizumab/ interferon (BI)	PFS: 8.2 months (BT), 8.2 months (S), 16.8 months (BI); increased toxicity with BT regimen	
VEGF + Other				
Bevacizumab + erlotinib	Phase I/II	Single arm	ORR 25%, PFS 11 months	69
Bevacizumab + erlotinib + imatinib	Phase I/II	Single arm	ORR 17%	68
Bevacizumab + IL-2	Phase I	Single arm	ORR 28%, PFS 9 months	73

VEGF, vascular endothelial growth factor; TKI, tyrosine kinase inhibitor; mTOR, mammalian target of rapamycin; PFS, progression-free survival; ORR, overall response rate; TTP, time to progression; NPR, nonprogression rate.

Forty-eight percent of patients had to discontinue treatment due to toxicity. The most common grade 3/4 toxicities included hypertension (60%), proteinuria (36%), and thrombocytopenia (24%). In addition, two patients developed microangiopathic hemolytic anemia (MAHA) and reversible posterior leukoencephalopathy syndrome (RPLS), and one patient suffered a fatal myocardial infarction. Based on these findings, it was felt that the combination of bevacizumab and sunitinib was too toxic to take forward.

In terms of VEGF-mTOR horizontal blockade, the largest reported study to-date has been the TORAVA trial, which was recently reported by Escudier et al. (67). In this study, 88 patients were randomized (3:1) to one of three arms: bevacizumab + temsirolimus (n = 88), bevacizumab + IFN (n = 40), or single-agent sunitinib (n = 42). This was a randomized, "pick-the-winner" phase II study with a primary endpoint of nonprogression rate at 48 weeks. The nonprogression rate for bevacizumab/temsirolimus, bevacizumab/IFN, and sunitinib were 30.7%, 65.9%, and 40.5%, respectively (ORRs were 25%, 34%, and 24%, respectively). The poorer than hoped for findings of the bevacizumab/temsirolimus combination were also overshadowed by increased toxicities as well. In the bevacizumab/temsirolimus arm, 38.5% of patients experienced grade 3/4 toxicities compared to 27.5% and 14.3% in the comparator arms. Two deaths occurred in the bevacizumab/temsirolimus arm, which were felt to be treatment related.

Other ongoing studies are also evaluating the combination of a VEGF and mTOR inhibitor. The BeST trial is a randomized phase II trial comparing the combination of bevacizumab + sorafenib, bevacizumab + temsirolimus, and temsirolimus + sorafenib (NCT00378703). The primary endpoint of this trial is PFS. The INTORACT trial is a randomized phase III study evaluating the combination of bevacizumab + temsirolimus compared to the standard bevacizumab/IFN combination in previously untreated patients (NCT00631371). Finally, CALGB 90802 is evaluating the combination of bevacizumab and the mTOR inhibitor everolimus versus standard everolimus alone in patients refractory to VEGFR TKI's.

Agents of other classes, such as imatinib (a c-kit TKI), erlotinib (epidermal growth factor receptor (EGFR) inhibitor), and everolimus (mTOR inhibitor), have also been combined with bevacizumab in prospective studies (68–72). These studies did not result in additional activity over that which would be expected with bevacizumab. Dandamudi et al. recently reported a phase II study of the combination of bevacizumab and high-dose IL-2 in 51 patients with clear cell metastatic renal carcinoma (73). The median PFS was 9.0 months and 2-year PFS frequency was 15%. In addition, there was a 28% response rate (including 8% complete responders) and 42% had stable disease. The toxicity profile was similar to that expected for bevacizumab or IL-2 alone. Although this combination is appealing for select patients, a randomized study will be required to compare this approach to single-agent VEGF inhibition. Other anti-angiogenesis agents are also being combined with VEGF pathway inhibitors in current ongoing trials. AMG-386, a novel peptibody, which binds and clears angiopoeitin 1 and 2, is being combined with sorafenib in a blinded, placebo controlled phase II trial (n = 150) (NCT00467025). In this study, two combination arms (two different AMG-386 dosings with sorafenib) are being compared to single-agent sorafenib in the treatment-naïve setting. In addition, in a separate single-arm phase II, AMG-386 is being combined with sunitinib in prior cytokine-treated or treatment-naïve renal carcinoma patients (NCT00853372). Finally, BNC105P, which represents a new class of vascular disrupting agents, is being evaluated in combination with everolimus in a phase I/II study compared to everolimus alone in previously VEGF TKI treated renal carcinoma patients (NCT01034631). BNC105P is felt to disrupt newly forming blood vessels within tumors by binding to tubulin in endothelial cells with the net result of tumor vascular endothelium disruption and tumor ischemia. The development of novel agents continues to create interest in testing combination regimens with the available active agents. However, in order for a combination therapy to be adopted, it should result in an improved survival outcomes compared to sequential therapy with an acceptable toxicity profile.

■ PROGNOSTIC AND PREDICTIVE BIOMARKERS OF VEGF THERAPIES

Prognostic Markers

A prognostic marker or a group of prognostic markers should give the clinician information regarding the patient's potential outcome independent of therapeutic choices. Prognostic markers are essential for not only designing well-balanced trials but also directing physician-patient discussions. Prognostic scoring systems such as the previously described MSKCC criteria (4) as well as other systems such as the UCLA Integrated survival score (UISS) (74) and SSIGN score (Stage Size Grade Necrosis, Mayo clinic) (75) were developed in the era of cytokine therapy. Interestingly, the recent landmark studies, which led to the approval of all of the current VEGF-targeted therapies, included inclusion/exclusion criteria based on these previously established MSKCC prognostic criteria. It may be that these prognostic criteria are still adequate in predicting prognosis with current renal carcinoma patients treated with VEGF pathway (59) and mTOR inhibitors (44); however, this has yet to be determined in a prospective fashion.

In an attempt to modernize the current clinical prognostic criteria, several retrospective analyses have explored clinical markers that may be important for determining prognosis with currently available agents. Clinical factors that have been shown to correlate with poorer outcomes include poor performance status (76), time to diagnosis to systemic treatment < 1 year (76,77), anemia (76), hypercalcemia (76), elevated neutrophil count (76), elevated platelet count (76), age > 60 (77), and brain metastases (77). These current clinical prognostic markers share striking similarity with previous markers discovered in the cytokine therapy era, suggesting that utilization of prior prognostic systems are still relevant today and may be employed.

Several molecularly based biomarkers have also been explored with most being focused on the known dysfunctional pathway in most clear cell renal carcinomas, the VHL-HIF-VEGF pathway. Exploration of *VHL* gene status has been explored in many studies with some in support of VHL as a prognostic/predictive factor (78–83) and others against (84–88). In addition, evaluation of HIF and its genetic targets have also been explored as candidate biomarkers. It has been shown that VHL-deficient clear cell renal carcinoma tumors differentially express HIF-1 and HIF-2 with readily identifiable phenotypes, HIF-1/HIF-2 expressing, HIF-2 only expressing (89,90). Although these HIF phenotypes may have prognostic implications, prospective evaluation has not been performed in patients. Other candidate markers down stream of HIF activation have also been examined in retrospective fashion, including CAIX expression (91–93) VEGF levels (64,94,95), genetic signatures (96–98), and a variety of other molecules (99–104); however, no single-candidate prognostic biomarker has been prospectively validated.

Predictive Markers

With the panoply of new agents that have been approved in the past several years and the host of other agents that are in the pipeline, the practical management of renal carcinoma has become quite complex. Establishment of markers which may predict response to an agent or class of agents would be extremely useful in providing patients with a therapy that is most likely to help them but also avoiding therapies which can have significant toxicity that are unlikely to help them. Currently, the development of molecular predictive biomarkers is in its infancy. A number of different molecular markers are being explored for their potential as predictive biomarkers; although no one or group of biomarkers has been prospectively validated to predict response to any of the available targeted therapies. Examples of some candidate predictive markers for VEGF-directed therapy include IL-8 (105), alterations in t-regulatory cells (106), VEGF (107), TNF-alpha (108), MMP-9 (108), HGF (109), IL-6 (109), e-selectin (109), and infiltration of tumors with myeloid cells. Prospective validation of candidate predictive markers is important for advancing the field toward an individualized medicine approach.

■ INCORPORATION OF VEGF THERAPIES IN THE PERIOPERATIVE SETTING

Preoperative VEGF Therapy Approaches

Use of VEGF-targeted therapies in the preoperative setting for both localized and metastatic renal carcinoma have been explored in several small nonrandomized studies, and it appears that preoperative VEGF inhibition is safe and can result in shrinkage of the primary tumor (110–113). There are multiple potential benefits of implementing preoperative therapy prior to cytoreductive or curative nephrectomy. Shrinkage of large tumors may result in easier operations and anecdotal reports of significant downstaging of renal carcinoma tumors have been reported. More importantly, preoperative therapy gives the opportunity for the clinician to evaluate tumor response while *in vivo*, which has direct implications to subsequent treatment choices for the patient. In scenarios where widespread metastatic disease exists and the clinician is uncertain of the pace of disease progression and potential sensitivity to front-line VEGF therapy, a course of systemic therapy makes sense prior to subjecting the patient to nephrectomy.

Cytoreductive nephrectomy has become the standard of care in renal carcinoma based on studies showing improvement in survival endpoints in the context of IFN therapy (114,115). Unfortunately, it remains unknown if cytoreductive nephrectomy is necessary with the use of VEGF or mTOR pathway–targeted therapies. Several studies are underway, which may help

answer these questions. In a randomized phase III EORTC study (NCT01099423), 458 patients are planned to be enrolled and undergo randomization to immediate cytoreductive nephrectomy or treatment with sunitinib followed by cytoreductive nephrectomy (primary endpoint, PFS). In another trial (NCT00930033), patients (*n* = 576) will be randomized to cytoreductive nephrectomy followed by sunitinib therapy or to sunitinib therapy alone with a primary endpoint of PFS.

Adjuvant VEGF Therapy Approaches

Patients with localized renal carcinoma who have undergone surgical resection are at risk of recurrence and later development of incurable metastatic disease. Therefore, the adjuvant utility of VEGF inhibitors following a curative-intent surgical resection of localized renal carcinoma is being explored in multiple large randomized phase III trials. The S-TRAC study is an ongoing phase III study of 1 year of sunitinib therapy versus placebo following nephrectomy for localized clear cell or non–clear cell renal carcinoma (NCT00375674). In the ASSURE trial, two adjuvant treatment arms (sorafenib vs. sunitinib) are being compared to placebo with a primary endpoint of disease-free survival (NCT00326898). Both the S-TRAC and ASSURE trials are designed to administer the study agents for a 1-year period of time. The phase III SORCE trial is evaluating 1 and 3 years of adjuvant sorafenib compared to placebo (NCT00492258). These trials will hopefully answer the key questions of whether VEGF-directed therapy can eradicate microscopic disease and if so of the duration of therapy that is necessary.

■ CONCLUSION

Angiogenesis plays a critical role in renal carcinoma and hypervascular tumors are a hallmark of this disease. The discovery of the *VHL* gene and its relationship to HIF and hypoxia-inducible genes, such as VEGF, has accelerated the development of therapeutics, which have drastically changed the landscape of renal carcinoma therapy. Six agents, including four VEGF inhibitors, have been approved for use since 2005 with more potent agents currently in the later stages of development. A variety of studies are ongoing, which should shed light on the proper use of existing agents in terms of optimal sequence, activity of combination strategies, and use as adjuvant therapies. Although VEGF pathway inhibitors have had dramatic impacts on patient outcomes, metastatic renal carcinoma remains an incurable disease and the cancer invariably becomes resistant to VEGF-directed therapy. An in-depth understanding of the mechanisms of resistance to VEGF inhibition is crucial in taking steps toward the development of novel agents to bypass these pathways. Several agents that may play a role in overcoming VEGF resistance are in development, including FGF and angiopoietin inhibitors. Perhaps the most important challenge for the next years in renal carcinoma clinical research is the identification and validation of potential candidate predictive biomarkers for selecting amongst an increasing number of treatment options.

■ REFERENCES

1. Jemal A, Siegel R, Xu J, Ward E. Cancer statistics, 2010. *CA Cancer J Clin* 2010;60(5):277–300.
2. Frank I, Blute ML, Leibovich BC, Cheville JC, Lohse CM, Zincke H. Independent validation of the 2002 American Joint Committee on cancer primary tumor classification for renal cell carcinoma using a large, single institution cohort. *J Urol* 2005;173(6):1889–1892.
3. Motzer RJ, Russo P. Systemic therapy for renal cell carcinoma. *J Urol* 2000;163(2):408–417.
4. Motzer RJ, Mazumdar M, Bacik J, Berg W, Amsterdam A, Ferrara J. Survival and prognostic stratification of 670 patients with advanced renal cell carcinoma. *J Clin Oncol* 1999;17(8):2530–2540.
5. Cowey CL, Rathmell WK. Using Molecular Biology to Develop Drugs for Renal Cell Carcinoma. *Expert Opin Drug Discov* 2008;3(3):311–327.
6. Kim WY, Kaelin WG. Role of VHL gene mutation in human cancer. *J Clin Oncol* 2004;22(24):4991–5004.
7. Lonser RR, Glenn GM, Walther M, et al. von Hippel-Lindau disease. *Lancet* 2003;361(9374):2059–2067.
8. Latif F, Tory K, Gnarra J, et al. Identification of the von Hippel-Lindau disease tumor suppressor gene. *Science* 1993;260(5112):1317–1320.
9. Iliopoulos O, Levy AP, Jiang C, Kaelin WG Jr, Goldberg MA. Negative regulation of hypoxia-inducible genes by the von Hippel-Lindau protein. *Proc Natl Acad Sci USA* 1996;93(20):10595–10599.
10. Maxwell PH, Wiesener MS, Chang GW, et al. The tumour suppressor protein VHL targets hypoxia-inducible factors for oxygen-dependent proteolysis. *Nature* 1999;399(6733):271–275.
11. Iwai K, Yamanaka K, Kamura T, et al. Identification of the von Hippel-lindau tumor-suppressor protein as part of an active E3 ubiquitin ligase complex. *Proc Natl Acad Sci USA* 1999;96(22):12436–12441.
12. Cowey CL, Rathmell WK. VHL gene mutations in renal cell carcinoma: role as a biomarker of disease outcome and drug efficacy. *Curr Oncol Rep* 2009;11(2):94–101.
13. Wiesener MS, Münchenhagen PM, Berger I, et al. Constitutive activation of hypoxia-inducible genes related to overexpression of hypoxia-inducible factor-1alpha in clear cell renal carcinomas. *Cancer Res* 2001;61(13):5215–5222.
14. Semenza GL. Targeting HIF-1 for cancer therapy. *Nat Rev Cancer* 2003;3(10):721–732.
15. Michaelson IC. The mode of development of the vascular system of the retina with some observations on its significance for certain retinal disorders. *Trans Ophthalmol Soc UK* 1948;68:137–180.
16. Fukumura D, Xavier R, Sugiura T, et al. Tumor induction of VEGF promoter activity in stromal cells. *Cell* 1998;94(6):715–725.
17. Edgren M, Lennernäs B, Larsson A, Nilsson S. Serum concentrations of VEGF and b-FGF in renal cell, prostate and urinary bladder carcinomas. *Anticancer Res* 1999;19(1B):869–873.
18. Tischer E, Mitchell R, Hartman T, et al. The human gene for vascular endothelial growth factor. Multiple protein forms are encoded through alternative exon splicing. *J Biol Chem* 1991;266(18):11947–11954.
19. Mendel DB, Laird AD, Xin X, et al. *In vivo* antitumor activity of SU11248, a novel tyrosine kinase inhibitor targeting vascular endothelial growth factor

and platelet-derived growth factor receptors: determination of a pharmacokinetic/pharmacodynamic relationship. *Clin Cancer Res* 2003;9(1):327–337.

20. Faivre S, Delbaldo C, Vera K, et al. Safety, pharmacokinetic, and antitumor activity of SU11248, a novel oral multitarget tyrosine kinase inhibitor, in patients with cancer. *J Clin Oncol* 2006;24(1):25–35.

21. Motzer RJ, Michaelson MD, Redman BG, et al. Activity of SU11248, a multitargeted inhibitor of vascular endothelial growth factor receptor and platelet-derived growth factor receptor, in patients with metastatic renal cell carcinoma. *J Clin Oncol* 2006;24(1):16–24.

22. Motzer RJ, Rini BI, Bukowski RM, et al. Sunitinib in patients with metastatic renal cell carcinoma. *JAMA* 2006;295(21):2516–2524.

23. Motzer RJ, Michaelson MD, Rosenberg J, et al. Sunitinib efficacy against advanced renal cell carcinoma. *J Urol* 2007;178(5):1883–1887.

24. Motzer RJ, Hutson TE, Tomczak P, et al. Sunitinib versus interferon alfa in metastatic renal-cell carcinoma. *N Engl J Med* 2007;356(2):115–124.

25. Motzer RJ, Hutson TE, Tomczak P, et al. Overall survival and updated results for sunitinib compared with interferon alfa in patients with metastatic renal cell carcinoma. *J Clin Oncol* 2009;27(22):3584–3590.

26. Strumberg D, Richly H, Hilger RA, et al. Phase I clinical and pharmacokinetic study of the Novel Raf kinase and vascular endothelial growth factor receptor inhibitor BAY 43–9006 in patients with advanced refractory solid tumors. *J Clin Oncol* 2005;23(5):965–972.

27. Clark JW, Eder JP, Ryan D, Lathia C, Lenz HJ. Safety and pharmacokinetics of the dual action Raf kinase and vascular endothelial growth factor receptor inhibitor, BAY 43–9006, in patients with advanced, refractory solid tumors. *Clin Cancer Res* 2005;11(15):5472–5480.

28. Moore M, Hirte HW, Siu L, et al. Phase I study to determine the safety and pharmacokinetics of the novel Raf kinase and VEGFR inhibitor BAY 43–9006, administered for 28 days on/7 days off in patients with advanced, refractory solid tumors. *Ann Oncol* 2005;16(10):1688–1694.

29. Awada A, Hendlisz A, Gil T, et al. Phase I safety and pharmacokinetics of BAY 43–9006 administered for 21 days on/7 days off in patients with advanced, refractory solid tumours. *Br J Cancer* 2005;92(10):1855–1861.

30. Ratain MJ, Eisen T, Stadler WM, et al. Phase II placebo-controlled randomized discontinuation trial of sorafenib in patients with metastatic renal cell carcinoma. *J Clin Oncol* 2006;24(16):2505–2512.

31. Escudier B, Eisen T, Stadler WM, et al. Sorafenib in advanced clear-cell renal-cell carcinoma. *N Engl J Med* 2007;356(2):125–134.

32. Escudier B, Eisen T, Stadler WM, et al. Sorafenib for treatment of renal cell carcinoma: Final efficacy and safety results of the phase III treatment approaches in renal cancer global evaluation trial. *J Clin Oncol* 2009;27(20):3312–3318.

33. Presta LG, Chen H, O'Connor SJ, et al. Humanization of an anti-vascular endothelial growth factor monoclonal antibody for the therapy of solid tumors and other disorders. *Cancer Res* 1997;57(20):4593–4599.

34. Escudier B, Pluzanska A, Koralewski P, et al. Bevacizumab plus interferon alfa-2a for treatment of metastatic renal cell carcinoma: a randomised, double-blind phase III trial. *Lancet* 2007;370(9605):2103–2111.

35. Escudier B, Bellmunt J, Negrier S, et al. Phase III trial of bevacizumab plus interferon alfa-2a in patients with metastatic renal cell carcinoma (AVOREN): final analysis of overall survival. *J Clin Oncol.* 2010;28(13):2144–2150.

36. Rini BI, Halabi S, Rosenberg JE, et al. Bevacizumab plus interferon alfa compared with interferon alfa monotherapy in patients with metastatic renal cell carcinoma: CALGB 90206. *J Clin Oncol* 2008;26(33):5422–5428.

37. Rini BI, Halabi S, Rosenberg JE, et al. Phase III trial of bevacizumab plus interferon alfa versus interferon alfa monotherapy in patients with metastatic renal cell carcinoma: final results of CALGB 90206. *J Clin Oncol* 2010;28(13):2137–2143.

38. Kumar R, Knick VB, Rudolph SK, et al. Pharmacokinetic-pharmacodynamic correlation from mouse to human with pazopanib, a multikinase angiogenesis inhibitor with potent antitumor and antiangiogenic activity. *Mol Cancer Ther* 2007;6(7):2012–2021.

39. Hurwitz HI, Dowlati A, Saini S, et al. Phase I trial of pazopanib in patients with advanced cancer. *Clin Cancer Res* 2009;15(12):4220–4227.

40. Sternberg CN, Davis ID, Mardiak J, et al. Pazopanib in locally advanced or metastatic renal cell carcinoma: results of a randomized phase III trial. *J Clin Oncol* 2010;28(6):1061–1068.

41. Hudes G, Carducci M, Tomczak P, et al. Temsirolimus, interferon alfa, or both for advanced renal-cell carcinoma. *N Engl J Med* 2007;356(22):2271–2281.

42. McDermott DF, Ghebremichael MS, Signoretti S, et al. The high-dose aldesleukin (HD IL-2) "SELECT"

trial in patients with metastatic renal cell carcinoma (mRCC). *J Clin Oncol (Meeting Abstracts)* 2010;28(15 suppl):4514.

43. Motzer RJ, Escudier B, Oudard S, et al. Efficacy of everolimus in advanced renal cell carcinoma: a double-blind, randomised, placebo-controlled phase III trial. *Lancet* 2008;372(9637):449–456.

44. Motzer RJ, Escudier B, Oudard S, et al. Phase 3 trial of everolimus for metastatic renal cell carcinoma: final results and analysis of prognostic factors. *Cancer* 2010;116(18):4256–4265.

45. Golshayan AR, George S, Heng DY, et al. Metastatic sarcomatoid renal cell carcinoma treated with vascular endothelial growth factor-targeted therapy. *J Clin Oncol* 2009;27(2):235–241.

46. Choueiri TK, Lim ZD, Hirsch MS, et al. Vascular endothelial growth factor-targeted therapy for the treatment of adult metastatic Xp11.2 translocation renal cell carcinoma. *Cancer.* 2010;116(22):5219–5225.

47. Hu-Lowe DD, Zou HY, Grazzini ML, et al. Nonclinical antiangiogenesis and antitumor activities of axitinib (AG-013736), an oral, potent, and selective inhibitor of vascular endothelial growth factor receptor tyrosine kinases 1, 2, 3. *Clin Cancer Res* 2008;14(22):7272–7283.

48. Rixe O, Bukowski RM, Michaelson MD, et al. Axitinib treatment in patients with cytokine-refractory metastatic renal-cell cancer: a phase II study. *Lancet Oncol* 2007;8(11):975–984.

49. Rini BI, Wilding G, Hudes G, et al. Phase II study of axitinib in sorafenib-refractory metastatic renal cell carcinoma. *J Clin Oncol* 2009;27(27):4462–4468.

50. Eskens F, de Jonge M, Esteves B, et al. Updated results from a Phase I study of AV-951 (KRN951), a potent and selective VEGFR-1, -2 and -3 tyrosine kinase inhibitor, in patients with advanced solid tumors. *AACR Meeting Abstracts* 2008;2008 (1_Annual_Meeting):LB-201.

51. Bhargava P, Esteves B, Nosov DA, et al. Updated activity and safety results of a phase II randomized discontinuation trial (RDT) of AV-951, a potent and selective VEGFR1, 2, and 3 kinase inhibitor, in patients with renal cell carcinoma (RCC). *J Clin Oncol (Meeting Abstracts)* 2009;27(15S):5032.

52. Angevin E, Lin C, Pande AU, et al. A phase I/II study of dovitinib (TKI258), a FGFR and VEGFR inhibitor, in patients (pts) with advanced or metastatic renal cell cancer: Phase I results. *J Clin Oncol (Meeting Abstracts)* 2010;28(15 suppl):3057.

53. Wong CI, Koh TS, Soo R, et al. Phase I and biomarker study of ABT-869, a multiple receptor tyrosine kinase inhibitor, in patients with refractory solid malignancies. *J Clin Oncol* 2009;27(28):4718–4726.

54. Tannir N, Wong Y, Kollmannsberger C, et al. Phase II trial of ABT-869 in advanced renal cell cancer (RCC) after sunitinib failure: efficacy and safety results. *J Clin Oncol (Meeting Abstracts)* 2009;27(15S):5036.

55. Dupont J, Rothenberg ML, Spriggs DR, et al. Safety and pharmacokinetics of intravenous VEGF Trap in a phase I clinical trial of patients with advanced solid tumors. *J Clin Oncol (Meeting Abstracts)* 2005;23(16 suppl):3029.

56. Horowitz JR, Rivard A, van der Zee R, et al. Vascular endothelial growth factor/vascular permeability factor produces nitric oxide-dependent hypotension. Evidence for a maintenance role in quiescent adult endothelium. *Arterioscler Thromb Vasc Biol* 1997;17(11):2793–2800.

57. Cumurciuc R, Martinez-Almoyna L, Henry C, Husson H, de Broucker T. Posterior reversible encephalopathy syndrome during sunitinib therapy. *Rev Neurol (Paris)* 2008;164(6–7):605–607.

58. Rini BI, Atkins MB. Resistance to targeted therapy in renal-cell carcinoma. *Lancet Oncol* 2009;10(10):992–1000.

59. Huang D, Ding Y, Zhou M, et al. Interleukin-8 mediates resistance to antiangiogenic agent sunitinib in renal cell carcinoma. *Cancer Res.* 2010; 70(3):1063–1071.

60. Sablin MP, Negrier S, Ravaud A, et al. Sequential sorafenib and sunitinib for renal cell carcinoma. *J Urol* 2009;182(1):29–34; discussion 34.

61. Dudek AZ, Zolnierek J, Dham A, Lindgren BR, Szczylik C. Sequential therapy with sorafenib and sunitinib in renal cell carcinoma. *Cancer* 2009; 115(1):61–67.

62. Eichelberg C, Heuer R, Chun FK, et al. Sequential use of the tyrosine kinase inhibitors sorafenib and sunitinib in metastatic renal cell carcinoma: a retrospective outcome analysis. *Eur Urol* 2008;54(6): 1373–1378.

63. Tamaskar I, Garcia JA, Elson P, et al. Antitumor effects of sunitinib or sorafenib in patients with metastatic renal cell carcinoma who received prior antiangiogenic therapy. *J Urol* 2008;179(1):81–86; discussion 86.

64. Rini BI, Michaelson MD, Rosenberg JE, et al. Antitumor activity and biomarker analysis of sunitinib in patients with bevacizumab-refractory metastatic renal cell carcinoma. *J Clin Oncol* 2008;26(22): 3743–3748.

65. Di Lorenzo G, Cartenì G, Autorino R, et al. Phase II study of sorafenib in patients with sunitinib-refractory metastatic renal cell cancer. *J Clin Oncol* 2009;27(27):4469–4474.

66. Feldman DR, Baum MS, Ginsberg MS, et al. Phase I trial of bevacizumab plus escalated doses of sunitinib in patients with metastatic renal cell carcinoma. *J Clin Oncol* 2009;27(9):1432–1439.

67. Escudier BJ, Negrier S, Gravis G, et al. Can the combination of temsirolimus and bevacizumab improve the treatment of metastatic renal cell carcinoma (mRCC)? Results of the randomized TORAVA phase II trial. *J Clin Oncol (Meeting Abstracts)* 2010;28(15 suppl):4516.

68. Hainsworth JD, Sosman JA, Spigel DR, et al. Bevacizumab, erlotinib, and imatinib in the treatment of patients (pts) with advanced renal cell carcinoma (RCC): A Minnie Pearl Cancer Research Network phase I/II trial. *J Clin Oncol (Meeting Abstracts)* 2005;23(16_suppl):4542.

69. Hainsworth JD, Sosman JA, Spigel DR, Edwards DL, Baughman C, Greco A. Treatment of metastatic renal cell carcinoma with a combination of bevacizumab and erlotinib. *J Clin Oncol* 2005;23(31):7889–7896.

70. Sosman JA, Flaherty KT, Atkins MB, et al. Updated results of phase I trial of sorafenib (S) and bevacizumab (B) in patients with metastatic renal cell cancer (mRCC). *J Clin Oncol (Meeting Abstracts)* 2008;26(15 suppl):5011.

71. Merchan JR, Liu G, Fitch T, et al. Phase I/II trial of CCI-779 and bevacizumab in stage IV renal cell carcinoma: Phase I safety and activity results. *J Clin Oncol (Meeting Abstracts)* 2007;25(18 suppl):5034.

72. Hainsworth JD, Spigel DR, Burris HA 3rd, Waterhouse D, Clark BL, Whorf R. Phase II trial of bevacizumab and everolimus in patients with advanced renal cell carcinoma. *J Clin Oncol* 2010;28(13):2131–2136.

73. Dandamudi UB, Ghebremichael MS, Sosman JA, et al. A phase II study of bevacizumab (B) and high-dose aldesleukin (IL-2) in patients (p) with metastatic renal cell carcinoma (mRCC): a Cytokine Working Group Study (CWGS). *J Clin Oncol (Meeting Abstracts)* 2010;28(15 suppl):4530.

74. Zisman A, Pantuck AJ, Dorey F, et al. Mathematical model to predict individual survival for patients with renal cell carcinoma. *J Clin Oncol* 2002;20(5):1368–1374.

75. Frank I, Blute ML, Cheville JC, Lohse CM, Weaver AL, Zincke H. An outcome prediction model for patients with clear cell renal cell carcinoma treated with radical nephrectomy based on tumor stage,

76. Heng DY, Xie W, Regan MM, et al. Prognostic factors for overall survival in patients with metastatic renal cell carcinoma treated with vascular endothelial growth factor-targeted agents: results from a large, multicenter study. *J Clin Oncol* 2009; 27(34):5794–5799.

77. Elfiky AA, Cho DC, McDermott DF, et al. Predictors of response to sequential sunitinib and the impact of prior VEGF-targeted drug washout in patients with metastatic clear-cell renal cell carcinoma. *Urol Oncol.* 2010;Epub ahead of print: PMID 20451414.

78. Brauch H, Weirich G, Brieger J, et al. VHL alterations in human clear cell renal cell carcinoma: association with advanced tumor stage and a novel hot spot mutation. *Cancer Res* 2000;60(7):1942–1948.

79. Yao M, Yoshida M, Kishida T, et al. VHL tumor suppressor gene alterations associated with good prognosis in sporadic clear-cell renal carcinoma. *J Natl Cancer Inst* 2002;94(20):1569–1575.

80. Schraml P, Struckmann K, Hatz F, et al. VHL mutations and their correlation with tumour cell proliferation, microvessel density, and patient prognosis in clear cell renal cell carcinoma. *J Pathol* 2002; 196(2):186–193.

81. Patard JJ, Fergelot P, Karakiewicz PI, et al. Low CAIX expression and absence of VHL gene mutation are associated with tumor aggressiveness and poor survival of clear cell renal cell carcinoma. *Int J Cancer* 2008;123(2):395–400.

82. Kim JH, Jung CW, Cho YH, et al. Somatic VHL alteration and its impact on prognosis in patients with clear cell renal cell carcinoma. *Oncol Rep* 2005;13(5):859–864.

83. Choueiri TK, Vaziri SA, Jaeger E, et al. von Hippel-Lindau gene status and response to vascular endothelial growth factor targeted therapy for metastatic clear cell renal cell carcinoma. *J Urol* 2008;180(3):860–865; discussion 865–866.

84. Kondo K, Yao M, Yoshida M, et al. Comprehensive mutational analysis of the VHL gene in sporadic renal cell carcinoma: relationship to clinicopathological parameters. *Genes Chromosomes Cancer* 2002; 34(1):58–68.

85. Giménez-Bachs JM, Salinas-Sánchez AS, Sánchez-Sánchez F, et al. Determination of vhl gene mutations in sporadic renal cell carcinoma. *Eur Urol* 2006;49(6):1051–1057.

86. Smits KM, Schouten LJ, van Dijk BA, et al. Genetic and epigenetic alterations in the von hippel-lindau

size, grade and necrosis: the SSIGN score. *J Urol* 2002;168(6):2395–2400.

gene: the influence on renal cancer prognosis. *Clin Cancer Res* 2008;14(3):782–787.

87. Gad S. S-AV, Meric JB, Izzedine H, Khayat, D, Richard S, Rixe, O. Somatic von Hippel-Lindau (VHL) gene analysis and clinical outcome under antiangiogenic treatment in metastatic renal cell carcinoma: preliminary results. *Targeted Oncol* 2007;2:3–6.

88. Hutson TE, Davis ID, Machiels JH, et al. Biomarker analysis and final efficacy and safety results of a phase II renal cell carcinoma trial with pazopanib (GW786034), a multi-kinase angiogenesis inhibitor. *J Clin Oncol (Meeting Abstracts)* 2008;26 (15 suppl):5046.

89. Gordan JD, Simon MC. Hypoxia-inducible factors: central regulators of the tumor phenotype. *Curr Opin Genet Dev* 2007;17(1):71–77.

90. Gordan JD, Lal P, Dondeti VR, et al. HIF-alpha effects on c-Myc distinguish two subtypes of sporadic VHL-deficient clear cell renal carcinoma. *Cancer Cell* 2008;14(6):435–446.

91. Sandlund J, Oosterwijk E, Grankvist K, Oosterwijk-Wakka J, Ljungberg B, Rasmuson T. Prognostic impact of carbonic anhydrase IX expression in human renal cell carcinoma. *BJU Int* 2007; 100(3):556–560.

92. Leibovich BC, Sheinin Y, Lohse CM, et al. Carbonic anhydrase IX is not an independent predictor of outcome for patients with clear cell renal cell carcinoma. *J Clin Oncol* 2007;25(30):4757–4764.

93. Li G, Feng G, Gentil-Perret A, Genin C, Tostain J. Serum carbonic anhydrase 9 level is associated with postoperative recurrence of conventional renal cell cancer. *J Urol* 2008;180(2):510–513; discussion 513–514.

94. Choueiri TK, Regan MM, Rosenberg JE, et al. Carbonic anhydrase IX and pathological features as predictors of outcome in patients with metastatic clear-cell renal cell carcinoma receiving vascular endothelial growth factor-targeted therapy. *BJU Int* 2010;106(6):772–778.

95. Peña C, Lathia C, Shan M, Escudier B, Bukowski RM. Biomarkers predicting outcome in patients with advanced renal cell carcinoma: Results from sorafenib phase III Treatment Approaches in Renal Cancer Global Evaluation Trial. *Clin Cancer Res* 2010;16(19):4853–4863.

96. Arai E, Ushijima S, Tsuda H, et al. Genetic clustering of clear cell renal cell carcinoma based on array-comparative genomic hybridization: its association with DNA methylation alteration and patient outcome. *Clin Cancer Res* 2008;14(17):5531–5539.

97. Brannon AR, Reddy A, Seiler M, et al. Molecular Stratification of Clear Cell Renal Cell Carcinoma by Consensus Clustering Reveals Distinct Subtypes and Survival Patterns. *Genes Cancer* 2010; 1(2):152–163.

98. Rini BI, Zhou M, Aydin H, et al. Identification of prognostic genomic markers in patients with localized clear cell renal cell carcinoma (ccRCC). *J Clin Oncol (Meeting Abstracts)* 2010;28(15 suppl):4501.

99. Campbell L, Jasani B, Edwards K, Gumbleton M, Griffiths DF. Combined expression of caveolin-1 and an activated AKT/mTOR pathway predicts reduced disease-free survival in clinically confined renal cell carcinoma. *Br J Cancer* 2008;98(5):931–940.

100. Klatte T, Seligson DB, Leppert JT, et al. The chemokine receptor CXCR3 is an independent prognostic factor in patients with localized clear cell renal cell carcinoma. *J Urol* 2008;179(1):61–66.

101. Crispen PL, Sheinin Y, Roth TJ, et al. Tumor cell and tumor vasculature expression of B7-H3 predict survival in clear cell renal cell carcinoma. *Clin Cancer Res* 2008;14(16):5150–5157.

102. Seligson DB, Rajasekaran SA, Yu H, et al. Na, K-adenosine triphosphatase alpha1-subunit predicts survival of renal clear cell carcinoma. *J Urol* 2008;179(1):338–345.

103. Lim SD, Young AN, Paner GP, Amin MB. Prognostic role of CD44 cell adhesion molecule expression in primary and metastatic renal cell carcinoma: a clinicopathologic study of 125 cases. *Virchows Arch* 2008;452(1):49–55.

104. Lee HJ, Kim DI, Kwak C, Ku JH, Moon KC. Expression of CD24 in clear cell renal cell carcinoma and its prognostic significance. *Urology* 2008;72(3): 603–607.

105. Huang D, Ding Y, Zhou M, et al. Interleukin-8 mediates resistance to antiangiogenic agent sunitinib in renal cell carcinoma. *Cancer Res* 2010;70(3): 1063–1071.

106. Adotevi O, Pere H, Ravel P, et al. A decrease of regulatory T cells correlates with overall survival after sunitinib-based antiangiogenic therapy in metastatic renal cancer patients. *J Immunother* 2010;33(9):991–998.

107. Porta C, Paglino C, De Amici M, et al. Predictive value of baseline serum vascular endothelial growth factor and neutrophil gelatinase-associated lipocalin in advanced kidney cancer patients receiving sunitinib. *Kidney Int* 2010;77(9):809–815.

108. Perez-Gracia JL, Prior C, Guillén-Grima F, et al. Identification of TNF-alpha and MMP-9 as

potential baseline predictive serum markers of sunitinib activity in patients with renal cell carcinoma using a human cytokine array. *Br J Cancer* 2009;101(11):1876–1883.

109. Tran HT, Liu Y, Lin Y, et al. Use of a multiplatform analysis of plasma cytokines and angiogenic factors (CAFs) to identify baseline CAFs associated with pazopanib response and tumor burden in renal cell carcinoma (RCC) patients. *J Clin Oncol (Meeting Abstracts)* 2010;28(15 suppl):4522.

110. Cowey CL, Amin C, Pruthi RS, et al. Neoadjuvant clinical trial with sorafenib for patients with stage II or higher renal cell carcinoma. *J Clin Oncol* 2010: JCO.2009.2024.7759.

111. Thomas AA, Rini BI, Lane BR, et al. Response of the primary tumor to neoadjuvant sunitinib in patients with advanced renal cell carcinoma. *J Urol* 2009;181(2):518–523; discussion 523.

112. Jonasch E, Wood CG, Matin SF, et al. Phase II pre-surgical feasibility study of bevacizumab in untreated patients with metastatic renal cell carcinoma. *J Clin Oncol.* 2009;27(25):4076–4081.

113. Bex A, van der Veldt AA, Blank C, et al. Neoadjuvant sunitinib for surgically complex advanced renal cell cancer of doubtful resectability: initial experience with downsizing to reconsider cytoreductive surgery. *World J Urol.* 2009;27(4):533–539.

114. Mickisch GH, Garin A, van Poppel H, de Prijck L, Sylvester R. Radical nephrectomy plus interferon-alfa-based immunotherapy compared with interferon alfa alone in metastatic renal-cell carcinoma: a randomised trial. *Lancet* 2001;358(9286):966–970.

115. Flanigan RC, Salmon SE, Blumenstein BA, et al. Nephrectomy followed by interferon alfa-2b compared with interferon alfa-2b alone for metastatic renal-cell cancer. *N Engl J Med* 2001;345(23):1655–1659.

116. Vogelzang NJ, Hutson TE, Samlowski W, et al. Phase II study of perifosine in metastatic renal cell carcinoma (RCC) progressing after prior therapy (Rx) with a VEGF receptor inhibitor. *J Clin Oncol (Meeting Abstracts)* 2009;27(15S):5034.

117. Shepard DR, Rini BI, Garcia JA, et al. A multicenter prospective trial of sorafenib in patients (pts) with metastatic clear cell renal cell carcinoma (mccRCC) refractory to prior sunitinib or bevacizumab. *J Clin Oncol (Meeting Abstracts)* 2008;26(15 suppl):5123.

118. Zimmermann K, Schmittel A, Steiner U, et al. Sunitinib treatment for patients with advanced clear-cell renal-cell carcinoma after progression on sorafenib. *Oncology* 2009;76(5):350–354.

119. Feldman DR, Ginsberg MS, Baum M, et al. Phase I trial of bevacizumab plus sunitinib in patients with metastatic renal cell carcinoma. *J Clin Oncol (Meeting Abstracts)* 2008;26(15 suppl):5100.

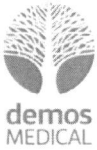

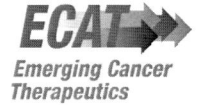

mTOR Pathway–Directed Agents in Renal Cell Carcinoma

Janice P. Dutcher*

St. Luke's Roosevelt Hospital Center, Continuum Cancer Centers, New York, NY

■ ABSTRACT

Mammalian target of rapamycin (mTOR) is a critical signaling protein in cellular biology. It is critical for cell proliferation, protein synthesis, nutrient utilization, and angiogenesis. Components of this pathway are dysregulated in more than 50% of tumors, to varying degrees, and therefore this pathway becomes of great interest in the development of anti-tumor strategies. Early clinical trials identified renal cell cancer (RCC) as potentially sensitive to inhibition of this pathway, which has led to the approval of two agents for treatment of metastatic RCC. Further elucidation of this pathway, possibly through clarification in RCC, becomes important for further development of anti-cancer therapies in general.

Keywords: renal cancer, mTOR inhibition, rapamycin, TORC1, TORC2

■ THE mTOR PATHWAY COMPONENTS

The biology of renal cell cancer (RCC), with particular emphasis on the highly active angiogenic drive in VHL inactivated clear cell renal tumors (see Chapter 1), has led to tremendous interest in inhibiting components of the angiogenesis pathway. A large part of this focus has been directed toward inhibition of signaling through vascular endothelial growth factor (VEGF) receptor tyrosine kinase inhibitors and direct binding to VEGF itself, as discussed in a previous chapter (1,2). However, it is clear that other pathways of cell cycle regulation and cellular metabolism are also important in renal cancer and may be targets for anti-tumor therapy. Although we identify multiple subtypes of renal cancer, and presume that there are varying impacts of multiple pathways on tumor growth, it is also clear that many of the growth-stimulating

---

*Corresponding author, Professor, St. Luke's Roosevelt Hospital Center, Continuum Cancer Centers, 1000 Amsterdam Ave, Ste 11C02, New York, NY 10019
  E-mail address: Jpd4401@aol.com

Emerging Cancer Therapeutics 2:1 (2011) 137–144.
DOI: 10.5003/2151–4194.2.1.137

pathways that have been identified are not unique to RCC, and in fact are aberrantly over or under active in other tumors as well. Protein kinases have been identified as important signaling switches for stimulation or inhibition of growth, utilization of nutrients, and proliferation.

The mammalian target of rapamycin (mTOR) is one such important and often key serine-threonine protein kinase that is central to regulation of cell growth, protein synthesis, and metabolism, as well as impacting angiogenesis (3). This pathway has been the subject of intense investigation and has been found to be aberrant in a number of malignancies including RCC. The impact of alterations both upstream and downstream from mTOR is continuing to be elucidated but appears to be critical in a number of tumor types (3).

The evaluation of the impact of mTOR inhibition began with the discovery of rapamycin, initially developed as an anti-fungal antibiotic, that is a natural product derived from *Streptomyces hygroscopicus* (4,5). This agent is currently utilized as an immunosuppressive agent in solid-organ transplantation (6,7). Rapamycin binds to immunophilin, FK-binding protein (FKBP12), and by doing so utilizes a different immunosuppressive pathway in comparison to other immunosuppressive agents used in the transplant setting, such as cyclosporine A or FK506 (6,7). The rapamycin/FKBP12 complex initiates a series of interactions that have been the subject of intense investigation for several decades. This has become all the more interesting in view of the relatively recent observations of clinical anti-tumor activity in humans.

The anti-proliferative properties and the potential for anti-cancer activity were demonstrated relatively early in the evaluation of rapamycin (6,7). The rapamycin/FKBP12 complex was demonstrated to interact with mTOR and inhibit its activation, thus impacting protein synthesis, cellular proliferation, and angiogenesis (8). The mechanism for inhibiting cellular proliferation was demonstrated to be due to interference from the G1 to S cell cycle transition (9). It was also shown that mTOR inhibition blocked protein synthesis through inhibition of the eukaryotic translation initiation factor, 4E binding protein-1 (4E-BP1), and through the 40S ribosomal protein p70 S5 kinase (8–11). The subtleties of this control system continue to be investigated (10,11). Other pathways dependent on mTOR activity include signaling through cyclin D3 and MYC, and angiogenesis (12,13). This potential for multiple levels of regulation led to further development of mTOR inhibition as an important mechanism for antiproliferative and anti-cancer therapy (8,14).

Just as downstream signaling affects the outcome of mTOR stimulation and mTOR inhibition, there are many upstream mTOR regulators that impact cellular function. Most relevant to cancer are Akt and *PTEN*. Akt is activated by phosphatidylinositol 3-kinase (PI3K), which in turn is controlled by *PTEN* (a tumor suppressor gene).

Aberrations of this entire series of regulatory interactions are identified in malignancies, and PTEN-inactivating mutations have been associated with more aggressive phenotypes (15). PTEN-mutated tumors have dysregulated mTOR activity and numerous other dysregulated pathways (15). In vitro studies demonstrate enhanced sensitivity of PTEN-deficient tumors to inhibition of mTOR, and this is being tested clinically (16,17). In addition, stimulation through insulin receptor signaling interacts with both the PI3K/Akt/mTOR pathway and PTEN (18).

More recently, it has become apparent that there are two binding complexes for mTOR: mTORC1 and mTORC2 (10,19–21). The mTORC1 complex is inhibited by the current agents in clinical use (22–24). This complex is composed of raptor, PRAS40, and mLST8. This complex is thought to primarily control protein translation through its effects on S6K1 and 4EBP1, which upon phosphorylation, lead to transcription and translation (22–24). This complex appears to be the major tumor-promoting pathway (19). However, it is important to recognize mTORC2 as well, which is a complex composed of rictor, proctor, mSINI, and mLST8 (21). mTORC2 activation has effects on actin cytoskeleton organization and appears to provide an escape regulatory route for additional Akt activation, following inhibition of mTORC1 (19–21).

■ CLINICAL ACTIVITY OF mTOR INHIBITION IN RCC

Two mTOR inhibitors, temsirolimus and everolimus, have been approved within the past 2 years for treatment of RCC. Both are chemical modifications of rapamycin (sirolimus) (23,24). In fact, temsirolimus is metabolized by serum esterases to sirolimus, the active moiety, while everolimus has activity as the intact molecule (23,24).

Temsirolimus is an intravenous preparation that in the phase I setting was evaluated at a weekly dose schedule and as a daily times 5 schedule every 2 weeks (25,26). In both phase I studies, partial responses were noted, including in RCC, breast cancer, non–small cell lung cancer, and in a neuroendocrine tumor. There was a broad dose range in the study of weekly dosing (7.5–220 mg/m^2/week), and there was no dose-limiting toxicity noted (25). Because the weekly dosing was very well tolerated, this schedule was utilized in phase II studies.

A large randomized phase II study of temsirolimus was conducted in metastatic RCC patients, who were previously treated with cytokines or were not eligible for cytokines (27). This study evaluated three flat dose levels of temsirolimus, 25 mg, 75 mg, and 250 mg, since no maximally tolerated dose had been identified in the phase I study of weekly administration. This study found all three doses tolerable, and most toxicity being grade 1 or 2. The most common grade 3 or 4 adverse events were hyperglycemia and anemia. The median time to progression was 5.8 months and the median overall survival was 15 months. Clinical benefit in terms of complete and partial response and stable disease greater than 24 weeks was observed in 51% of these patients (27).

In a retrospective analysis, stratifying patients by Memorial Sloan Kettering Cancer Center risk categories, it was observed that patients in the poor-risk category had a significantly better outcome than expected on the basis of historical controls. In fact, there was no difference in outcome among the three risk categories, unlike what was previously observed with interferon-treated patients (27). Thus, there was a suggestion of a potential role for mTOR inhibition in poor-risk patients who had progressed after cytokines or who were unlikely to benefit from cytokines (27). As a result, the pivotal phase III trial was conducted in poor-risk patients. In addition, a dose-response relationship was not observed in the phase II trial, and therefore, the phase III trial utilized a flat 25 mg per dose.

In the phase III trial, patients were randomized to temsirolimus alone, interferon alone, or a combination of temsirolimus and interferon, both given at lower doses than in the single-agent arms (22). As expected, both interferon-related and temsirolimus-related toxicities were observed, and both of the interferon-containing arms had greater toxicity than the temsirolimus alone arm (22). There were more dose adjustments and discontinuations in the interferon-containing arms. There was a significant survival benefit for temsirolimus compared to interferon in this poor-risk group of patients, with a hazard ratio for death of 0.73 ($P = 0.008$) (22). The median survival for the temsirolimus groups was 10.9 months compared to 7.3 months for the interferon group. This was the first clinical trial in RCC to demonstrate a survival benefit and led to approval of temsirolimus for treatment of patients with advanced RCC.

Of interest, in this study, unlike the studies with anti-angiogenesis inhibitors, patients with non–clear cell RCC were allowed. The histologic subtype was recorded at study entry, according to evaluation by the treating institutions. There was no central pathology review. Approximately 20% of patients entered were coded as non–clear cell RCC, with the majority being called papillary RCC. Among patients treated with temsirolimus, those patients with clear cell or other histologies had comparable median overall survival, 10.7 months for clear cell and 11.6 months for those with other histologies. For patients treated with interferon, those with histologies other than clear cell demonstrated a shorter median overall survival than did patients with clear cell histology, 4.3 months for other compared to 8.2 months for clear cell (28). This was consistent with previous impressions of the activity of cytokines in non–clear cell RCC. However, it was of interest that temsirolimus maintained activity in the non–clear cell histology patients.

Everolimus (RAD001) is an orally administered mTOR inhibitor that is administered as a single daily dose continuously. As a rapamycin analog, this agent was first used in solid-organ transplantation as immunosuppressive therapy. However, it has significant anti-tumor activity, which has directed its subsequent development. The development of this agent in RCC treatment occurred at a later date and after the regulatory approval of the VEGFR tyrosine kinase inhibitors sorafenib and sunitinib. As a result, it was evaluated in patients with RCC, previously treated with anti-angiogenesis therapy.

More specifically, the pivotal phase III trial enrolled metastatic RCC patients who had been previously treated and then progressed on treatment with an anti-VEGFR TKI (23). This study was placebo controlled, with a 2:1 randomization and the allowance of a cross-over to everolimus for patients who progressed on the placebo arm. In the report of the final results, the median progression-free survival was 4.9 months for the everolimus group compared to 1.9 months for the placebo group, with a hazard ratio of 0.33 ($P < 0.001$) (29). The median overall survival was 14.8 months for the everolimus group and 14.4 months for the placebo group, with 80% of patients in the placebo arm able to cross-over to everolimus. Further statistical analysis corrected the survival analysis (rank-preserving structural failure time model) and suggested a 1.9-fold longer survival with everolimus compared to placebo (29).

A third mTOR inhibitor (ap23573) (deforolimus, now called ridaforolimus) with activity against the TORC1 complex is also in clinical trials but not specifically in RCC (30). This agent is being evaluated as a single agent in sarcomas and brain tumors and has demonstrated activity. Clinical evaluation in combination with chemotherapy in more common tumors and in hematologic malignancies is ongoing.

■ EVALUATION OF COMBINATION THERAPY WITH CURRENT mTOR INHIBITORS

Developing combination therapy with the newer targeted therapies has not been straightforward. The combination of temsirolimus with interferon that was utilized in the phase III trial in RCC required that both agents be dose reduced, as determined by the phase I/II clinical trial that preceded the phase III trial (22,31). In addition, in RCC studies, combinations of temsirolimus with sunitinib were too toxic, and the tolerable combination of temsirolimus with sorafenib required dose reductions, as is currently being utilized in the ongoing Eastern Cooperative Oncology first-line RCC clinical trial.

However, both temsirolimus and everolimus have been successfully studied in combination with bevacizumab, a monoclonal antibody that binds to VEGF (32,33). This combination is directed toward an anti-angiogenesis approach as well as the other growth inhibiting properties of mTOR inhibition. Randomized trials are currently ongoing, comparing bevacizumab plus interferon-α to bevacizumab plus an mTOR inhibitor, either temsirolimus or everolimus. According to early phase II data, the combination does not appear to produce prohibitive toxicity (32,33), although in a recent report at the American Society of Clinical Oncology meeting, there were more dose interruptions with this combination compared to single-agent sunitinib (34). Nevertheless, these are important randomized trials in terms of evaluating both efficacy and safety.

As stated earlier, there are ongoing studies evaluating the safety and efficacy of the combination of mTOR inhibitors with chemotherapy, primarily in patients with tumors other than RCC (35–37). These combinations appear to be tolerable, and it is yet to be determined if these provide additive or synergistic efficacy (35–37).

■ INHIBITION OF OTHER COMPONENTS OF THE mTOR PATHWAY

Despite the fact reports indicate that the mTOR/Akt/PI3K signaling pathway is dysregulated in as many as 50% of human malignancies, the clinical trials of temsirolimus and everolimus to date in tumor types other than RCC have been of limited success (19,38). Ongoing laboratory work in preclinical models has demonstrated significant antitumor activity of mTOR inhibition with these agents. This has led to closer scrutiny of the signaling pathway components, and as noted in the introduction, the recognition of the formation of a second complex involving mTOR—mTORC2. It is now apparent that mTORC2 can provide positive regulation via hyperphosphorylation and activation of AKT via a feedback loop, and thus provide a potential proliferative escape even when mTORC1 is inhibited (19,39). In addition, mTORC2 can also provide feedback activation of PI3K and or ERK/MAPK signaling, again leading to activation of proliferative signals (39).

Based on the increased understanding of the PI3K/AKT/TOR pathway and the complex formation of mTORC1 and mTORC2, several strategies are currently under investigation, to attempt to block these pathways at multiple sites. One strategy that is entering clinical trials is dual mTORC1/mTORC2 blockade. The second strategy is to attempt vertical blockade of the PI3K/AKT pathway.

■ mTORC1 AND mTORC2 BLOCKADE

After preclinical investigations elucidated the complex interaction of mTORC1 and mTORC2 complexes, and the feedback phosphorylation of Akt leading to activation and mTORC1 inhibition

escape, the goal was to develop and investigate dual mTORC1 and mTORC2 inhibitors. The research group at Wyeth Research, developers of CCI-779, have recently reported activity of a newly developed dual inhibitor compound, WYE-132, and compared its activity in cell lines to that of CCI-779 (39). It has shown substantially stronger inhibition of cancer cell growth and survival, as well as stronger inhibition of protein synthesis, cell size, bioenergetic metabolism, and adaptation to hypoxia compared to CCI-779 (39). They have also investigated its potency in human xenograft models in tumor-bearing mice and have shown more potent single-agent antitumor activity against a variety of human tumors (39). They view these findings as substantiating the critical role of mTOR in tumor growth and proliferation, and that the more potent inhibition of mTOR complexes will have major effects on clinical outcome of cancer (39). Other compounds with similar activity are also in early clinical trials, such as OSI-027, which is being evaluated in phase I human clinical trials (40). These compounds have shown equivalent inhibition of downstream targets of mTORC1, such as S6K and 4EBP1, as the mTORC1 inhibitors, while also inhibiting the mTORC2 signaling loop to phosphorylated Akt/Scr473 (39,40). Phase I clinical data for OSI-027 was reported at the 2010 American Society of Clinical Oncology meeting and demonstrated clear pharmacodynamic activity in inhibition of downstream targets of both mTORC1 and mTORC2 (41). This initial study was conducted in patients with solid tumors and lymphomas who had failed numerous prior therapy. Stable disease lasting 12 or more weeks was reported. Dose-limiting toxicities reported were fatigue and decreased cardiac ejection fraction (41). Janes et al. evaluated the potency of two TORC1/2 inhibitors in a leukemia cell model harboring the Philadelphia translocation (41). PP242 delayed leukemia onset and seemed to potentiate current frontline tyrosine kinase inhibitors, and rapamycin did not produce these effects (41). This compound was less immunosuppressive than rapamycin (41). These types of preclinical studies will try to identify compounds that are able to separate the anti-tumor activities from the immunosuppressive activities and focus the former on cancer therapy.

■ TARGETING PI3K/Akt/TOR

The other promising strategy being investigated to inhibit the control produced by mTOR inhibition is what is called "vertical" inhibition, where the upstream signaling molecules are also inhibited. This has proven prohibitively toxic for much of the VEGFR pathway, but is being explored in the mTOR pathway (19). Two such compounds in preclinical and clinical development are BEZ235 and XL765. BEZ235 is a PI3K and Akt inhibitor that was reported in a phase I study at the 2010 American Society of Clinical Oncology meeting (42). Patients with a variety of solid tumors were treated, and this was a reasonably well-tolerated medication. There were responses observed in patients with PI3K pathway dysregulated tumors, such that this may be a very specific inhibitor (42). However, further evaluation is underway, as well as the development of a new formulation with improved bioavailability and pharmacokinetic properties (42). Additional preclinical data have been reported with this compound. There appears to be substantial anti-leukemic activity when evaluated in primary acute myeloid leukemia (AML) cells and human leukemic cell lines (43). There was significant inhibition of protein translation in AML cells, causing a reduction in proliferative rate and apoptosis (43).

XL765 (SAR245409) is a PI3K/TORC1/2 inhibitor and a phase I study was presented at the 2010 American Society of Clinical Oncology meeting (44). This compound is quite potent and selective and produces tumor inhibition in human xenograft models (44). Again, the downstream pharmacodynamic modulation demonstrates a major inhibitory effect.

The mechanism of resistance to mTOR inhibition is currently unknown. There is some evidence that deregulation of the PI3K and KRAS-signaling pathways may impact on sensitivity of tumors to the rapalog mTOR inhibitors (45). Although this requires further investigation, it is interesting to speculate that differential sensitivity to various components of the pathway may lead to varying degrees of sensitivity and resistance. Others have suggested that genetic variations in the PI3K-Akt-mTOR pathway impact on clinical outcome and sensitivity to the various inhibitors under investigation (46).

■ ROLE OF INSULIN-LIKE GROWTH FACTOR AND mTOR

In addition, there is interest in investigating the mTOR pathway as a metabolic pathway, with dysregulation of metabolic factors leading to tumor growth (3). The insulin-like growth factor family has been implicated in tumor development and growth, and mTOR is integral in the metabolism of both glucose and lipids (47). These growth factors play a major role in regulation of cell proliferation, differentiation, and apoptosis. Therefore, their interaction with mTOR is also critical to cell growth. Laboratory investigations suggest that mTOR inhibition can interfere or block insulin-mediated tumor progression (48). Others have linked the connection between malignancy and obesity through mTOR signaling. Further investigation is clearly needed.

■ SUMMARY

In summary, mTOR is a key signaling protein involved in cancer development and proliferation. It is key to a number of cellular processes, related to nutrient metabolism, protein synthesis, proliferation, and angiogenesis. The pathway, both upstream and downstream, is complex and it appears that all components enter into the systematic development of many cellular aberrancies. We look forward to the next generation of clinical trials focused on the mTOR pathway in an attempt to improve efficacy and sort out the most critical components of this signaling pathway.

■ REFERENCES

1. Hutson T. VEGF directed therapies. In: Stadler W (ed). *Emerging Cancer Therapeutics, Renal Cancer.* Chapter 8. New York: Demos Medical Publishing; 2010.

2. Yang JC, Haworth L, Sherry RM, et al. A randomized trial of bevacizumab, an anti-vascular endothelial growth factor antibody, for metastatic renal cancer. *N Engl J Med* 2003;349(5):427–434.

3. Meric-Bernstam F, Gonzalez-Angulo AM. Targeting the mTOR signaling network for cancer therapy. *J Clin Oncol* 2009;27(13):2278–2287.

4. Baker H, Sidorowicz A, Sehgal SN, Vézina C. Rapamycin (AY-22,989), a new antifungal antibiotic. III. *In vitro* and *in vivo* evaluation. *J Antibiot* 1978;31(6):539–545.

5. Sehgal SN, Baker H, Vézina C. Rapamycin (AY-22,989), a new antifungal antibiotic. II. Fermentation, isolation and characterization. *J Antibiot* 1975;28(10):727–732.

6. Luan FL, Hojo M, Maluccio M, Yamaji K, Suthanthiran M. Rapamycin blocks tumor progression: unlinking immunosuppression from antitumor efficacy. *Transplantation* 2002;73(10):1565–1572.

7. Husain S, Singh N. The impact of novel immunosuppressive agents on infections in organ transplant recipients and the interactions of these agents with antimicrobials. *Clin Infect Dis* 2002;35(1):53–61.

8. Hidalgo M, Rowinsky EK. The rapamycin-sensitive signal transduction pathway as a target for cancer therapy. *Oncogene* 2000;19(56):6680–6686.

9. Wiederrecht GJ, Sabers CJ, Brunn GJ, Martin MM, Dumont FJ, Abraham RT. Mechanism of action of rapamycin: new insights into the regulation of G1-phase progression in eukaryotic cells. *Prog Cell Cycle Res* 1995;1:53–71.

10. Choo AY, Yoon SO, Kim SG, Roux PP, Blenis J. Rapamycin differentially inhibits S6Ks and 4E-BP1 to mediate cell-type-specific repression of mRNA translation. *Proc Natl Acad Sci USA* 2008; 105(45):17414–17419.

11. Choo AY, Blenis J. Not all substrates are treated equally: implications for mTOR, rapamycin-resistance and cancer therapy. *Cell Cycle* 2009;8(4):567–572.

12. Yu K, Toral-Barza L, Discafani C, et al. mTOR, a novel target in breast cancer: the effect of CCI-779, an mTOR inhibitor, in preclinical models of breast cancer. *Endocr Relat Cancer* 2001;8(3):249–258.

13. Humar R, Kiefer FN, Berns H, Resink TJ, Battegay EJ. Hypoxia enhances vascular cell proliferation and angiogenesis *in vitro* via rapamycin (mTOR)-dependent signaling. *FASEB J* 2002;16(8):771–780.

14. Gibbons JJ, Discafani C, Peterson R, et al. The effect of CCI-779, a novel macrolide antitumor agent, on the growth of human tumor cells in vitro and in nude mouse xenograft in vivo. *Proc Am Assoc Cancer Res* 2000;40:301.

15. Tamura M, Gu J, Tran H, Yamada KM. PTEN gene and integrin signaling in cancer. *J Natl Cancer Inst* 1999;91(21):1820–1828.

16. Neshat MS, Mellinghoff IK, Tran C, et al. Enhanced sensitivity of PTEN-deficient tumors to inhibition of FRAP/mTOR. *Proc Natl Acad Sci USA* 2001;98(18):10314–10319.

17. Podsypanina K, Lee RT, Politis C, et al. An inhibitor of mTOR reduces neoplasia and normalizes p70/S6 kinase activity in Pten+/- mice. *Proc Natl Acad Sci USA* 2001;98(18):10320–10325.

18. Ozes ON, Akca H, Mayo LD, et al. A phosphatidylinositol 3-kinase/Akt/mTOR pathway mediates and PTEN antagonizes tumor necrosis factor inhibition of insulin signaling through insulin receptor substrate-1. *Proc Natl Acad Sci USA* 2001;98(8):4640–4645.

19. Wacheck V. mTOR pathway inhibitors in cancer therapy: moving past rapamycin. *Pharmacogenomics* 2010;11(9):1189–1191.

20. Foster KG, Fingar DC. Mammalian target of rapamycin (mTOR): conducting the cellular signaling symphony. *J Biol Chem* 2010;285(19):14071–14077.

21. Guertin DA, Sabatini DM. The pharmacology of mTOR inhibition. *Sci Signal* 2009;2(67):pe24.

22. Hudes G, Carducci M, Tomczak P, et al. Temsirolimus, interferon alfa, or both for advanced renal-cell carcinoma. *N Engl J Med* 2007;356(22):2271–2281.

23. Motzer RJ, Escudier B, Oudard S, et al. Efficacy of everolimus in advanced renal cell carcinoma: a double-blind, randomised, placebo-controlled phase III trial. *Lancet* 2008;372(9637):449–456.

24. Clackson T, Metcalf CCA, Rivera VM, et al. Broad anti-tumor activity of ap23573, an mTOR inhibitor in clinical development. *Proc Am Soc Clin Oncol* 2003;22:220: abst 882.

25. Raymond E, Alexandre J, Faivre S, et al. Safety and pharmacokinetics of escalated doses of weekly intravenous infusion of CCI-779, a novel mTOR

inhibitor, in patients with cancer. *J Clin Oncol* 2004;22(12):2336–2347.

26. Hidalgo M, Buckner JC, Erlichman C, et al. A phase I and pharmacokinetic study of temsirolimus (CCI-779) administered intravenously daily for 5 days every 2 weeks to patients with advanced cancer. *Clin Cancer Res* 2006;12(19):5755–5763.

27. Atkins MB, Hidalgo M, Stadler WM, et al. Randomized phase II study of multiple dose levels of CCI-779, a novel mammalian target of rapamycin kinase inhibitor, in patients with advanced refractory renal cell carcinoma. *J Clin Oncol* 2004; 22(5):909–918.

28. Dutcher JP, de Souza P, McDermott D, et al. Effect of temsirolimus versus interferon-alpha on outcome of patients with advanced renal cell carcinoma of different tumor histologies. *Med Oncol* 2009; 26(2):202–209.

29. Motzer RJ, Escudier B, Oudard S, et al. Phase 3 trial of everolimus for metastatic renal cell carcinoma: final results and analysis of prognostic factors. *Cancer* 2010;116(18):4256–4265.

30. Hartford CM, Desai AA, Janisch L, et al. A phase I trial to determine the safety, tolerability, and maximum tolerated dose of deforolimus in patients with advanced malignancies. *Clin Cancer Res* 2009;15(4): 1428–1434.

31. Motzer RJ, Hudes GR, Curti BD, et al. Phase I/II trial of temsirolimus combined with interferon alfa for advanced renal cell carcinoma. *J Clin Oncol* 2007;25(25):3958–3964.

32. Hainsworth JD, Spigel DR, Burris HA 3rd, Waterhouse D, Clark BL, Whorf R. Phase II trial of bevacizumab and everolimus in patients with advanced renal cell carcinoma. *J Clin Oncol* 2010;28(13):2131–2136.

33. Merchan JR, Liu G, Fitch T, et al. Phase I/II trial of CCI-779 and bevacizumab in stage IV renal cell carcinoma. Phase I safety and activity results. *J Clin Oncol* 2008;25:18s: abst 5034.

34. Escudier BJ, Negrier S, Gravis G, et al. Can the combination of temsirolimus and bevacizumab improve the treatment of metastatic renal cell carcinoma? Results of the randomized TORAVA phase II trial. *J Clin Oncol* 2010;28 (15s): abst 4516.

35. Perotti A, Locatelli A, Sessa C, et al. Phase IB study of the mTOR inhibitor ridaforolimus with capecitabine. *J Clin Oncol* 2010;28(30):4554–4561.

36. Phase Ib study of weekly mammalian target of rapamycin inhibitor ridaforolimus (AP23573; MK-8669) with weekly paclitaxel. *Ann Oncol* 2010;21:15–22.

37. Coiffier B, Ribrag V. Exploring mammalian target of rapamycin (mTOR) inhibition for treatment of mantle cell lymphoma and other hematologic malignancies. *Leuk Lymphoma* 2009;50(12):1916–1930.

38. Carracedo A, Pandolfi PP. The PTEN-PI3K pathway: of feedbacks and cross-talks. *Oncogene* 2008;27(41):5527–5541.

39. Yu K, Shi C, Toral-Barza L, et al. Beyond rapalog therapy: preclinical pharmacology and antitumor activity of WYE-125132, an ATP-competitive and specific inhibitor of mTORC1 and mTORC2. *Cancer Res* 2010;70(2):621–631.

40. Tan DS, Dumez H, Olmos D, et al. First-in-human phase I study exploring three schedules of OSI-027, a novel small molecule TORC1/TORC2 inhibitor, in patients with advanced solid tumors and lymphoma. *J Clin Oncol* 2010; 28, 15s, 2010.

41. Janes MR, Limon JJ, So L, et al. Effective and selective targeting of leukemia cells using a TORC1/2 kinase inhibitor. *Nat Med* 2010;16(2):205–213.

42. Burris H, Rodon J, Sharma S, et al. First-in-human phase I study of the oral PI3K inhibitor BEZ235 in patients with advanced solid tumors. *J Clin Oncol* 2010;28:15s (abst 3005).

43. Chapuis N, Tamburini J, Green AS, et al. Dual inhibition of PI3K and mTORC1/2 signaling by NVP-BEZ235 as a new therapeutic strategy for acute myeloid leukemia. *Clin Cancer Res* 2010; 16(22):5424–5435.

44. Brana I, LoRusso P, Baselga J, et al. A phase I dose-escalation study of the safety, pharmacokinetics and pharmacodynamics of XL765 (SAR245409) a PI3K/TORC1/TORC2 inhibitor administered orally to patients with advanced malignancies. *J Clin Oncol* 2010;28:15s (abst 3030).

45. Di Nicolantonio F, Arena S, Tabernero J, et al. Deregulation of the PI3K and KRAS signaling pathways in human cancer cells determines their response to everolimus. *J Clin Invest* 2010;120(8):2858–2866.

46. Chen M, Gu J, Delclos GL, et al. Genetic variations of the PI3K-AKT-mTOR pathway and clinical outcome in muscle invasive and metastatic bladder cancer patients. *Carcinogenesis* 2010;31(8):1387–1391.

47. Yu H, Rohan T. Role of the insulin-like growth factor family in cancer development and progression. *J Natl Cancer Inst* 2000;92(18):1472–1489.

48. Fierz Y, Novosyadlyy R, Vijayakumar A, Yakar S, LeRoith D. Mammalian target of rapamycin inhibition abrogates insulin-mediated mammary tumor progression in type 2 diabetes. *Endocr Relat Cancer* 2010;17(4):941–951.

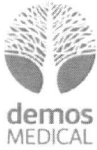

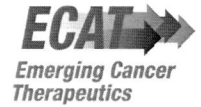

Emerging and Novel Therapeutic Targets in Renal Cancer

Kevin D. Courtney, Daniel C. Cho, and Toni K. Choueiri*

Kidney Cancer Program, Dana-Farber/Harvard Cancer Center, Boston, MA

■ ABSTRACT

For nearly 20 years, high-dose interleukin-2 (IL-2) was the only FDA-approved treatment offering potentially meaningful clinical benefit for a very small subset of patients with metastatic renal carcinoma. However, in the past 5 years, six new drugs have demonstrated improved progression-free survival (PFS) or overall survival (OS) and have been approved for the treatment of patients with advanced renal carcinoma. These new drugs fall into the general categories of tyrosine kinase inhibitors and antibodies that target vascular endothelial growth factor (VEGF) ligands and their receptors to impair angiogenesis, and analogues of rapamycin that inhibit mTOR and the translation of several proteins including VEGF and alter cancer cell proliferation and metabolism. The introduction of each of these new therapies was guided by our growing understanding of the proliferative and angiogenic signaling pathways underlying the pathogenesis of clear cell renal carcinoma. The challenge before us is to build on these successes to develop more potent inhibitors of these pathways with fewer and less severe associated toxicities and to identify new targets for intervention both within these signaling cascades and through independent processes that correlate with renal carcinoma viability. Here, we discuss such emerging and novel therapeutic targets for the treatment of renal carcinoma.

Keywords: angiogenesis, tyrosine kinase inhibitors, phosphatidylinostiol 3-kinase pathway, resistance, synthetic lethality

---

*Corresponding author, The Lank Center for Genitourinary Oncology, Dana-Farber Cancer Institute, DANA 1230, 450 Brookline Ave., Boston, MA 02215
   E-mail address: toni_choueiri@dfci.harvard.edu

Emerging Cancer Therapeutics 2:1 (2011) 145–156.
© 2011 Demos Medical Publishing LLC. All rights reserved.
DOI: 10.5003/2151–4194.2.1.145

■ INTRODUCTION

More than 57,000 new cases of kidney cancer and nearly 13,000 deaths related to kidney cancer were estimated to have occurred in the United States in 2009 (1). Conventional or clear cell renal carcinoma is the most common histologic subtype of kidney cancer, accounting for about 80% of cases. Cytotoxic chemotherapy is ineffective in the treatment of metastatic renal carcinoma, with response rates of less than 5% and no impact on overall survival (OS) (2,3). For two decades, immune modulating therapy, in the form of aldesleukin or interferon-α (IFN-α), was the principal treatment option. High-dose aldesleukin (interleukin-2, IL-2) can rarely cause durable complete responses (4,5) and remains a viable frontline treatment option for a highly select group of patients with favorable-prognosis metastatic disease. However, its application is limited by both its potentially severe toxicity and availability only in specialized centers. Furthermore, only a limited subset of patients appears to sustain benefit from immunotherapy (6).

Improved understanding of the pathogenesis of renal carcinoma, in particular the role of angiogenesis in kidney cancer, has led to a recent explosion in the development of targeted therapies for the treatment of patients with advanced disease. In particular, our growing understanding of the roles played by the von Hippel-Lindau tumor suppressor gene *VHL* and the phosphatidylinositol 3-kinase (PI3K)/mammalian target of rapamycin (mTOR) signaling pathway in regulating renal carcinoma growth and vascularization has spurred the generation of inhibitors with efficacy in the treatment of this cancer. *VHL* is silenced in most cases of sporadic renal carcinoma (7). A VHL-containing E3 ubiquitin ligase targets hypoxia-inducible factor α (HIFα) proteins for degradation under conditions of normal oxygen tension. Under hypoxic conditions, or if *VHL* function is silenced, HIFα proteins heterodimerize with HIFβ to promote transcription of multiple hypoxia-inducible genes involved in proliferation, angiogenesis, and

metabolism, including VEGF, platelet-derived growth factor (PDGF), epidermal growth factor receptor (EGFR), and many others (7). Sunitinib, sorafenib, and pazopanib are U.S. Food and Drug Administration (FDA)–approved multikinase inhibitors for the treatment of metastatic renal carcinoma. These tyrosine kinase inhibitors (TKIs) block receptors for VEGF and PDGF (including VEGFR-1, VEGFR-2, VEGFR-3, and PDGFR-β), to inhibit tumor angiogenesis. In addition, a combination of the anti-VEGF monoclonal antibody bevacizumab and IFN-α demonstrated efficacy in two phase III studies in the treatment of patients with metastatic renal carcinoma (8,9). Temsirolimus and everolimus are approved allosteric inhibitors of the mTOR/Raptor complex (mTORC1) (10). mTOR is a serine/threonine kinase in the phosphatidylinositol 3-kinase (PI3K) pathway that plays multiple critical roles in cell metabolism, proliferation, and survival, including regulation of HIF expression. While these approved agents can slow the progression of renal carcinoma and in some cases improve OS, the vast majority of patients will eventually experience disease progression (11–14). In addition, the toxicities associated with these treatments can be significant, Consequently, there remains a pressing need for additional and better therapeutic options for patients with metastatic renal carcinoma, both from the standpoint of efficacy as well as tolerability. Here, we will review novel agents for targeting these pathways and discuss new targets for intervention in renal carcinoma.

■ NOVEL TYROSINE KINASE INHIBITORS OF VEGFR FAMILY MEMBERS

Several TKIs designed to impede angiogenesis by blocking the activity of VEGFR family members are being evaluated in clinical trials. These therapies seek to improve on the toxicity profiles of approved agents such as sunitinib, pazopanib, and sorafenib without hopefully sacrificing efficacy.

Two novel TKIs, axitinib and tivozanib, have demonstrated efficacy and relative safety in the treatment of patients with metastatic renal carcinoma in large phase II studies and are under evaluation in phase III clinical trials. The clinical efficacy and side-effects profile of these two agents, as well as a discussion of other VEGFR TKIs under development, are reviewed extensively by Cowey and Hutson in Chapter 8 (15).

■ NOVEL ANTIBODY THERAPIES TARGETING VEGF AND VEGFR

Bevacizumab is an antibody against VEGF. Alternative antibody-based therapies are under evaluation and offer different approaches to targeting the VEGF-VEGFR axis. Ramucirumab (IMC-1121B) is a monoclonal antibody that recognizes VEGFR-2. A phase II trial of ramucirumab in 40 patients with metastatic renal carcinoma following failure or intolerance of TKI therapy showed a preliminary PFS of 6 months with good side-effects profile. Aflibercept is a fusion protein composed of extracellular domains of VEGFR-1 and VEGFR-2 with Fc of IgG1 (16,17). In a phase I study involving 38 patients with advanced solid tumors, including 9 with renal carcinoma, aflibercept was well tolerated and resulted in stable disease of ≥ 18 weeks in 18 patients (17). A phase II study of aflibercept with a planned enrollment of 120 patients with metastatic or unresectable kidney cancer is underway (clinicaltrials.gov ID: NCT00357760).

■ INHIBITORS OF PROTEINS INVOLVED IN SECONDARY RESISTANCE TO VEGF-TARGETED THERAPY

Determining the mechanisms by which tumors develop resistance to VEGF-targeted therapies ("adaptive" or secondary resistance) remains an area of active investigation (18). However, a number of potential mediators of resistance to antiangiogenic

therapies have already emerged from preclinical studies, several of which offer viable targets for therapeutic intervention.

The angiopoietins (ANG1, 2, 3, and 4) form a class of growth factors that interact with Tie receptor tyrosine kinases (19). The angiopoietin/Tie-signaling unit plays critical roles in vascular homeostasis. ANG1 was identified as a TIE2 agonist, whereas ANG2 was found to be a TIE2 antagonist (19). In a preclinical pancreatic islet tumor model, resistance to VEGFR2 inhibition was associated with resumption of angiogenesis and upregulation of angiopoietin, fibroblast growth factor (FGF), and ephrin family members (18). ANG1 activation promoted blood vessel survival and xenograft tumor growth in mice being treated with aflibercept to block VEGF (20). ANG2 inhibition has been shown not only to decrease tumor growth and the number of tumor-associated blood vessels but also to induce vascular normalization (21). Blockade of both ANG1 and ANG2 prevented this blood vessel normalization (21). This dichotomy has direct implications for therapeutic intervention by blocking the angiopoietin-TIE2 axis. Inhibition of VEGFR signaling results in vascular normalization, and there is evidence that ANG1 mediates the blood vessel normalization induced by blocking VEGF signaling (19,21). Consequently, it is possible that targeting ANG1 and ANG2 in the context of VEGF/VEGFR inhibition could impair both tumor neovascularization and VEGF-inhibition-induced vessel normalization with therapeutic effect. AMG 386 is a peptibody that blocks the interaction of ANG1 and ANG2 with TIE2 (22,23). A phase I study of 51 patients with advanced solid tumors evaluated the safety and efficacy of AMG 386 administered in conjunction with three different VEGF-targeted therapies: motesanib (AMG 706, a VEGF TKI), bevacizumab, or sorafenib. The combination of AMG 386 and sorafenib resulted in partial responses for 5 of 17 patients (29%) with renal carcinoma (22,23). A subsequent randomized phase II study of sorafenib with or without AMG 386 in patients with renal carcinoma who had received no prior VEGF-targeted treatment completed accrual (22,23). In addition, a phase II studies of sunitinib plus AMG 386 (clinicaltrials.gov ID: NCT 00853372) and a phase Ib/II trial of sunitinib +/– CVX-060 (a peptibody targeting ANG2; clinicaltrials.gov ID: NCT00982657) are ongoing.

As noted above, Casanovas and colleagues observed that expression of several FGF family members was induced following short-term VEGFR2 inhibition (18). The authors concluded that hypoxia-mediated changes in the expression of other proangiogenic proteins promoted resistance to VEGF/VEGFR pathway inhibition (18). Indeed, inhibition of FGF family signaling in conjunction with continued anti-VEGFR2 treatment impaired revascularization and tumor regrowth otherwise observed with resistance to VEGFR2 therapy (18). Dovitinib (TKI258), a TKI that inhibits FGFR1–3, as well as other RTKs, including VEGFR and PDGFR members, is being evaluated in a phase I/II study involving patients with refractory advanced and metastatic renal carcinoma (clinicaltrials.gov ID: NCT00715182). Preliminary data in VEGF TKI refractory patients showed that 2 of 20 patients experienced a PR, whereas 7 of 20 had stable disease with dovitinib treatment (24). In addition, BAY 73–4506 is an inhibitor of VEGFR, fibroblast growth factor receptor (FGFR), PDGFR, c-Kit, RET tyrosine kinases, Raf, mitogen-activated protein kinase (MAPK), and serine/threonine kinases that have been evaluated in a single-arm phase II study (clinicaltrials.gov ID: NCT00664326). The trial enrolled 49 patients with previously untreated advanced renal carcinoma. Preliminary results from 33 patients evaluable for efficacy showed 27% achieved a PR and 42% had stable disease with manageable side effects (25).

Hypoxia has been shown to activate transcription of the Met tyrosine kinase and to activate signaling through the Met ligand hepatocyte growth factor (HGF) in vitro 26. More recently, preclinical in vivo studies demonstrated that antiangiogenic treatment with sunitinib, a VEGFR2 antibody,

or the selective VEGFR inhibitor SU10944 promoted increased local tumor invasion and distant metastasis formation (27). This has led to the hypothesis that inhibition of VEGF signaling could lead to disinhibition of HGF/Met–mediated tumor invasion (27,28). In addition, Bommi-Reddy and colleagues performed a synthetic lethal screen employing multiple short hairpin RNAs (shRNAs) to preferentially kill *VHL*–/– renal cell carcinoma cell lines compared with isogenic lines in which VHL function had been reconstituted (29). Multiple shRNAs against Met were preferentially cytotoxic toward the *VHL*-deficient renal carcinoma cells (29). Consequently, Met presents another attractive therapeutic target in cancers that initially respond to antiangiogenic therapy.

Interleukin-8 (IL-8) has also been associated with resistance to antiangiogenic therapy. Employing human renal carcinoma cell lines in xenograft tumor studies, Huang and colleagues observed increased levels of secreted IL-8 following the development of resistance to sunitinib treatment (30). Introduction of an IL-8 antibody restored sunitinib sensitivity (30). Whether IL-8 will serve as a useful biomarker to predict sunitinib resistance or a viable therapeutic target in patients remains to be seen.

■ NOVEL INHIBITORS OF THE PI3K/ mTOR SIGNALING PATHWAY

Although drugs that target VEGF signaling have had a significant impact on the treatment of metastatic renal carcinoma, there are notable limitations to this approach. Although these agents impair angiogenesis, they appear to have little direct impact on the growth of renal carcinoma tumor cells. For example, using renal carcinoma xenografts, Huang and colleagues observed that sunitinib impaired tumor angiogenesis as early as 12 hours after beginning treatment but failed to significantly inhibit tumor-cell proliferation or promote apoptosis out to 3 days (31). One approach to impairing both cell autonomous renal carcinoma proliferation and survival and tumor angiogenesis is through targeted inhibition of the PI3K/mTOR signaling pathway. PI3K signaling is a critical regulator of normal cell proliferation, metabolism, vascularization, and survival. Constitutive activation of this pathway is a frequent event in human cancer, and several components of this signaling cascade offer targets for therapeutic intervention.

Class IA PI3Ks (hereafter referred to as "PI3K") are the most widely studied in mammalian systems and have been directly linked to cancer. Activation of certain RTKs by growth factor stimulation recruits PI3K to the plasma membrane, where it catalyzes the phosphorylation of phosphatidylinositol 4,5-bisphosphate (PI-4,5-P$_2$) to PI-3,4,5-P$_3$ (32,33). The tumor-suppressor phosphatase and tensin homolog deleted on chromosome 10 (PTEN) counters the activity of PI3K by dephosphorylating PI(3,4,5)P$_3$ to PI(4,5)P$_2$. PI(3,4,5)P$_3$ and PI(3,4)P$_2$ bind to pleckstrin homology (PH) domains of signaling proteins, including the serine/threonine kinases phosphoinositide-dependent kinase 1 (PDK1) and Akt (34). PI(3,4,5)P$_3$ binding stimulates PDK1 to phosphorylate and activate Akt (35–37). Akt regulates several proteins that mediate cell growth and survival. Included among these are the tuberous sclerosis complex TSC1/TSC2. Akt inhibits TSC1/TSC2-mediated negative regulation of Rheb (38). Rheb can then activate mTORC1 (39). Activated mTORC1 promotes synthesis through regulation of eukaryotic initiation factor 4E (eIF-4E) and p70 S6 kinase (p70S6K) (40,41). In addition, Akt can inhibit apoptosis through regulation of the Bcl-2 family member BAD, NF-kB, Mdms, and forkhead transcription factors (FOXO) (34,39,42).

The rapamycin analogues temsirolimus and everolimus block the activity of the mTOR-containing multiprotein complex mTORC1 and have been approved for use in the treatment of metastatic renal carcinoma (43). Although mTORC1 inhibitors typically offer only modest clinical benefit, our growing understanding of the PI3K/mTOR signaling axis provides insight into potential means to improve on the outcomes achieved

by rapamycin analogue treatment (41). For example, mTOR is present in two protein complexes within the cell, mTORC1 and mTORC2, that have distinct regulatory roles. Whereas mTORC1 relays signals downstream of PI3K/Akt, mTORC2 phosphorylate promotes Akt activation (44,45). Rapamycin analogues may not effectively inhibit mTORC2 activity (46). In addition, the mTORC1 target p70S6K can feedback to inhibit upstream activation of PI3K (47,48). Treatment with rapamycin analogues can block this negative feedback loop, which can lead to Akt activation (46). In addition, mTORC1 and mTORC2 have differential effects on HIF1α and HIF2α expression (41,49). Whereas HIF1α expression by renal carcinoma cells is dependent on both complexes, HIF2α expression relies on mTORC2 and is less sensitive to treatment with rapamycin (41,49). HIF2α appears to be the critical HIF species in clear cell renal carcinoma (41,50). Consequently, compounds that directly inhibit PI3K or Akt or are ATP-competitive inhibitors that block mTOR in both mTORC1 and mTORC2 may be more effective treatments for patients with renal carcinoma than rapaloges.

Several novel drugs that target the PI3K/Akt/mTOR signaling cascade are in preclinical development, and a number of these have entered clinical trials (51). They include pan-PI3K inhibitors that selectively block the catalytic subunit of multiple Class IA PI3Ks; isoform-specific PI3K inhibitors; dual PI3K-mTOR inhibitors; Akt active site inhibitors; allosteric inhibitors of Akt; and mTOR catalytic site inhibitors (51–54). These agents may be particularly effective in treating tumors that are dependent on PI3K pathway activation. However, in addition to the cell autonomous antiproliferative or cytotoxic potential of these drugs, PI3K inhibition has also been demonstrated to impair vascular development and tumor neovascularization (55,56). Consequently, these agents have generated excitement as potential novel therapies for renal carcinoma.

The potential efficacy of some of these novel PI3K pathway inhibitors in the treatment of renal carcinoma has been reported. Cho and colleagues observed that the dual PI3K/mTOR inhibitor NVP-BEZ235 was more effective than rapamycin (at doses at which both agents block S6 phosphorylation) at impairing proliferation of renal carcinoma cell lines both in vitro and in vivo (41). In addition, two phase II studies of the Akt inhibitor perifosine have demonstrated modest efficacy in the treatment of patients with renal carcinoma (57,58). Perifosine is a heterocyclic alkylphospholipid that is proposed to block Akt activity by disrupting membrane phospholipid binding (57,58). A trial involving 46 patients who had received prior treatment with either a VEGFR inhibitor (Group A, N = 31) or a VEGFR inhibitor and an mTOR inhibitor (Group B, N = 15) resulted in 1 PR in Group A and 1 in Group B, with 19 of 44 evaluable patients experiencing stable disease for greater than 12 weeks (58). The second study involved 24 patients with metastatic renal carcinoma who had failed prior sunitinib or sorafenib treatment. Two of 24 patients experienced a PR, and 10 had stable disease for more than 12 weeks, with a median PFS of 19 weeks (57).

■ NOVEL IMMUNOMODULATORY AGENTS

High-dose IL-2 remains a valid first-line option for a highly select group of patients with metastatic renal carcinoma. However, acute toxicities associated with high-dose IL-2 treatment can be severe and novel immunomodulatory agents are needed (4). Rosenblatt and McDermott provide an extensive review of conventional and novel immunotherapy approaches in Chapter 7 (59). Here, we briefly discuss two approaches to targeting tumor infiltrating immune cells that have generated particular excitement as potential renal carcinoma therapies.

Programmed Death 1 (PD-1) is an inhibitory receptor found on T and B cells that is proposed to suppress antitumor activity (60,61). The presence of PD-1-expressing tumor-infiltrating immune cells in patients with renal carcinoma is associated with poor clinical outcomes (61). The principal ligand for PD-1, B7-H1, is expressed by renal carcinomas and is also associated with aggressive tumors and decreased survival. Phase I clinical trials involving two different antibodies targeting PD-1 (MDX-1106 and ONO-4538) are recruiting patients with solid tumors, and a third (CT-011) is being evaluated in the treatment of myeloma (clinicaltrials.gov). Of 39 patients with advanced, refractory solid tumors enrolled in a phase I trial involving intermittent dosing of MDX-1106, one had renal carcinoma, and that patient experienced a PR with treatment (60). This was one of three responses (1 CR, 2 PR) reported (60). In addition, in a phase I study of biweekly MDX-1106 treatment in patients with advanced solid malignancies, 6 of 16 evaluable patients experienced objective tumor responses, including 2 patients with renal carcinoma.

Several studies in animal models investigating tumor-induced immune suppression and angiogenic escape have proposed that immature myeloid cells, characterized by coexpression of CD11b and Gr1, may play a critical role in the development of resistance to VEGF-targeted therapies (62). Shojaei and Ferrara recently showed that tumors resistant to VEGF-targeted therapy were associated with an increase in CD11b/Gr-1+ infiltrating cells compared with sensitive tumors (63). Therapeutic strategies that might deplete these myeloid cells or prevent their infiltration of tumor stroma are topics of active investigation.

■ EMERGING AND FUTURE THERAPEUTIC TARGETS

All of the therapeutic approaches described so far in this chapter take advantage of unique genotypic and phenotypic features of renal cell carcinoma. The development of novel VEGF-targeted therapies, PI3K/mTOR pathway inhibitors, and immunomodulatory agents builds on our current understanding of the underlying pathophysiology of renal carcinoma. In this section, we will introduce additional exciting new directions that may lead to effective treatments for metastatic renal carcinoma that extend beyond the broad categories previously introduced.

■ NOVEL TUMOR-ASSOCIATED ANTIGENS AS TARGETS FOR ANTIBODY-DEPENDENT CELL-MEDIATED CYTOTOXICITY

The ideal tumor-associated antigen (TAA) is one that is overexpressed exclusively at the membrane of the cancer cell of interest and not in normal tissue. Few TAAs have been identified in renal carcinoma that are sufficiently restricted in their expression as to provide viable therapeutic targets. Carbonic anhydrase IX (CAIX) is frequently overexpressed in clear cell renal carcinoma, a fact that has been exploited for both diagnostic and attempted therapeutic purposes (64,65). For example, a radiolabeled antibody recognizing CAIX has been used for detecting metastatic disease and as an antitumor agent in clinical trials involving patients with metastatic renal carcinoma (64,65). More recently, AGS-16 was identified as a novel transmembrane antigen expressed in kidney and liver cancers (66). AGS-16 was detected by immunohistochemistry in better than 90% or clear cell renal carcinoma samples (and 80% of papillary renal carcinomas) (66). A monoclonal antibody against AGS-16 was conjugated to monomethyl auristatin F, an antimicrotubule agent, to yield AGS-16M8F (66). AGS-16M8F demonstrated antitumor efficacy in vivo in renal carcinoma xenograft models and has entered phase I clinical testing in patients with advanced kidney cancer (clinicaltrials.gov ID: NCT01114230). Similarly, CD70 is highly expressed in renal cancer. SGN-75 is an antibody-drug conjugate (ADC) targeted to CD70. A phase I study in renal cancer and non-Hodgkin lymphoma was recently reported. The most common adverse events were fatigue, nausea, and peripheral edema (67). Best clinical response among RCC patients included one patient with a partial response, three patients with stable disease, and five patients with progressive disease (67).

■ NEW APPROACHES TO TARGETING HIFs

A central component of the pathogenesis of the majority of clear cell renal carcinomas is dysregulation of HIF signaling due to *VHL* loss of function. This provided the rationale for the use of rapamycin analogues that impair HIF translation and angiogenesis inhibitors that target VEGF species and their receptors in the treatment of renal carcinoma. Alternative approaches are being investigated to disrupt HIF function. These include promoting HIF degradation and disrupting HIF binding to DNA or coregulatory proteins to prevent transcriptional activation of HIF target genes (68). However, blocking protein degradation or preventing protein-protein interactions or DNA binding with necessary specificity to provide clinical utility poses a significant challenge (69).

The molecular chaperone Hsp90 has been shown to bind to HIF-1α, -2α, and 3α and is proposed to play a role in regulating the stabilization of HIF-α proteins as well as several other transcription factors and oncoproteins (68,70). Inhibition of Hsp90 was shown to promote proteasome-mediated HIF-1 degradation independent of VHL (68). Hsp90 inhibitors are in clinical development and have entered clinical trials (68). Histone deacetylases also regulate HIF activity and degradation (68,71). For example, the deacetylase sirtuin 1 (Sirt1) selectively stimulates HIF-2α-mediated transcription under hypoxic conditions (68,72). Histone deacetylase inhibitors are under clinical development and have entered clinical trials (clinicaltrials.gov). In addition, using small interfering RNA (siRNA) to decrease HIF levels is an attractive approach that is under investigation. Although effective delivery of siRNAs to tumor cells poses a challenge, novel methods to improve on this are being developed, and siRNAs have entered clinical trials in the treatment of solid tumors (clinicaltrials.gov). Although agents that promote HIF degradation warrant further investigation in the treatment of renal carcinoma, it should be noted that the proteasome inhibitor bortezomib failed to elicit a significant clinical response in a phase II study involving 37 patients with metastatic renal carcinoma (4 of 37 patients experienced a PR) (73).

A number of compounds that prevent HIF-1α DNA binding or HIF-1α/HIFβ dimerization have been described, as discussed in recent reviews by Onnis and colleagues and Koehler (68,69). For example, the antibiotic echinomycin inhibits HIF-1 binding to DNA with some degree of specificity (68). Although echinomycin failed to show significant clinical activity in phase I and phase II studies, it provides a proof-of-principle example that it may be possible to design small molecules to more selectively hinder transcription factor–DNA binding (68,69). Semenza and colleagues also recently identified acriflavine as a compound that binds HIF-1α and HIF-2α and prevents HIF-1 dimerization and impairs tumor growth in xenograft studies using mice (74).

When considering targeting HIF in the treatment of renal carcinoma, an important consideration is whether to block all HIF-α species or only HIF-2α. In many cancers, inhibition of HIF-1α blocks tumor growth and vascularization (71). However, there is growing evidence that in VHL-deficient tumors like most clear cell renal carcinomas, HIF-2α is the more critical HIF (75). For example, HIF-2α loss is sufficient to block the growth of VHL–/– tumors (75). Furthermore, in some circumstances, HIF-1α appears to have tumor-suppressor activity (76–78). For example, BNIP3 (Bcl-2/adenovirus E1B 19 kDa interacting protein 3) is a HIF-1α-inducible pro-cell death gene (78–80). BNIP3 expression correlates with hypoxia- or hypoxia-mimetic-mediated cell death in cancer cell lines (78–80). HIF-1α positively regulates BNIP3, while HIF-2α negatively regulates BNIP3 (78). HIF-1α also antagonizes the activity of the c-Myc oncoprotein in certain settings, in opposition to the role of HIF-2α (76). Interestingly, analysis of primary tumors from patients with renal carcinoma led to the identification of three subtypes of renal carcinoma distinguished by VHL and HIF-α expression: those expressing wild-type VHL protein (VHL WT), tumors deficient in VHL that express both HIF-1α and HIF-2α (H1H2), and VHL-deficient tumors that express only HIF-2α (H2) (76). Whereas VHL WT and H1H2 tumors showed activation of the Akt/mTOR and Erk/MAPK signaling pathways, proliferation of H2 tumors appeared to be driven by c-Myc activation. Characterization of the HIF status of renal carcinoma tumors from individual patients may therefore assist in tailoring an appropriate treatment regimen. Perhaps patients with VHL WT and H1H2 tumors will be better candidates for treatment with TKIs or PI3K/mTOR pathway inhibitors than those with H2 tumors (76,77).

■ DRUGS SELECTED FOR TOXICITY AGAINST VHL–/– CELLS

Two recent synthetic lethal screens identified novel targets that selectively impair the survival of *VHL*–/– renal carcinoma cells. Synthetic lethality makes use of combining two otherwise nonlethal mutations or conditions that are cytotoxic in combination (81). Bommi-Reddy and colleagues screened a short hairpin RNA (shRNA) library against 88 kinases in *VHL*-deficient renal carcinoma cells and in isogenic cells with reconstituted pVHL function (29). Following introduction of the shRNAs by lentiviral infection, cell viability was assayed and the relative cytotoxicity toward VHL–/– and VHL-restored cells was scored (29). VHL-deficiency was associated with increased sensitivity to depletion of a number of kinases. In particular, multiple shRNAs against the kinases cyclin-dependent kinase 6 (CDK6), MET, and MAP2K1 (MEK1) preferentially killed VHL-deficient renal carcinoma cells (29). Interestingly, the selective cytotoxicity imparted by depletion of these kinases was HIF-independent. Providing proof of principle for the potential clinical utility of this synthetic lethal screen, the authors also demonstrated that a small molecule inhibitor of CDK4/6 preferentially killed VHL-deficient cells (29). In a second screen for synthetic lethality with VHL-deficiency, Turcotte et al. screened 64,000 compounds against VHL-deficient and VHL-wild type renal carcinomas using a fluorescence-based approach (82). They identified the compound STF-62247 to be selectively toxic to VHL-deficient cells. STF-62247 was found to induce cell death via autophagy through a HIF-independent mechanism involving proteins associated with Golgi trafficking (82). STF-62247 is a 4-pyridyl-2-anilinothiazole that now serves as a lead compound for the development of possible clinically viable drugs (83).

■ REFERENCES

1. Society AC. *Cancer Facts & Figures 2009*. Atlanta: American Cancer Society; 2009.
2. Cohen HT, McGovern FJ. Renal-cell carcinoma. *N Engl J Med* 2005;353(23):2477–2490.
3. Coppin C, Le L, Porzsolt F, Wilt T. Targeted therapy for advanced renal cell carcinoma. *Cochrane Database Syst Rev* 2008:CD006017.
4. Fyfe G, Fisher RI, Rosenberg SA, Sznol M, Parkinson DR, Louie AC. Results of treatment of 255 patients with metastatic renal cell carcinoma who received high-dose recombinant interleukin-2 therapy. *J Clin Oncol* 1995;13(3):688–696.
5. McDermott DF, Atkins MB. Interleukin-2 therapy of metastatic renal cell carcinoma–predictors of response. *Semin Oncol* 2006;33(5):583–587.
6. Negrier S, Perol D, Ravaud A, et al.. Medroxyprogesterone, interferon alfa-2a, interleukin 2, or combination of both cytokines in patients with metastatic renal carcinoma of intermediate prognosis: results of a randomized controlled trial. *Cancer* 2007;110(11):2468–2477.
7. Kaelin WG Jr. The von Hippel-Lindau tumor suppressor gene and kidney cancer. *Clin Cancer Res* 2004;10(18 Pt 2):6290S–6295S.
8. Escudier B, Bellmunt J, Négrier S, et al. Phase III trial of bevacizumab plus interferon alfa-2a in patients with metastatic renal cell carcinoma (AVOREN): final analysis of overall survival. *J Clin Oncol* 2010;28(13):2144–2150.
9. Rini BI, Halabi S, Rosenberg JE, et al. Phase III trial of bevacizumab plus interferon alfa versus interferon alfa monotherapy in patients with metastatic renal cell carcinoma: final results of CALGB 90206. *J Clin Oncol* 2010;28(13):2137–2143.
10. Le Tourneau C, Faivre S, Serova M, Raymond E. mTORC1 inhibitors: is temsirolimus in renal cancer telling us how they really work? *Br J Cancer* 2008;99(8):1197–1203.
11. Escudier B, Eisen T, Stadler WM, et al. Sorafenib for treatment of renal cell carcinoma: final efficacy and safety results of the phase III treatment approaches in renal cancer global evaluation trial. *J Clin Oncol* 2009;27(20):3312–3318.
12. Hudes G, Carducci M, Tomczak P, et al.. Temsirolimus, interferon alfa, or both for advanced renal-cell carcinoma. *N Engl J Med*. 2007;356(22):2271–2281.
13. Motzer RJ, Escudier B, Oudard S, et al.. Efficacy of everolimus in advanced renal cell carcinoma: a double-blind, randomised, placebo-controlled phase III trial. *Lancet* 2008;372(9637):449–456.
14. Motzer RJ, Hutson TE, Tomczak P, et al. Sunitinib versus interferon alfa in metastatic renal-cell carcinoma. *N Engl J Med* 2007;356(2):115–124.
15. Cowey CL, Hutson TE. VEGF directed therapies. Emerging Cancer Therapeutics.
16. Holash J, Davis S, Papadopoulos N, et al. VEGF-Trap: a VEGF blocker with potent antitumor effects. *Proc Natl Acad Sci USA* 2002;99(17):11393–11398.
17. Tew WP, Gordon M, Murren J, et al. Phase 1 study of aflibercept administered subcutaneously to patients with advanced solid tumors. *Clin Cancer Res* 2010;16(1):358–366.
18. Casanovas O, Hicklin DJ, Bergers G, Hanahan D. Drug resistance by evasion of antiangiogenic targeting of VEGF signaling in late-stage pancreatic islet tumors. *Cancer Cell* 2005;8(4):299–309.
19. Augustin HG, Koh GY, Thurston G, Alitalo K. Control of vascular morphogenesis and homeostasis through the angiopoietin-Tie system. *Nat Rev Mol Cell Biol* 2009;10(3):165–177.
20. Huang J, Bae JO, Tsai JP, et al. Angiopoietin-1/Tie-2 activation contributes to vascular survival and tumor growth during VEGF blockade. *Int J Oncol* 2009;34(1):79–87.

21. Saharinen P, Bry M, Alitalo K. How do angiopoietins Tie in with vascular endothelial growth factors? *Curr Opin Hematol* 2010;17(3):198–205.

22. Rini BI. AMG 386 plus sorafenib in metastatic renal cell carcinoma. *Community Oncol* 2008;5:1–4.

23. Rini BI. New strategies in kidney cancer: therapeutic advances through understanding the molecular basis of response and resistance. *Clin Cancer Res* 2010;16(5):1348–1354.

24. Angevin E, Lin C, Pande AU, et al. A phase I/II study of dovitinib (TKI258), a FGFR and VEGFR inhibitor, in patients (pts) with advanced or metastatic renal cell cancer: Phase I results. *J Clin Oncol* 2010;28:abstr 3057.

25. Eisen T, Joensuu H, Nathan P, et al. Phase II study of BAY 73–4506, a multikinase inhibitor, in previously untreated patients with metastatic or unresectable renal cell cancer. *J Clin Oncol* 2009;27:abstr 5033.

26. Pennacchietti S, Michieli P, Galluzzo M, Mazzone M, Giordano S, Comoglio PM. Hypoxia promotes invasive growth by transcriptional activation of the met protooncogene. *Cancer Cell* 2003;3(4):347–361.

27. Pàez-Ribes M, Allen E, Hudock J, et al. Antiangiogenic therapy elicits malignant progression of tumors to increased local invasion and distant metastasis. *Cancer Cell* 2009;15(3):220–231.

28. Schmidt C. Why do tumors become resistant to antiangiogenesis drugs? *J Natl Cancer Inst* 2009;101(22):1530–1532.

29. Bommi-Reddy A, Almeciga I, Sawyer J, et al. Kinase requirements in human cells: III. Altered kinase requirements in VHL–/– cancer cells detected in a pilot synthetic lethal screen. *Proc Natl Acad Sci USA* 2008;105(43):16484–16489.

30. Huang D, Ding Y, Zhou M, et al. Interleukin-8 mediates resistance to antiangiogenic agent sunitinib in renal cell carcinoma. *Cancer Res* 2010;70(3):1063–1071.

31. Huang D, Ding Y, Li Y, et al. Sunitinib acts primarily on tumor endothelium rather than tumor cells to inhibit the growth of renal cell carcinoma. *Cancer Res* 2010;70(3):1053–1062.

32. Carpenter CL, Auger KR, Chanudhuri M, et al. Phosphoinositide 3-kinase is activated by phosphopeptides that bind to the SH2 domains of the 85-kDa subunit. *J Biol Chem* 1993;268(13):9478–9483.

33. Zhao L, Vogt PK. Class I PI3K in oncogenic cellular transformation. *Oncogene* 2008;27(41):5486–5496.

34. Cantley LC. The phosphoinositide 3-kinase pathway. *Science* 2002;296(5573):1655–1657.

35. Alessi DR, James SR, Downes CP, et al. Characterization of a 3-phosphoinositide-dependent protein kinase which phosphorylates and activates protein kinase B-alpha. *Curr Biol* 1997;7(4):261–269.

36. Currie RA, Walker KS, Gray A, et al. Role of phosphatidylinositol 3,4,5-trisphosphate in regulating the activity and localization of 3-phosphoinositide-dependent protein kinase-1. *Biochem J* 1999;337 (Pt 3):575–583.

37. Majumder PK, Sellers WR. Akt-regulated pathways in prostate cancer. *Oncogene* 2005;24(50):7465–7474.

38. Huang J, Manning BD. The TSC1-TSC2 complex: a molecular switchboard controlling cell growth. *Biochem J* 2008;412(2):179–190.

39. Engelman JA, Luo J, Cantley LC. The evolution of phosphatidylinositol 3-kinases as regulators of growth and metabolism. *Nat Rev Genet* 2006;7(8):606–619.

40. Cho D, Signoretti S, Regan M, Mier JW, Atkins MB. The role of mammalian target of rapamycin inhibitors in the treatment of advanced renal cancer. *Clin Cancer Res* 2007;13(2 Pt 2):758s–763s.

41. Cho DC, Cohen MB, Panka DJ, et al. The efficacy of the novel dual PI3-kinase/mTOR inhibitor NVP-BEZ235 compared with rapamycin in renal cell carcinoma. *Clin Cancer Res* 2010;16(14):3628–3638.

42. Duronio V. The life of a cell: apoptosis regulation by the PI3K/PKB pathway. *Biochem J* 2008;415(3):333–344.

43. Courtney KD, Choueiri TK. Updates on novel therapies for metastatic renal cell carcinoma. *Ther Adv Med Oncol* 2010;2:209–219.

44. Hresko RC, Mueckler M. mTOR.RICTOR is the Ser473 kinase for Akt/protein kinase B in 3T3-L1 adipocytes. *J Biol Chem* 2005;280(49):40406–40416.

45. Sarbassov DD, Guertin DA, Ali SM, Sabatini DM. Phosphorylation and regulation of Akt/PKB by the rictor-mTOR complex. *Science* 2005;307 (5712):1098–1101.

46. Meric-Bernstam F, Gonzalez-Angulo AM. Targeting the mTOR signaling network for cancer therapy. *J Clin Oncol* 2009;27(13):2278–2287.

47. Carracedo A, Pandolfi PP. The PTEN-PI3K pathway: of feedbacks and cross-talks. *Oncogene* 2008;27(41):5527–5541.

48. O'Reilly KE, Rojo F, She QB, et al. mTOR inhibition induces upstream receptor tyrosine kinase signaling and activates Akt. *Cancer Res* 2006;66(3):1500–1508.

49. Toschi A, Lee E, Gadir N, Ohh M, Foster DA. Differential dependence of hypoxia-inducible factors 1 alpha and 2 alpha on mTORC1 and mTORC2. *J Biol Chem* 2008;283(50):34495–34499.

50. Kondo K, Kim WY, Lechpammer M, Kaelin WG Jr. Inhibition of HIF2alpha is sufficient to suppress pVHL-defective tumor growth. *PLoS Biol* 2003;1(3):E83.

51. Yuan TL, Cantley LC. PI3K pathway alterations in cancer: variations on a theme. *Oncogene* 2008; 27(41):5497–5510.

52. Courtney KD, Corcoran RB, Engelman JA. The PI3K pathway as drug target in human cancer. *J Clin Oncol* 2010;28(6):1075–1083.

53. Garcia-Echeverria C, Sellers WR. Drug discovery approaches targeting the PI3K/Akt pathway in cancer. *Oncogene* 2008;27(41):5511–5526.

54. Ma WW, Adjei AA. Novel agents on the horizon for cancer therapy. *CA Cancer J Clin* 2009;59(2):111–137.

55. Graupera M, Guillermet-Guibert J, Foukas LC, et al. Angiogenesis selectively requires the p110alpha isoform of PI3K to control endothelial cell migration. *Nature* 2008;453(7195):662–666.

56. Yuan TL, Choi HS, Matsui A, et al. Class 1A PI3K regulates vessel integrity during development and tumorigenesis. *Proc Natl Acad Sci USA* 2008; 105(28):9739–9744.

57. Cho DC, Figlin RA, Flaherty KT, et al. A phase II trial of perifosine in patients with advanced renal cell carcinoma (RCC) who have failed tyrosine kinase inhibitors (TKI). *J Clin Oncol* 2009;27:5101 (abstr).

58. Volgelzang NJ, Hutson TE, Samlowski W, Somer BA, Richards PD, Sportelli P. Phase II study of perifosine in metastatic RCC (clear and non-clear) progressing after one prior therapy (Rx) with a VEGF receptor inhibitor. *ASCO 2009 Genitourinary Cancers Symp* 2009:302 (abstr).

59. Rosenblatt J, McDermott DF. IL-2 and other immunotherapy. Emerging Cancer Therapeutics.

60. Brahmer JR, Drake CG, Wollner I, et al. Phase I study of single-agent anti-programmed death-1 (MDX-1106) in refractory solid tumors: safety, clinical activity, pharmacodynamics, and immunologic correlates. *J Clin Oncol* 2010;28(19):3167–3175.

61. Thompson RH, Dong H, Lohse CM, et al. PD-1 is expressed by tumor-infiltrating immune cells and is associated with poor outcome for patients with renal cell carcinoma. *Clin Cancer Res* 2007;13(6): 1757–1761.

62. Shojaei F, Ferrara N. Refractoriness to antivascular endothelial growth factor treatment: role of myeloid cells. *Cancer Res* 2008;68(14):5501–5504.

63. Shojaei F, Wu X, Malik AK, et al. Tumor refractoriness to anti-VEGF treatment is mediated by CD11b+Gr1+ myeloid cells. *Nat Biotechnol* 2007;25(8):911–920.

64. Lamers CH, Sleijfer S, Vulto AG, et al. Treatment of metastatic renal cell carcinoma with autologous T-lymphocytes genetically retargeted against carbonic anhydrase IX: first clinical experience. *J Clin Oncol* 2006;24(13):e20–e22.

65. Stillebroer AB, Oosterwijk E, Oyen WJ, Mulders PF, Boerman OC. Radiolabeled antibodies in renal cell carcinoma. *Cancer Imaging* 2007;7:179–188.

66. Gudas JM, Torgov M, An Z, et al. AGS-16M8F: a novel antibody drug conjugate (ADC) for treating renal and liver cancers. *ASCO 2010 Genitourinary Cancers Symp*; 2010. abstr 328.

67. Ansell SM, Thompson JA, Infante J, et al. Targeting CD70 in non-Hodgkin lymphoma and renal cell carcinoma: a phase I study of the antibody drug conjugate SGN-75. *Ann Oncol* 2010;21:abstr 532P.

68. Onnis B, Rapisarda A, Melillo G. Development of HIF-1 inhibitors for cancer therapy. *J Cell Mol Med* 2009;13(9A):2780–2786.

69. Koehler AN. A complex task? Direct modulation of transcription factors with small molecules. *Curr Opin Chem Biol* 2010;14(3):331–340.

70. Katschinski DM, Le L, Schindler SG, Thomas T, Voss AK, Wenger RH. Interaction of the PAS B domain with HSP90 accelerates hypoxia-inducible factor-1alpha stabilization. *Cell Physiol Biochem* 2004;14(4–6):351–360.

71. Semenza GL. Defining the role of hypoxia-inducible factor 1 in cancer biology and therapeutics. *Oncogene* 2010;29(5):625–634.

72. Dioum EM, Chen R, Alexander MS, et al. Regulation of hypoxia-inducible factor 2alpha signaling by the stress-responsive deacetylase sirtuin 1. *Science* 2009;324(5932):1289–1293.

73. Kondagunta GV, Drucker B, Schwartz L, et al. Phase II trial of bortezomib for patients with advanced renal cell carcinoma. *J Clin Oncol* 2004; 22(18):3720–3725.

74. Lee K, Zhang H, Qian DZ, Rey S, Liu JO, Semenza GL. Acriflavine inhibits HIF-1 dimerization, tumor growth, and vascularization. *Proc Natl Acad Sci USA* 2009;106(42):17910–17915.

75. Kaelin WG Jr. SDH5 mutations and familial paraganglioma: somewhere Warburg is smiling. *Cancer Cell* 2009;16(3):180–182.

76. Gordan JD, Lal P, Dondeti VR, et al. HIF-alpha effects on c-Myc distinguish two subtypes of sporadic VHL-deficient clear cell renal carcinoma. *Cancer Cell* 2008;14(6):435–446.

77. Kaelin WG Jr. Kidney cancer: now available in a new flavor. *Cancer Cell* 2008;14(6):423–424.

78. Raval RR, Lau KW, Tran MG, et al. Contrasting properties of hypoxia-inducible factor 1 (HIF-1) and HIF-2 in von Hippel-Lindau-associated renal cell carcinoma. *Mol Cell Biol* 2005;25(13):5675–5686.

79. Farrall AL, Whitelaw ML. The HIF1alpha-inducible pro-cell death gene BNIP3 is a novel target of SIM2s repression through cross-talk on the hypoxia response element. *Oncogene* 2009;28(41):3671–3680.

80. Tracy K, Dibling BC, Spike BT, Knabb JR, Schumacker P, Macleod KF. BNIP3 is an RB/E2F target gene required for hypoxia-induced autophagy. *Mol Cell Biol* 2007;27(17):6229–6242.

81. Kaelin WG Jr. The concept of synthetic lethality in the context of anticancer therapy. *Nat Rev Cancer* 2005;5(9):689–698.

82. Turcotte S, Chan DA, Sutphin PD, Hay MP, Denny WA, Giaccia AJ. A molecule targeting VHL-deficient renal cell carcinoma that induces autophagy. *Cancer Cell* 2008;14(1):90–102.

83. Hay MP, Turcotte S, Flanagan JU, et al. 4-Pyridylanilinothiazoles that selectively target von Hippel-Lindau deficient renal cell carcinoma cells by inducing autophagic cell death. *J Med Chem* 2010; 53(2):787–797.

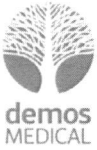

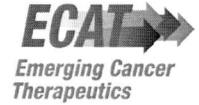

Management of Central Nervous System Metastases from Renal Cancer

Rimas V. Lukas*, Steven Chmura, and Martin Kelly Nicholas

University of Chicago, Chicago, IL

■ **ABSTRACT**

The central nervous system (CNS) is a frequent site for metastatic spread of renal cancer. The morbidity and mortality associated with CNS metastases is high. Surgery, radiation, and chemotherapy all play roles in the therapeutic management of CNS metastases. This review will address the existing data for the treatment of renal cancer CNS metastases. Symptom management will also be discussed.

Keywords: brain metastases, renal cancer, spinal cord compression, surgery, radiation, chemotherapy

■ **INTRODUCTION**

The central nervous system (CNS) is a common site of solid tumor metastases, associated with both high morbidity and mortality. Although less common than lung, breast, and melanoma, renal cancer (RC) is an important contributor to CNS metastases. In this review, we will cover the epidemiology of RC CNS metastases before delving into management. We will briefly touch on symptomatic management before discussing in greater detail therapeutic management and the roles of surgery, radiation (both whole brain [WBRT] and stereotactic radiosurgery [SRS]), and chemotherapy. Although the focus will center on brain metastases as these are the best studied, spinal cord and leptomeningeal metastases (LM) will also be discussed. The majority of data regarding RC involving the CNS deals with clear cell histology. Outcome-based reports that include other histologies are typically classified only as renal cancer. However, many believe that investigating CNS metastases in a histology-specific manner is important to the rational development of future therapies.

*Corresponding author, 5841 South Maryland Avenue, MC 2030, Chicago, IL 60637

E-mail address: rlukas@neurology.bsd.uchicago.edu

Emerging Cancer Therapeutics 2:1 (2011) 157–168.
DOI: 10.5003/2151–4194.2.1.157

■ EPIDEMIOLOGY

CNS metastases are thought to occur in approximately 10% to 30% of patients with solid tumors (1). The incidence appears to be increasing due to a number of factors. Overall survival rates are increasing in many cancers. There is thus more time for metastases to spread to other organs including the CNS. Furthermore, with improved survival, early previously undetected spread to the CNS may become apparent. In addition increased use of more sensitive imaging modalities may lead to earlier detection. Regarding CNS metastases in particular, conventional cancer screening tools such as whole body PET and CT scans of chest/abdomen/pelvis often miss clinically silent CNS disease. Indeed, many instances of presumed late metastases to CNS from solid tumors may have been present at diagnosis. A high percentage of patients have metastatic disease at diagnosis and many without metastases at presentation go on to develop them (2). Reports of the incidence of CNS metastases in patients with RC vary from < 2% to 11% (2–5). The highest incidence is from autopsy series and likely represents both clinically silent and late metastases. Rarely is the CNS involved as the solitary site (2,6). CNS metastases in RC usually develop metachronously (7). Unlike in lung and breast cancer, the relationship between diagnosis of the RC primary and the brain metastasis is less clear (8). There appears to be an association with increased stage at diagnosis and shorter interval to the development of brain metastases (7). The natural history of RC brain metastases can reflect potentially indolent disease (9).

The effect of brain metastases in RC on survival is significant. Untreated, the overall survival (OS) is between 1 and 3 months. This increases to approximately 8 months with radiation therapy (RT) and up to 13.8 months with surgery (10). This notable improvement in the surgical group is potentially due to selection bias. Patients undergoing surgical intervention are most often those with single brain metastases and stable systemic disease. Higher Karnofsky performance status (KPS),

younger age, controlled primary tumor, and fewer number of brain metastases have been demonstrated to be favorable prognostic factors for brain metastases from solid tumors in general (11,12). When looked at in a histology-specific fashion, KPS and the number of brain metastases were the most significant prognostic factors in RC (13). There is some controversy regarding the importance of systemic disease burden in overall prognosis of RC patients with brain metastases (14).

■ RADIOGRAPHIC DIAGNOSIS

The radiographic appearance of RC metastases is similar to those from other solid tumors (Figure 1). Like melanoma, there is an increased incidence of associated intracranial hemorrhage (ICH). Almost 50% of all RC brain metastases develop some degree of ICH (3). Symptomatic ICH is much lower at 9% (3). Noninfused head CT is a rapid

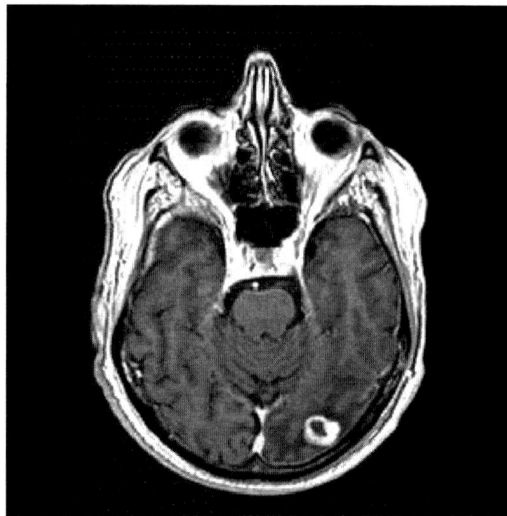

FIGURE 1

Renal cancer brain metastasis. A T1 post-contrast axial sequence MRI demonstrating a ring-enhancing lesion at the gray-white interface with surrounding peritumoral edema represented by the area of low signal subcortically surrounding the metastasis.

way to evaluate for intracranial hemorrhage or significant cerebral edema associated with brain metastases. MRI provides a more detailed picture and may detect metastases that would be below the resolution of CT imaging. Certain sequences such as the T2* and T1 precontrast have high sensitivity for evidence of prior ICH. There is no consensus on surveillance protocols for RC (2). Brain surveillance in asymptomatic patients is not recommended as part of standard evaluations (2).

■ SYMPTOMATIC MANAGEMENT

Symptomatic management of RC CNS metastases depends significantly on location of tumor as well as its associated edema. Neurologic symptoms can be classified in a number of ways. One way to categorize them is focal deficits and global deficits. Focal deficits are due to the location and size of tumor/edema. Global deficits are often due to increased intracranial pressure (ICP). These nonlocalizable deficits include headaches and decreased level of consciousness. Headaches associated with increased ICP are often more pronounced when lying down, may be present when first awakening in the morning, awake the patient from sleep, worsen with Valsalva, be associated with nausea and vomiting, and be associated with diplopia. Increased ICP is often due to significant cerebral edema and/or cerebrospinal fluid (CSF) involvement of malignancy causing decreased CSF reabsorption or blockage of CSF flow leading to hydrocephalus. Both focal and global tumor symptomatology are most often treated with steroids, often dexamethasone. There is no evidence to support the use of steroids in asymptomatic patients without mass effect. It is recommended that steroids be tapered slowly on an individualized basis (15). There is some evidence in brain metastases from solid tumors in general that response to steroids is a favorable prognostic factor (8). In acute scenarios, hypertonic agents such as mannitol or hypertonic saline can be used in the short term to decrease cerebral edema.

Of special note are symptoms caused by metastases in the spinal region. When discussing "spinal" metastases, it is important to clearly define the exact location of the lesion: spinal cord parenchyma versus paraspinal intradural metastases (as can be seen with CSF involvement) versus epidural (which can be seen in bony vertebral body involvement or in adjacent soft tissue). It is necessary for the treating physician to understand if there is nervous system involvement of cancer (cord or CSF) or if there are CNS symptoms due to mechanical effects of systemic cancer. This provides the overarching framework within which the acute decision making is made. It is important to evaluate the entire cord since, in approximately one third of patients with epidural cord compression, multiple sites are involved (16).

Whether the spinal cord pathology is due to CNS involvement of cancer or extra-CNS compression of the cord, the initial intervention is typically acute initiation of high-dose steroids. There is no specific data on RC-associated cord compression so the data we will refer to are for systemic cancer in general. The steroid most often used is dexamethasone. The only randomized trial evaluating the role of steroids in symptomatic cord compression due to solid tumors used very high-dose dexamethasone in combination with focal RT to 28 Gy (4 Gy fractions for 7 consecutive days). The group which received 96 mg intravenous (IV) dexamethasone followed by 24 mg four times a day for 3 days, followed by a taper, had a better ambulatory status at the conclusion of therapy and at 6 months compared with the patients who only received RT. There was only one patient with RC in the steroid arm and none in the RT-only arm (17). Other evaluations of high-dose (96–100 mg dexamethasone) versus moderate-dose (10–16 mg dexamethasone) steroids in similar settings found higher complication rates and no improvement in outcome with the higher doses (18,19). The role of surgery and RT in this setting will be discussed in the separate subsections.

Patients with central nervous system involvement of cancer are at increased risk of seizures. In patients with brain metastases who develop seizures, treatment with antiepileptic drugs (AEDs) is recommended. There are a number of AEDs which are appropriate. It is important for the clinician to consider efficacy of seizure control, side-effect profile, and interaction with other medications, particularly VEGF pathway inhibitors and anticoagulants. A number of the more traditional AEDs are inducers and inhibitors of the cytochrome p450 (CYP) system which is important in the metabolism of agents typically used in renal cancer (Table 1). For example, both sunitinib and sorafenib are substrates for CYP3A4. There is recent evidence supporting efficacy of seizure control and tolerability of newer non-enzyme-inducing AEDs such as levitaracetam in a solid tumor brain metastases population (20). Prophylactic AEDs for patients with brain metastases but no history of seizures are not recommended due to the limited data in this setting (21).

■ SURGERY

Focal therapies such as surgery and SRS should be considered in the setting of single or limited number of brain or spinal cord or paraspinal metastases. More than half of all RC patients with brain metastases have more than two lesions (14). In turn, a significant number of RC brain metastases patients would not be ideal candidates for focal therapies. The randomized data directly addressing the appropriate role for surgery is not specific for RC. The available level 1 evidence was obtained in unselected solid tumor metastases, the majority being from lung and breast cancer. We will first discuss the role for surgery in metastatic brain tumors from RC and then discuss the role of surgical intervention for spinal lesions in RC.

The first two prospective randomized trials looking at surgery for single brain metastases from solid tumors followed by WBRT to either 36 Gy

TABLE 1   Antiepileptic medication induction and inhibition of cytochrome p450 enzymes

Antiepileptic Medication	Enzyme Induction	Enzyme Inhibition
Carbamazepine	1A2, 2B6, 2C9, 2C19, 3A4	NA
Ethosuximide	3A4	3A4
Felbamate	3A4	2C19
Gabapentin	NA	NA
Lacosamide	NA	NA
Lamotrigine	NA	NA
Levitaracetam	NA	NA
Oxcarbazepine	3A4	2C19
Phenobarbital	1A2, 2A6, 2B6, 2C8, 2C9, 3A4	NA
Phenytoin	2B6, 2C8, 2C9, 2C19, 3A4	NA
Pregabalin	NA	NA
Primidone	1A2, 2B6, 2C8, 2C9, 3A4	NA
Tiagabine	NA	NA
Topiramate	3A4	2C19
Valproic acid	2A6	2C9, 2C19, 2D6, 3A4
Zonisamide	NA	NA

NA, not applicable.

(3 Gy × 12 fractions) or 40 Gy (2 Gy twice a day for total of 10 days) compared with WBRT alone demonstrated improved OS and functional independence. OS in the surgical arms was approximately 10 months in both studies compared with less than 4 to 6 months in the WBRT-only arms. Disseminated or progressive systemic disease was associated with poorer OS. These two studies included a limited number of patients with RC (4/63 in Vecht et al. and 2/48 nonspecified genitourinary in Patchell et al.) (22,23). A third randomized trial for single brain metastases comparing surgery followed by slightly lower dose WBRT (30 Gy, 3 Gy × 10 fractions) to WBRT alone found no benefit with the addition of surgery. This trial also included only a small number of RC patients (n = 3/41) (24). These studies appear to demonstrate that aggressive local control may improve OS; however, the state of systemic disease is an important variable in determining outcome.

In patients with good performance status, limited/stable extra-CNS disease, and a single resectable brain metastasis surgery followed by WBRT is recommended (25). These guidelines are based on the data from all solid tumors and are not specific to RC. In acknowledgement of this as well as RC's relative radioresistance, it can be reasoned that surgery may be of particular benefit in RC. More recently, there has been significant interest in the use of SRS alone in an attempt to avoid or delay the use of WBRT. However, patients with brain metastases from RC often have other systemic metastases, although this may not be as important a prognostic factor as it is in other solid tumors (13). One potential benefit of SRS over surgery is the potential to more quickly move forward with initiation of systemic chemotherapy, particularly with agents which have antiangiogenic mechanisms and in turn may be associated with delayed wound healing. Thus far, there have been no prospective trials specifically addressing the role of surgery for brain metastases from RC.

There has been comparison of surgery followed by WBRT versus SRS alone for patients with single solid tumor metastases. Poor accrual led to early termination of the study. Analysis of enrolled patients revealed no statistical difference in local tumor control (82% with surgery, 96.8% with SRS) but, unsurprisingly, poorer distant CNS tumor control in the SRS arm. At 1-year distant, recurrence in the brain was 3% in the surgery + WBRT arm compared with 25.8% in the SRS arm (P < 0.05). OS demonstrated no significant difference (9.5 months with surgery vs. 10.3 months with SRS). This trial included a higher percentage of patients (~15%) with nonspecified genitourinary cancer compared with the two previously discussed trials (26).

The role of surgery or other treatment modalities such as RT for the treatment of spinal cord lesions due to RC depends on the location of the metastases, as discussed in the section on Symptomatic Management. It is important to delineate whether the lesion is within the cord parenchyma itself (uncommon) versus in the CSF space causing compression of the cord versus in the extradural soft tissue versus within the bony structures of the vertebral column to allow for rational management. Intraparenchymal spinal cord lesions are most often addressed with focal RT, although surgery may be an option in select cases. The management of extraaxial lesions can include surgery and/or RT.

The lifetime incidence of extradural spinal cord compression in RC patients is higher than in many other tumor types and is estimated to be almost 20% (27). As in brain metastases, the sole randomized prospective study comparing surgery versus RT for spinal cord compression from metastatic cancer included patients with solid tumors with RC only composing a small proportion of patients included. Eleven of 101 patients had nonprostate genitourinary cancers with the exact histologies not specified. Patients with symptomatic epidural cord compression from a single lesion were randomized in nonblinded fashion to either surgical decompression of the cord followed by focal RT (30 Gy in 10 fractions) or focal RT alone. The primary endpoint of ambulatory rate after treatment (84% vs. 57%, P = 0.001) favored the surgical arm. This could be influenced by the slower response that would be expected with RT. Other endpoints, however, also favored surgery: OS (126 days vs. 100 days, $P = 0.033$), maintenance of continence (156 days vs. 17 days, $P = 0.016$), and duration of retained ability to walk (122 days vs. 13 days, $P = 0.003$) (28). The beneficial role of surgery + RT over RT may be more pronounced in relatively radioresistant tumors such as RC. However, this has not been clearly demonstrated in the literature (27). The surgical approach should be made on a case-by-case basis as data demonstrating clear superiority of one approach over others are lacking. The randomized data do not address the role for surgical intervention for spinal cord compression at multiple levels.

■ RADIATION THERAPY

Radiation therapy has long been a cornerstone of treating CNS metastases. WBRT was initially the modality most often employed as it can address multiple radiographically evident metastases as well as micrometastases which are beyond the resolution of our current imaging studies. There is evidence that metastases from RC respond to higher doses of RT or, alternatively, with modern particles and fraction sizes, a higher biologically effective dose (29). In turn, for relatively radioresistant tumors such as RC, there is significant ongoing investigation of alternate dosing and fractionation of radiation particularly for patients with single or oligometastases. Much of this has been performed using SRS as the treatment modality. The varying inclusion/exclusion criteria and differing RT schemes limit the comparability of many of these radiation studies.

We will begin our discussion with the role of WBRT. In patients with multiple brain metastases, this is the treatment modality most often employed. WBRT is most often administered in 3 Gy fractions to a total dose of 30 Gy. There have been conflicting data concerning improved outcomes with alternate dosing schedules for patients

with solid tumor brain metastases (30). The role of WBRT in RC specifically has only been evaluated retrospectively. Comparisons of 30 Gy in 10 fractions against higher dose schedules (40 Gy in 20 fractions and 45 Gy in 15 fractions) for patients with brain metastases from RC suggest improved 6-month and 12-month survival with the higher dose schedules (31). Another retrospective study comparing 30 Gy in 10 fractions with lower (5–20 Gy) and higher doses (36–40.05 Gy) demonstrated improved OS in the higher dose group (32). These studies are confounded by the factors which plague all retrospective studies, including unequal distribution of patient characteristics with prognostic significance. Currently doses of 30 to 40 Gy in 10 or 15 fractions appear to be the norm.

The role of radiation after surgical resection of a single brain metastasis has been evaluated in a randomized prospective trial. The majority of patients had non–small cell lung cancer with 8 (8.4%) of the patients having a nonspecified genitourinary cancer. Patients were randomized to receive WBRT to a comparatively higher dose of 50.4 Gy (1.8 Gy × 28 fractions) within 28 days of surgery. There was no significant improvement in OS (48 weeks vs. 43 weeks, $P = 0.39$) comparing WBRT with observation. There was, however, a significant decrease in neurologic death, yet interestingly no prolongation of independent functioning in the WBRT arm (33). The number of patients with genitourinary cancer is too small to draw any RC specific conclusions from this study. Since this pivotal trial, there has been continued reevaluation of the role of postsurgical RT. One recent single-institution retrospective study looking at patients with single brain metastases status post resection treated with WBRT (30 Gy in 10–15 fractions) versus without WBRT included a substantial number of patients with renal cancer (71/358, 20%), the majority of whom ($n = 70$) were not treated with WBRT based on the relatively radioresistant nature of the tumor. When looking at all histologies, it was noted that WBRT decreased recurrence at the initial tumor site as well as elsewhere in the brain. An improvement in OS (14.7

months vs. 11.7 months, P = 0.02) was also noted. The tumor histology did not affect the benefit found with the use of WBRT (34). Studies such as this one again support the concept of additional benefit of postsurgical RT. This must be tempered with the potential for delayed toxicity with WBRT for brain metastases. WBRT schedules with varying doses schedules have all been reported to have delayed CNS toxicity. This toxicity ranges from what appears to be relatively asymptomatic radiographic brain atrophy to a progressive syndrome of leukoencephalopathy. Oftentimes, the neurologic toxicity evolves over months to years. There is also evidence that progressive brain metastases are equally likely to cause neurocognitive and quality-of-life symptomatology as is WBRT (35–37). This is of particular importance when considering the role of WBRT in metastatic renal cancer which can often follow an indolent course.

Treating CNS metastases with single large fractions using SRS has been evaluated by a number of groups over a period of years. Favorable prognostic factors for patients with solid tumor brain metastases treated with SRS are similar to those treated with surgical resection of a single lesion and include limited number of brain metastases, good performance status, no additional systemic metastases, as well as limited size of the metastasis (< 10 mL) and SRS dose of > 18 Gy (38,39). RC is one of the tumor histologies where this treatment paradigm has most actively been investigated. As noted earlier, both the optimal and maximum number of lesions which can safely receive SRS is unknown. As the size of the lesion increases, the dose which can safely be administered decreases. As dose decreases, control rates may decrease as well. SRS role in the treatment of brain metastases has been evaluated alone, in combination with WBRT and in combination with surgery. Good local tumor control rates have been reported using SRS in all of the above settings. All of the studies were limited to single or oligometastases and in turn may not be applicable to patients with a greater number of brain metastases. The randomized controlled trial comparing SRS alone with

surgery followed by WBRT has already been discussed in the Surgery section of this chapter (26). The other randomized controlled trials of SRS in brain metastases have compared it with WBRT alone. Two of these studies added SRS to WBRT. There were only a small number of RC patients (2%–4%) in these trials. In the first of these trials, patients with two to four newly diagnosed brain metastases were randomized to WBRT (30 Gy in 12 fractions) versus WBRT + SRS (16 Gy at the margin) (40). In the second trial, patients with one to three newly diagnosed brain metastases were randomized to a higher dose of WBRT (37.5 Gy in 15 fractions) versus WBRT + SRS (15–24 Gy at the margin) (41). Neither study demonstrated a statistically significant improvement in OS. The first trial was closed early due to a significant benefit in local control in the SRS arm at the interim analysis. After 12 months, local failure was 100% in the WBRT-only arm and 8% in the WBRT + SRS arm (40). Subgroup analysis of the second trial showed improved OS in patients with single brain (as opposed to 2 or 3) metastases who received SRS (41). The other randomized controlled trial evaluating the role of SRS in brain metastases had a higher percentage of RC patients (7.6%). In this trial of patients with one to four brain metastases, SRS (18–25 Gy at the margin) alone was compared with WBRT (30 Gy in 10 fractions) + SRS. There was no significant improvement in OS in the combined modality group. However, there was a significantly higher risk of recurrence elsewhere in the brain in patients who did not receive WBRT (42). These studies again demonstrate that aggressive local therapy with SRS, similar to surgery, is effective; however, omitting whole brain radiotherapy leads to more failures throughout the brain. Thus, in patients who wish to pursue such a strategy, close follow-up with MRI to detect new lesions is appropriate.

For RC, specifically there are no randomized data evaluating the role of RT in the treatment of brain metastases. Most studies to look specifically at brain metastases from RC are nonrandomized evaluations of focal therapies. Local control rates of

69% to 100% have been reported for RC patients with single and multiple brain metastases in retrospective case series using SRS alone (38,43–45). The higher control rates reported may reflect on the frequency and duration of radiographic follow-up. Focal RT modalities, unsurprisingly, do not improve control elsewhere in the brain. Complete responses ranging from 11% to 27% have been reported. These have been seen predominantly in the smaller lesions (38,46). Prospective data examining SRS in patients with a limited number (1–3) of newly diagnosed brain metastases from relatively radioresistant histologies (45% with RC, n = 14/31) demonstrate more conservative control rates. By 6 months, one third of patients had failed within the RT field and one third of patients had failed elsewhere in the brain. Median OS was 8.3 months. SRS has demonstrated good local control after progression post-WBRT (47). However, clinicians should move forward with reirradiation with caution as it is associated with a higher likelihood of radiation necrosis (48).

Focal RT has long been used in the treatment of spinal cord lesions. The lower tolerability of the cord for radiation must be considered when making management decisions. A number of technical factors limit the use of SRS for the treatment of spinal cord lesions. Newer frameless SRS systems have expanded the options available for treating the spinal cord. The majority of clinical research regarding the role of RT in metastatic spinal cord lesions evaluates tumors causing epidural cord compression. Functional improvement is best seen in patients with very radiosensitive tumors such as lymphoma (49). Patients with bony compression of the cord are much less likely to be ambulatory post-RT (27% vs. 66%, P = 0.025) (27). RT does provide some clear benefits. Most patients experience improvement in their pain, and deterioration of clinical functioning after RT is rare (50). Benefit of surgical resection followed by RT compared with RT alone has been discussed earlier (28). The role of RT in asymptomatic patients with asymptomatic cord compression or patients at risk for cord compression is not clear (27). As is the case with

RT for brain metastases, studies of spinal cord compression use varying doses and schedules of RT. There is no clear benefit of one schedule over others (27). There is no prospective data concerning RT for spinal cord compression due exclusively to RC. The relative radioresistance of RC must be considered when weighing the data which looks at all tumor histologies.

■ SYSTEMIC THERAPY

The role for chemo- and other systemic therapies in brain metastases is limited and is typically considered only after surgery and RT. Median survival of solid tumor patients treated with chemotherapy at time of CNS progression is 3.5 to 6.6 months (51). Many trials evaluating chemotherapies exclude patients with CNS metastases. We will begin our discussion of chemotherapies for RC in the CNS with agents approved for RC and then delve only briefly into other agents.

Interferon-alpha 2a in combination with bevacizumab, a monoclonal antibody to VEGF, is approved for upfront treatment of metastatic RC. There has been concern for increased risk of ICH in patients treated with antiangiogenic agents including bevacizumab. This agent has been used safely in highly vascular primary brain tumors such as glioblastoma (52). Review of data from a number of different solid tumor trials using bevacizumab found similar rates of ICH in patients with or without brain metastases (53). There have been no specific studies published prospectively evaluating the role of these agents in brain metastases from RC. Interferons are capable of crossing the blood–brain barrier (BBB). While bevacizumab does not cross the BBB in significant concentrations, this is of less significance as its effect is mediated by interactions on the luminal side of the vessels. As with all antiangiogenic agents, there is potential to significantly decrease cerebral edema and in turn improve symptomatology. This is a combination which warrants additional exploration in the treatment of CNS metastases.

Two oral small molecule agents approved for RC with antiangiogenic effects, sunitinib and sorafenib, have been considered in the treatment of CNS metastases from RC. Caution must be taken in interpreting radiographic response in antiangiogenic agents as blockade of VEGF pathway is associated with a decrease in cerebral edema and enhancement. This not only alters the appearance of the imaging studies but also may provide clinical benefit by decreasing edema (54). Data regarding CNS concentrations of these agents is limited to animal studies. There is evidence that small molecule tyrosine kinase inhibitors can cross the BBB at effective concentrations.

Sunitinib is a multikinase inhibitor of VEGFR-1, -2, PDGFR-ά, -β, c-Kit, Flt-3, and RET. Animal studies demonstrate uptake of the agent into the CNS in mice, rats, and monkeys. On repeat dosing schedules, the concentrations in brain are lower than in other tissues and more comparable with serum concentrations (55). Clinically, there have been reports with sunitinib of sustained partial (PR) and complete responses (CR) of RC brain metastasis (56,57). There has been a report of its use in combination with RT to bulky disease in a patient with parenchymal brain metastases from RC as well as CSF involvement. Survival was only 4 months, which is comparable with reports of patients with other solid tumor CSF metastases (58). Prospective studies include a large expanded access trial in RC in which 321 patients (7%) had brain metastases. In the brain metastases subgroup, objective response was 12% with < 1% CR. More than half of the brain metastases patients had stable disease at 3 months and almost two thirds reported clinical benefit. These responses are slightly less than those seen in all patients on study. The OS was markedly lower in the brain metastases subgroup (9.2 months) compared with the overall OS (18.4 months). This likely reflects the poorer overall prognosis in this patient population. Importantly, the risk of ICH in this subgroup appears to be low (1/321, grades 1–2). Details of prior RT in this study were not reported (59). Although there may be potential benefit of sunitinib in existing brain metastases, there is retrospective evidence that it may not decrease the development of brain metastases in RC patients without CNS involvement (54). This differs from sorafenib, which may potentially decrease their incidence.

Sorafenib, another multikinase inhibitor of VEGFR-1, -2, -3, PDGFR-ά, Flt-3, c-Kit, RET receptor, and RAF is approved for treating RC. Similar to sunitinib, there has been prolonged PR reported for an RC patient with brain metastases treated with sorafenib (60). A case report of a patient with RC involving the dura with possible leptomeningeal involvement describes treatment with sorafenib. This resulted in a decrease in the size of the dural-based lesion which remained sustained at over 2.5 months (61). A large expanded access trial of sorafenib in RC included 70 patients (2.8%) with brain metastases. Two thirds of these patients demonstrated stable disease at 8 weeks, with 4% demonstrating PR, and no CR. There were no ICH reported in the brain metastases subgroup and < 1% in the overall population, echoing the findings in sunitinib (62).

Other agents for treating CNS involvement of RC have been looked at in more limited settings. Intrathecal administration has been attempted for RC LM without clear evidence of efficacy, for example (63).

■ CONCLUSIONS

RC involvement of the CNS is associated with a poor prognosis, and additional research into its treatment is needed. Current management of acute symptomatology often involves the use of steroids to decrease edema within the CNS. Focal therapies, both surgery and focal RT, are employed, if possible in treating focal CNS disease. There is growing evidence for a beneficial role of chemotherapies in treating RC-associated CNS disease. It will be important to investigate the currently available agents as well as future agents for their efficacy on CNS disease, particularly in the setting of concurrent systemic metastases.

■ REFERENCES

1. Aragon-Ching JB, Zujewski JA. CNS metastasis: an old problem in a new guise. *Clin Cancer Res.* 2007;13(6):1644–1647.

2. Janzen NK, Kim HL, Figlin RA, Belldegrun AS. Surveillance after radical or partial nephrectomy for localized renal cell carcinoma and management of recurrent disease. *Urol Clin North Am.* 2003;30(4):843–852.

3. Muacevic A, Siebels M, Tonn JC, Wowra B. Treatment of brain metastases in renal cell carcinoma: radiotherapy, radiosurgery, or surgery? *World J Urol.* 2005;23(3):180–184.

4. Harada Y, Nonomura N, Kondo M, et al. Clinical study of brain metastasis of renal cell carcinoma. *Eur Urol.* 1999;36(3):230–235.

5. Saitoh H. Distant metastasis of renal adenocarcinoma. *Cancer.* 1981;48(6):1487–1491.

6. Maor MH, Frias AE, Oswald MJ. Palliative radiotherapy for brain metastases in renal carcinoma. *Cancer.* 1988;62(9):1912–1917.

7. Nieder C, Spanne O, Nordoy T, Dalhaug A. Treatment of brain metastases from renal cell cancer. *Urol Oncol* 2009; doi:10.1016/j.urolonc.2009.07.004. [epub ahead of print].

8. Lagerwaard FJ, Levendag PC, Nowak PJ, Eijkenboom WM, Hanssens PE, Schmitz PI. Identification of prognostic factors in patients with brain metastases: a review of 1292 patients. *Int J Radiat Oncol Biol Phys.* 1999;43(4):795–803.

9. Lauretti L, Fernandez E, Pallini R, et al. Long term survival in an untreated solitary choroid plexus metastasis from renal cell carcinoma: case report and review of the literature. *J Neurooncol.* 2005;71(2):157–160.

10. Graham PH, Bucci J, Browne L. Randomized comparison of whole brain radiotherapy, 20 Gy in four daily fractions versus 40 Gy in 20 twice-daily fractions, for brain metastases. *Int J Radiat Oncol Biol Phys.* 2010;77(3):648–654.

11. Gaspar L, Scott C, Rotman M, et al. Recursive partitioning analysis (RPA) of prognostic factors in three Radiation Therapy Oncology Group (RTOG) brain metastases trials. *Int J Radiat Oncol Biol Phys.* 1997;37(4):745–751.

12. Sperduto PW, Berkey B, Gaspar LE, Mehta M, Curran W. A new prognostic index and comparison to three other indices for patients with brain metastases: an analysis of 1,960 patients in the RTOG database. *Int J Radiat Oncol Biol Phys.* 2008;70(2):510–514.

13. Sperduto PW, Chao ST, Sneed PK, et al. Diagnosis-specific prognostic factors, indexes, and treatment outcomes for patients with newly diagnosed brain metastases: a multi-institutional analysis of 4,259 patients. *Int J Radiat Oncol Biol Phys.* 2010;77(3):655–661.

14. Vogl UM, Bojic M, Lamm W, et al. Extracerebral metastases determine the outcome of patients with brain metastases from renal cell carcinoma. *BMC Cancer.* 2010;10:480.

15. Ryken TC, McDermott M, Robinson PD, et al. The role of steroids in the management of brain metastases: a systematic review and evidence-based clinical practice guideline. *J Neurooncol.* 2010;96(1):103–114.

16. Chamberlain MC, Kormanik PA. Epidural spinal cord compression: a single institution's retrospective experience. *Neuro-oncology.* 1999;1(2):120–123.

17. Sørensen S, Helweg-Larsen S, Mouridsen H, Hansen HH. Effect of high-dose dexamethasone in carcinomatous metastatic spinal cord compression treated with radiotherapy: a randomised trial. *Eur J Cancer.* 1994;30A(1):22–27.

18. Vecht CJ, Haaxma-Reiche H, van Putten WL, de Visser M, Vries EP, Twijnstra A. Initial bolus of conventional versus high-dose dexamethasone in metastatic spinal cord compression. *Neurology.* 1989;39(9):1255–1257.

19. Heimdal K, Hirschberg H, Slettebø H, Watne K, Nome O. High incidence of serious side effects of high-dose dexamethasone treatment in patients with epidural spinal cord compression. *J Neurooncol.* 1992;12(2):141–144.

20. Maschio M, Dinapoli L, Gomellini S, et al. Antiepileptics in brain metastases: safety, efficacy and impact on life expectancy. *J Neurooncol.* 2010;98(1):109–116.

21. Mikkelsen T, Paleologos NA, Robinson PD, et al. The role of prophylactic anticonvulsants in the management of brain metastases: a systematic review and evidence-based clinical practice guideline. *J Neurooncol.* 2010;96(1):97–102.

22. Patchell RA, Tibbs PA, Walsh JW, et al. A randomized trial of surgery in the treatment of single metastases to the brain. *N Engl J Med.* 1990;322(8):494–500.

23. Vecht CJ, Haaxma-Reiche H, Noordijk EM, et al. Treatment of single brain metastasis: radiotherapy alone or combined with neurosurgery? *Ann Neurol.* 1993;33(6):583–590.

24. Mintz AH, Kestle J, Rathbone MP, et al. A randomized trial to assess the efficacy of surgery in addition

to radiotherapy in patients with a single cerebral metastasis. *Cancer*. 1996;78(7):1470–1476.

25. Kalkanis SN, Kondziolka D, Gaspar LE, et al. The role of surgical resection in the management of newly diagnosed brain metastases: a systematic review and evidence-based clinical practice guideline. *J Neurooncol*. 2010;96(1):33–43.

26. Muacevic A, Wowra B, Siefert A, Tonn JC, Steiger HJ, Kreth FW. Microsurgery plus whole brain irradiation versus Gamma Knife surgery alone for treatment of single metastases to the brain: a randomized controlled multicentre phase III trial. *J Neurooncol*. 2008;87(3):299–307.

27. Loblaw DA, Perry J, Chambers A, Laperriere NJ. Systematic review of the diagnosis and management of malignant extradural spinal cord compression: the Cancer Care Ontario Practice Guidelines Initiative's Neuro-Oncology Disease Site Group. *J Clin Oncol*. 2005;23(9):2028–2037.

28. Patchell RA, Tibbs PA, Regine WF, et al. Direct decompressive surgical resection in the treatment of spinal cord compression caused by metastatic cancer: a randomised trial. *Lancet*. 2005;366(9486):643–648.

29. DiBiase SJ, Valicenti RK, Schultz D, Xie Y, Gomella LG, Corn BW. Palliative irradiation for focally symptomatic metastatic renal cell carcinoma: support for dose escalation based on a biological model. *J Urol*. 1997;158(3 Pt 1):746–749.

30. Gaspar LE, Mehta MP, Patchell RA, et al. The role of whole brain radiation therapy in the management of newly diagnosed brain metastases: a systematic review and evidence-based clinical practice guideline. *J Neurooncol*. 2010;96(1):17–32.

31. Rades D, Heisterkamp C, Schild SE. Do patients receiving whole-brain radiotherapy for brain metastases from renal cell carcinoma benefit from escalation of the radiation dose? *Int J Radiat Oncol Biol Phys*. 2010;78(2):398–403.

32. Cannady SB, Cavanaugh KA, Lee SY, et al. Results of whole brain radiotherapy and recursive partitioning analysis in patients with brain metastases from renal cell carcinoma: a retrospective study. *Int J Radiat Oncol Biol Phys*. 2004;58(1):253–258.

33. Patchell RA, Tibbs PA, Regine WF, et al. Postoperative radiotherapy in the treatment of single metastases to the brain: a randomized trial. *JAMA*. 1998;280(17):1485–1489.

34. McPherson CM, Suki D, Feiz-Erfan I, et al. Adjuvant whole-brain radiation therapy after surgical resection of single brain metastases. Neuro Oncol, 2010; doi: 10.1093/neuonc/noq005. [epub ahead of print]

35. DeAngelis LM, Delattre JY, Posner JB. Radiation-induced dementia in patients cured of brain metastases. *Neurology*. 1989;39(6):789–796.

36. Chang EL, Wefel JS, Hess KR, et al. Neurocognition in patients with brain metastases treated with radiosurgery or radiosurgery plus whole-brain irradiation: a randomised controlled trial. *Lancet Oncol*. 2009;10(11):1037–1044.

37. Movsas B, Bae K, Meyers C, et al. Phase III study of prophylactic cranial irradiation (PCI) versus observation in patients with stage IIInon-small cell lung cancer (NSCLC): Nuerocognitive and quality of life (QOL) analysis of RTOG 0214. ASTRO 2009 [Abstract]

38. Hoshi S, Jokura H, Nakamura H, et al. Gamma-knife radiosurgery for brain metastasis of renal cell carcinoma: results in 42 patients. *Int J Urol*. 2002;9(11):618–25; discussion 626; author reply 627.

39. Boyd TS, Mehta MP. Stereotactic radiosurgery for brain metastases. *Oncology (Williston Park, NY)*. 1999;13(10):1397–409; discussion, 1409.

40. Kondziolka D, Patel A, Lunsford LD, Kassam A, Flickinger JC. Stereotactic radiosurgery plus whole brain radiotherapy versus radiotherapy alone for patients with multiple brain metastases. *Int J Radiat Oncol Biol Phys*. 1999;45(2):427–434.

41. Andrews DW, Scott CB, Sperduto PW, et al. Whole brain radiation therapy with or without stereotactic radiosurgery boost for patients with one to three brain metastases: phase III results of the RTOG 9508 randomised trial. *Lancet*. 2004;363(9422):1665–1672.

42. Aoyama H, Shirato H, Tago M, et al. Stereotactic radiosurgery plus whole-brain radiation therapy vs stereotactic radiosurgery alone for treatment of brain metastases: a randomized controlled trial. *JAMA*. 2006;295(21):2483–2491.

43. Shuto T, Matsunaga S, Suenaga J, Inomori S, Fujino H. Treatment strategy for metastatic brain tumors from renal cell carcinoma: selection of gamma knife surgery or craniotomy for control of growth and peritumoral edema. *J Neurooncol*. 2010;98(2):169–175.

44. Muacevic A, Kreth FW, Mack A, Tonn JC, Wowra B. Stereotactic radiosurgery without radiation therapy providing high local tumor control of multiple brain metastases from renal cell carcinoma. *Minim Invasive Neurosurg*. 2004;47(4):203–208.

45. Payne BR, Prasad D, Szeifert G, Steiner M, Steiner L. Gamma surgery for intracranial metastases from renal cell carcinoma. *J Neurosurg*. 2000;92(5):760–765.

46. Mehta MP, Rozental JM, Levin AB, et al. Defining the role of radiosurgery in the management of

brain metastases. *Int J Radiat Oncol Biol Phys.* 1992;24(4):619–625.

47. Amendola BE, Wolf AL, Coy SR, Amendola M, Bloch L. Brain metastases in renal cell carcinoma: management with gamma knife radiosurgery. *Cancer J.* 2000;6(6):372–376.

48. Jagannathan J, Bourne TD, Schlesinger D, et al. Clinical and pathological characteristics of brain metastasis resected after failed radiosurgery. *Neurosurgery.* 2010;66(1):208–217.

49. Kim RY, Smith JW, Spencer SA, Meredith RF, Salter MM. Malignant epidural spinal cord compression associated with a paravertebral mass: its radiotherapeutic outcome on radiosensitivity. *Int J Radiat Oncol Biol Phys.* 1993;27(5):1079–1083.

50. Maranzano E, Latini P, Beneventi S, et al. Radiotherapy without steroids in selected metastatic spinal cord compression patients. A phase II trial. *Am J Clin Oncol.* 1996;19(2):179–183.

51. Ammirati M, Cobbs CS, Linskey ME, et al. The role of retreatment in the management of recurrent/progressive brain metastases: a systematic review and evidence-based clinical practice guideline. *J Neurooncol.* 2010;96(1):85–96.

52. Friedman HS, Prados MD, Wen PY, et al. Bevacizumab alone and in combination with irinotecan in recurrent glioblastoma. *J Clin Oncol.* 2009;27(28):4733–4740.

53. Besse B, Lasserre SF, Compton P, Huang J, Augustus S, Rohr UP. Bevacizumab safety in patients with central nervous system metastases. *Clin Cancer Res.* 2010;16(1):269–278.

54. Helgason HH, Mallo HA, Droogendijk H, et al. Brain metastases in patients with renal cell cancer receiving new targeted treatment. *J Clin Oncol.* 2008;26(1):152–154.

55. Haznedar JO, Patyna S, Bello CL, et al. Single- and multiple-dose disposition kinetics of sunitinib malate, a multitargeted receptor tyrosine kinase inhibitor: comparative plasma kinetics in non-clinical species. *Cancer Chemother Pharmacol.* 2009;64(4):691–706.

56. Koutras AK, Krikelis D, Alexandrou N, Starakis I, Kalofonos HP. Brain metastasis in renal cell cancer responding to sunitinib. *Anticancer Res.* 2007; 27(6C):4255–4257.

57. Zeng H, Li X, Yao J, et al. Multifocal brain metastases in clear cell renal cell carcinoma with complete response to sunitinib. *Urol Int.* 2009;83(4):482–485.

58. Dalhaug A, Haukland E, Nieder C. Leptomeningeal carcinomatosis from renal cell cancer: treatment attempt with radiation and sunitinib (case report). *World J Surg Oncol.* 2010;8:36.

59. Gore ME, Szczylik C, Porta C, et al. Safety and efficacy of sunitinib for metastatic renal-cell carcinoma: an expanded-access trial. *Lancet Oncol.* 2009; 10(8):757–763.

60. Valcamonico F, Ferrari V, Amoroso V, et al. Long-lasting successful cerebral response with sorafenib in advanced renal cell carcinoma. *J Neurooncol.* 2009; 91(1):47–50.

61. Ranze O, Hofmann E, Distelrath A, Hoeffkes HG. Renal cell cancer presented with leptomeningeal carcinomatosis effectively treated with sorafenib. *Onkologie.* 2007;30(8–9):450–451.

62. Stadler WM, Figlin RA, McDermott DF, et al.. Safety and efficacy results of the advanced renal cell carcinoma sorafenib expanded access program in North America. *Cancer.* 2010;116(5):1272–1280.

63. Tippin DB, Reeves W, Vogelzang NJ. Diagnosis and treatment of leptomeningeal metastases in a patient with renal carcinoma responding to 5-fluorouracil and gemcitabine. *J Urol.* 1999;162(1):155–156.

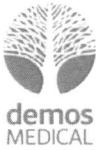

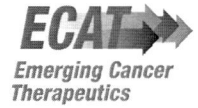

Evaluation and Management of Skeletal Metastases

Tessa Balach and Terrance D. Peabody*

University of Chicago Medical Center, Chicago, IL

■ ABSTRACT

Management of osseous metastases from kidney cancer presents treating physicians with unique challenges compared with those from other carcinomas. Evaluation of patients with bone disease includes x-rays with supplemental information provided by CT or MRI. Radiation therapy for management of local disease progression has proved to be unsuccessful, but may be useful as a treatment for pain from skeletal lesions. Embolization of lesions for which intralesional surgery is planned should be used to minimize intraoperative blood loss. In a patient with multifocal bone disease, intralesional curettage and internal fixation may be sufficient for skeletal stabilization. Solitary bone metastases should be resected with wide margins and reconstructed to facilitate rapid return to function and have a positive effect on disease progression. The treating surgeon must have knowledge of reconstruction techniques for various anatomic locations, such as the spine, humerus, femur, and tibia. Treating physicians must understand the unique characteristics of bony metastases from renal cell carcinomas to offer patients the best opportunity for skeletal stability, pain relief, and local disease control.

Keywords: carcinoma, kidney, surgery, resection, endoprosthetic reconstruction, embolization

*Corresponding author, Section of Orthopaedic Surgery and Rehabilitation Medicine, University of Chicago Medical Center, 5841 S. Maryland Ave, MC 3079, Chicago, IL 60637
E-mail address: tpeabody@surgery.bsd.uchicago.edu

Emerging Cancer Therapeutics 2:1 (2011) 169–182.
© 2011 Demos Medical Publishing LLC. All rights reserved.
DOI: 10.5003/2151–4194.2.1.169

■ INTRODUCTION

Metastases from renal cell carcinomas (RCCs) are common with 25% to 50% of patients having distant disease at the time of diagnosis. Bone is the second most common site of metastatic disease (1,2). Treatment goals for bone metastases, similar to that of other metastatic cancers, are management of pain, maintenance of function, and control of local disease progression. Unlike other carcinomas, however, the treatment of skeletal metastasis from kidney cancer presents treating physicians and surgeons with a different set of challenges, considerations, and therapeutic options.

Challenges have centered on the relative radioresistance of RCCs, the high recurrence rate of local disease that is not completely excised, and the historic lack of adequate systemic therapy to cure metastatic disease. These difficulties, along with morbidity associated with residual disease, have led surgeons to adopt a more aggressive approach to treatment of bone metastases, including, at times, a protocol focused on complete resection of lesions followed by reconstruction.

The effect of metastases on survival is not clear. Some studies have demonstrated a decreased length of survival in the presence of bony metastasis compared to patients with lung metastases alone (3–5). Others, meanwhile, have demonstrated that patients with metastatic disease involving bone alone have a better prognosis than those with pulmonary or visceral disease (6–8). These findings represent the unpredictable and uncertain natural history of metastatic kidney cancers.

Historically, the management of metastatic disease has included chemotherapy, cytokine therapy, and radiation. Improved treatment results and survival rates have been demonstrated with agents directed at vascular endothelial growth factor and mammalian target of rapamycin (see Chapters 8 and 9) (9,10). Despite these advances, there remain no curative systemic options for treatment of metastatic disease. The literature supports the idea that metastasectomy may have a role in overall management of disease burden, as well as providing a palliative benefit to the patient. Several groups have shown that patient survival is improved with complete resection of disease from all sources (7,8,11). A study performed at the Mayo Clinic demonstrated a 50% decrease in risk of death with complete resection of all sites of disease with 5-year survival of 49% compared to less than 20% survival in those with incomplete resection of disease (8). Though these data were based on resection of mostly solitary metastases, they underscore the potential benefit of complete metastasectomy on survival in these patients.

Metastases to bone can involve axial locations such as the pelvis and spine as well as appendicular sites like the femur and humerus. These lesions often cause significant pain and functional deficits requiring medical and often surgical intervention. The treatment of osseous metastases usually falls into one of four categories: observation, radiation alone, surgical stabilization, or resection with reconstruction. The treatment modality most appropriately applied is dependent upon several variables, including extent of local disease, resectability of lesions, the patient's overall condition, the ability to tolerate various surgical procedures, and the patient's expected survival. All patients' treatments are customized to manage their disease burden while maximizing pain relief and functional improvement. For example, observation of lesions in the upper extremity or spine may be prudent early in the course of treatment while the response to medical therapies is being measured. Alternatively, in a patient with solitary appendicular bone lesion, complete resection and reconstruction may offer the best outcome. Palliative management of impending fracture with intramedullary or internal fixation may be a useful alternative to complete resection and reconstruction in those patients who are medically unfit to undergo a more complicated procedure. Palliative treatment is also appropriate in cases where surgery is not an option for certain sites of disease that are neither resectable nor allow for reconstruction. Skeletal metastases in kidney cancers are common and a significant cause of morbidity. Their identification, evaluation, and management are essential in the treatment of associated symptoms and treatment of local disease.

■ EVALUATION OF SKELETAL METASTASES

Presentation

The most common mode of presentation of a patient with skeletal metastasis is pain in an extremity. Pain may be refractory to rest and exacerbated by activity, especially if the lesion is periarticular. Progressive pain that becomes present at all times, even at rest, should alert the physician that a large lesion with the possibility of impending fracture is likely.

Occasionally, a patient may present with a fracture through a pathologic lesion. This patient should be seen in an emergency department or outpatient office, routine fracture stabilization with splints or casts should be administered, and follow-up with an orthopedic surgeon should be arranged.

Metastatic lesions may be identified incidentally on routine imaging studies. Both staging studies and routine follow-up exams can identify lesions in the spine, proximal humerus, pelvis, and proximal femur. One should have a high degree of suspicion for the possibility of osseous metastasis, given their frequency in kidney cancers.

Regardless of their presentation, once identified, a patient with osseous metastases should be referred to an orthopedic surgeon for further evaluation and exploration of treatment options.

Radiologic Evaluation

X-Ray

Radiographic evaluation of a patient with musculoskeletal complaints is a simple, rapid, and cost-effective tool. All sites of pain should be imaged and evaluated for the presence of bony metastasis

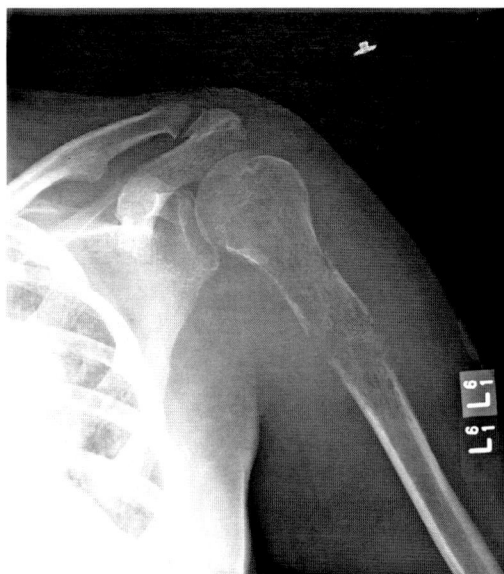

FIGURE 1

Anteroposterior x-ray of a patient with known kidney cancer who presented with left arm pain. This radiograph demonstrates a pathologic fracture through a permeative lesion with cortical destruction in the proximal humerus.

versus non-oncologic causes of pain (i.e., osteoarthritis). The entire bone should be evaluated radiographically to evaluate for multifocal disease within that bone. For example, a patient with complaints of hip pain should have x-rays of the entire femur. The x-ray appearance of lesions will typically be lytic or permeative with associated cortical expansion and destruction (Figure 1).

Although rare, a patient presenting with a new, solitary bone lesion in the absence of a diagnosis of a kidney cancer should be evaluated to determine whether this is a metastatic lesion or a primary bone tumor. The algorithm for evaluation of a solitary bone lesion in the absence of an oncologic diagnosis or in a patient with a remote history of cancer consists of laboratory examination, CT of the chest, abdomen, and pelvis, and a bone scan, as outlined by Simon and Bartucci (12) as well as Rougraff et al. (13). This method of assessment can identify the site of a primary carcinoma in 85%

with biopsy, identifying the carcinoma in another 8% of patients (13).

MRI

Although not completely necessary, MRI evaluation of a metastatic long bone lesion may provide the physician information about the extent of the lesion. This information may be helpful when resection and reconstruction are planned. When performed, an MRI for a metastatic lesion should evaluate the entirety of the involved bone, and the study should be performed with and without contrast to provide more detail about the soft tissue and intramedullary extent of tumor versus the reactive edema around the tumor.

MRI has the most utility in evaluating spine lesions and visualizing the mass effect of tumor on neurologic structures (Figure 2). These studies are essential when a patient presents with radicular symptoms such as radiating pain down the arm or leg consistent with spinal cord or nerve

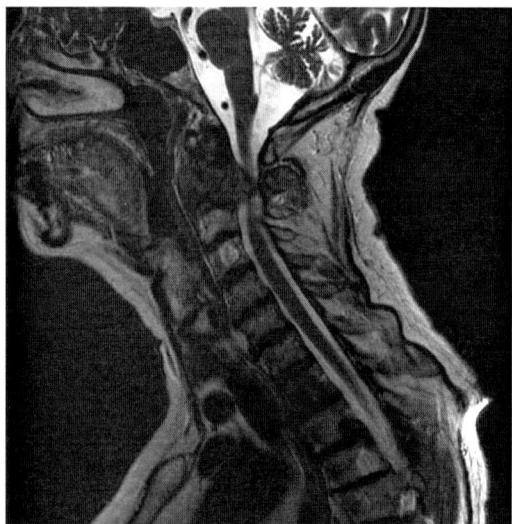

FIGURE 2
Cervical spine MRI of a patient previously treated with radiation to a cervical spine lesion. The MRI shows a mass within the vertebral body of C2 with extension into the spinal canal and encasement of the spinal cord.

root compression or if there is a concern for cauda equina syndrome, which can present with bilateral lower extremity weakness, saddle anesthesia, urinary retention, and bowel incontinence. MRI can provide great detail about the size of the lesion and its impingement on neurologic structures.

CT Scan

CT scans of metastatic lesions should be used for evaluation of those sites that are difficult to evaluate using plain radiographs, such as the spine, pelvis, and scapula. Detailed information garnered from a CT scan of the pelvis, for example, can provide the treating surgeon with information about periacetabular lesions that may alter a surgical plan made by evaluating plain x-rays alone.

When applied to evaluation of long bones, information from CT scans should be an adjunct and not a substitute for x-rays. These studies can provide more detailed information about the amount of cortical destruction and may provide information about an accompanying soft tissue mass. CT is superior to MRI or x-ray in providing important information about structural integrity and fracture risk. There are currently studies being conducted to evaluate the use of quantitative CT technology to predict fracture risk through bone lesions (14,15). The details of how such technology could be effectively applied to the cost-effective and routine evaluation of metastatic disease has not yet been completely evaluated.

Bone Scan

Radionucleotide bone scan is a part of the initial work-up and staging of a patient with a solitary bone lesion and selected other malignancies. Its role in the staging and evaluation of a patient with known kidney cancer is less important. Studies have confirmed the ability of radionucleotide bone scan to identify skeletal metastases in RCC (Figure 3). Several authors have examined the utility of bone scan in the evaluation of these patients. They have consistently shown that the routine use of bone scan is unnecessary given the fact that only a small number (one or two in each series)

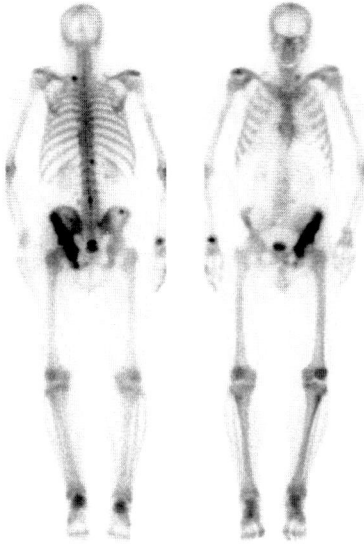

FIGURE 3

Bone scan of a patient with known metastatic kidney cancer. He presented with a left hip pathologic fracture. On the bone scan, metastatic lesions to the left pelvis, right iliac wing, upper thoracic spine, and the lumbar spine are seen.

identified lesions that were not already detected through other routine staging studies or via the presence of clinical signs (i.e., pain, fracture, neurologic symptoms) (16–20). Lindner et al. went so far as to say that "in no patient did the results of the scans influence or change the treatment plan" (20). Therefore, in the absence of skeletal complaints, bone scan has little utility in the routine evaluation of patients with RCC.

PET Scan

Positron emission tomography (PET) scans are becoming increasingly frequent in the evaluation, staging, and follow-up imaging of lymphomas and lung cancers. The application of this technology is currently being examined in the imaging of other carcinomas. While studies have demonstrated detectable activity with PET scan in the evaluation of metastatic RCC, the utility and efficacy of these studies in the evaluation of skeletal metastases are yet to be elucidated (21–23).

■ TREATMENT OF SKELETAL DISEASE

Skeletal metastases can be painful, disabling, and can contribute to the overall disease burden in a patient with kidney cancer. There are several modes of treatment for these lesions along with adjuvant therapies that may provide the orthopedic surgeon with tools to more effectively care for these patients.

Nonoperative Treatments

Radiation Therapy

Renal cancers have traditionally been thought of as being radioresistant relative to other malignancies. Halperin and Harisiadis demonstrated little improvement in symptoms and neurologic functions in their treatment of spinal cord compression (24). However, if effective, palliation of bone pain may be achieved for some months. In regard to eradication of metastatic skeletal disease, radiation therapy has no role.

Several studies have demonstrated that radiation therapy does little to affect disease progression. This finding may be related to the dose administered, suggesting that if radiation is to be an effective treatment, it should be administered at much higher doses such as those used for sarcoma. Groups like Tobisu et al. and Takashi et al. have demonstrated that surgical resection of metastatic lesions affords improved outcomes compared to radiation alone (7,25,26). In addition, other groups have shown that the addition of radiation therapy as an adjuvant to surgical treatment does little to affect local disease-free survival (3,27). Radiation therapy should be applied selectively with pain relief as its treatment goal.

Embolization

Bone metastases from renal cancers are notoriously hypervascular and surgical intervention on

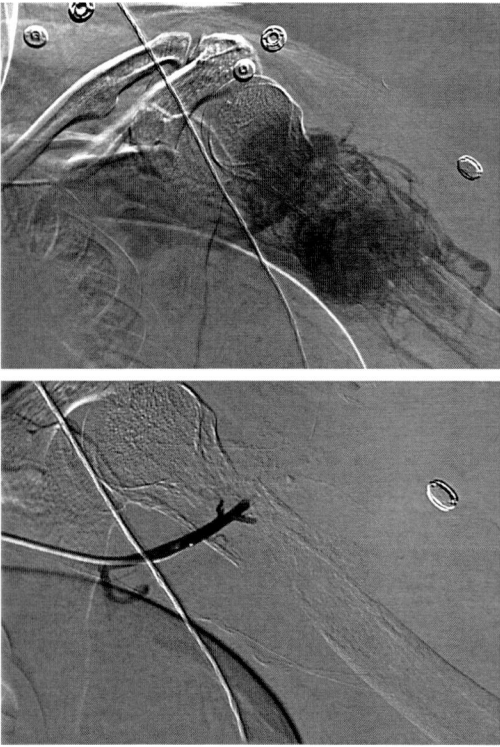

FIGURE 4

After the sudden onset of left arm pain, this woman with widely metastatic disease was found to have a pathologic fracture in the left humerus. Due to the extent of her disease, she was treated with preoperative embolization and intramedullary fixation of her fracture. The angiogram images demonstrate the large tumor blush and subsequent decrease in flow to the tumor after embolization.

such lesions can lead to significant blood loss. Embolization is an effective treatment for decreasing blood loss during the surgical resection of metastatic focus (28–32). Embolization is highly recommended for sites undergoing intralesional surgery, especially in the pelvis, spine, proximal femur, and humerus (Figure 4).

The goal of angiography and embolization of select arterial vessels should be to reduce tumor blush by at least 75% (29,32). The surgical procedure should follow within 24 hours of embolization to take maximum advantage of reduced blood flow

to the operative area. It has been demonstrated that flow to the area will begin to reconstitute through collateral vessels after 24 hours (32). Some authors caution against embolization for patients in whom a wide or radical resection is planned as it may increase blood flow to the area surrounding the embolized lesion (29).

There may be some role for embolization in the treatment of unresectable lesions. Barton et al. found success in providing pain relief in 11 cases of unresectable disease with pain relief lasting 2 to 8 months (29). While these finding also suggest embolization may not be useful for local disease control when used alone, the effectiveness of radiation in addition to embolization has not been studied extensively.

Embolization has proved to be a relatively safe procedure with few complications. There has been no evidence to support the development of a nonunion from ischemia due to embolization (30,32). When used for spinal lesions Manke et al. had no permanent neurologic deficits as a result of embolization (28). One of the most common side effects may be "postembolization syndrome" characterized by fever, pain, nausea, and vomiting. Symptomatic treatment is sufficient.

Operative Treatments

Multifocal Metastases

The disease burden in a certain patient and estimated life expectancy play a role in decision-making regarding treatment of skeletal metastases. Multiple bone and solid organ sites of disease have correlated with a poor prognosis and decreased survival rate compared to those with solitary bone metastases alone (3,5,33). In these situations, resection of all sites of disease with reconstructive procedures would be associated with significant morbidity for the patient.

Patients with multifocal disease who would benefit from surgical stabilization of impending fracture are candidates for internal fixation. Lin et al. achieved reasonable local control rates with curettage, cementing, and internal fixation equivalent to en block resection with reconstruction in their series. They caution that the small numbers in their study may not have been able to elucidate a difference (3). It can be extrapolated, though, that intralesional curettage and cementing in patients with multifocal disease may be adequate to offer some degree of local control (Figure 5). This local therapy combined with intramedullary or internal fixation would provide a means for skeletal stabilization in an area of impending fracture and pain relief from metastatic disease.

The treating oncologist and orthopedic surgeon should understand the indications for prophylactic fixation. Mirels' study is often referenced as a means of determining risk of pathologic fracture. This scoring system takes into account lesion size, pain, radiographic appearance, and size of the lesion. A score over 8 suggests risk of pathologic fracture, and prophylactic fixation is recommended (34). Over the years, many clinicians have found although the scoring system can suggest pathologic fracture, it is not absolute and must be considered in light of other clinical parameters (35–37). The other factors that would weigh into a decision regarding prophylactic fixation include functional status of the patient, anticipated life expectancy, and amount of cortical destruction.

Solitary Metastasis

In the treatment algorithms followed by many surgeons, patients with solitary osseous metastases are approached differently than those with multiple sites of disease. The goal in treating these patients is pain relief, maintenance of function, and prevention of local disease progression. It should be explicitly noted that the goal in treatment of these patients is not cure.

Currently, the mainstay of solitary bony metastasis is wide resection and reconstruction. Over the years, several groups have demonstrated improved local control and decreased rate of

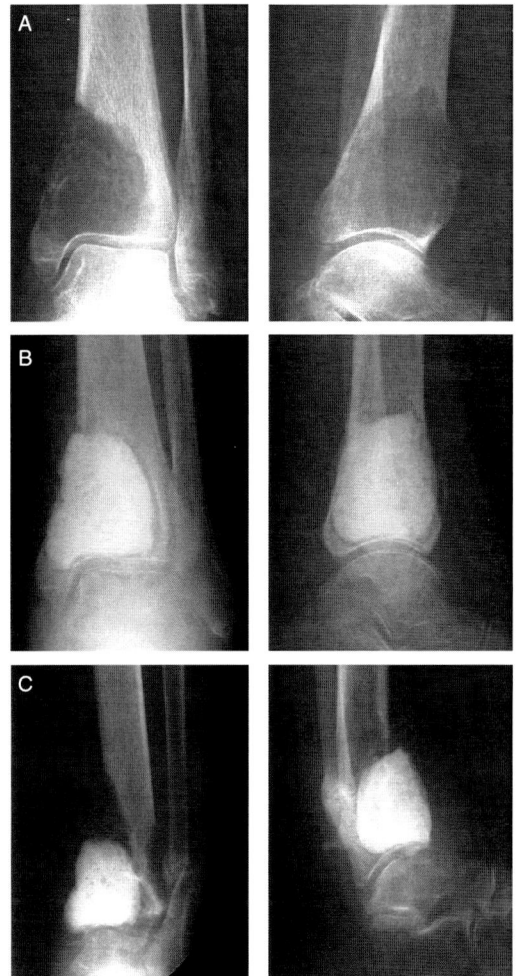

FIGURE 5
(A) Anteroposterior and lateral radiographs of the distal tibia demonstrating a lucent, expansile lesion of the distal tibia in a patient with metastatic RCC. The patient was taken to the operating room for curettage, intralesional adjuvant therapy with the argon beam coagulator, and placement of methylmethacrylate cement (B). Within 2 months of treatment, the lesion progressed to pathologic fracture (C). The patient's medical comorbidities were too significant to justify return to the operating room for stabilization.

reoperation in patients treated with resection and reconstruction compared to intralesional treatment and bony stabilization (3,5,7,27,38,39). Local recurrence in the face of intralesional surgery occurs commonly (27,38). Les et al. had a higher rate of return to the operating room and need for reoperation in their patients managed with intralesional surgery compared to their patients treated with resection (27). Fuchs et al. demonstrated a 15% implant failure rate as a result of local progression and advocated complete resection of a lesion with stable reconstruction in patients with solitary metastases (38).

Kollender et al. found resection and reconstruction with an endoprosthesis to be effective and safe for the treatment of skeletal instability, maintenance of function, and relief of pain in the setting of metastatic disease and asserted that "excising metastatic RCC of bone is associated with short hospital stay, good pain control, and functional outcome, as well as tolerable morbidity" (39). Takashi et al. also demonstrated improvement of Eastern Cooperative Oncology Group performance grade after surgical resection (7).

Survival rates after resection of solitary bone lesion vary from 35% to 60% at 5 years (6,8,38,40). Several authors have repeatedly demonstrated a survival advantage in patients with solitary disease who undergo resection of the metastatic focus (6,7,11,27,38,39,41). Whether this survival advantage is conferred through less aggressive tumor biology or an inherent advantage in the surgical procedure is yet to be determined conclusively (11,38).

Based on these available data and findings by the above authors, we recommend resection and reconstruction of solitary osseous metastases in an effort to maximize local control, preserve function, and possibly confer a survival advantage over treatment with intralesional procedures.

Anatomic Considerations

Resection and reconstruction are greatly dependent on anatomic location of a metastatic lesion and extent of bony involvement. Reconstruction is carried out in a similar fashion as for primary bone sarcomas.

Humerus

Proximal humerus lesions can be addressed with the use of a cemented proximal humerus replacement (42). Preservation of the deltoid and rotator cuff, if possible, will allow for improved postoperative function. If the tuberosities cannot be preserved, the endoprosthetic humeral head must be stabilized either through a capsular reconstruction with the remaining incised rotator cuff muscles or with synthetic vascular graft (Figure 6).

Diaphyseal lesions can be addressed with either endoprosthetic proximal or distal humerus replacement. The challenge in resection of mid-diaphyseal lesions is control and preservation of neurovascular structures.

Distal humerus lesions are best managed with endoprosthetic reconstruction in the form of a total elbow arthroplasty. Although range of motion and use of the arm is restored with adequate pain relief, the patient carries significant lifting and activity restrictions with the use of such endoprostheses. Lifting and carrying restrictions of 5 to 10 pounds are not uncommon.

Total humeral replacement can be considered the rare patient that has extensive disease within the humerus. Reconstruction incorporates principles

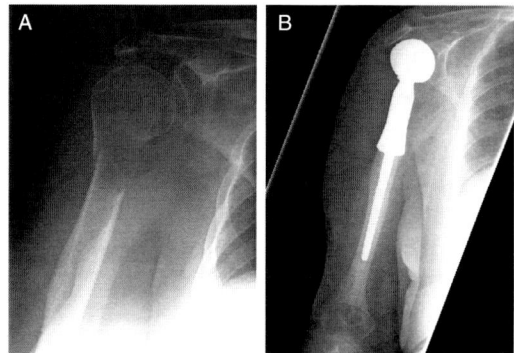

FIGURE 6

A 79-year-old woman presented with severe left arm pain for 1 week after turning over in bed. (A) Anteroposterior x-ray of pathologic fracture through a metastatic lesion in the proximal humerus. (B) Endoprosthetic reconstruction of the proximal humerus following resection.

inherent to proximal and distal humerus replacement. Stability must be achieved at both joints for the reconstruction to be successful. This would impose range of motion and activity restrictions for 6 to 8 weeks. Therefore, this procedure should be undertaken only in a patient whose expected survival allows for meaningful use of the extremity after recovery; otherwise, an alternative treatment should be sought.

Allograft reconstructions impose too many restrictions on patients to be useful in those with limited life expectancies whose main treatment goal is pain relief and near-immediate restoration of function. In addition, if radiation was used, the allograft reconstruction would be at high risk of failure.

Amputation for upper extremity lesions should be avoided, if at all possible. The functional loss resulting from an above elbow amputation or shoulder disarticulation to address a humeral lesion is significantly disabling. Amputation should be reserved for very limited indications such as symptomatic involvement of critical neurovascular structures by tumor that is refractory to other therapies, tumor fungation, infection, or intractable pain.

Spine

In addition to pain seen in the presence of bony metastases, lesions to the spine may present with neurologic dysfunction and decline with advancing disease. Beyond the goal of pain relief, spinal stability and preservation or restoration of neurologic function is of paramount importance in the treatment of these metastases.

Treatment of spinal metastases, according to several recent studies, has supported tumor resection and debulking, neural decompression, and stabilization (43–46). Current techniques often involve anterior or posterior approaches combined with vertebral reconstruction, stabilization, and instrumented fusion. Given the anatomic considerations of the spine and close proximity of vital neurovascular structures, wide resection, as would be possible in the extremities, is not always feasible.

In a series of 33 patients presented by King et al. pain relief was achieved in 88%, and 60% had improved neurologic function after surgical decompression and stabilization. They had a significant portion of nonambulatory patients regain their ability to walk and no cases of neurologic deterioration as a result of preoperative embolization (43).

When several series about surgical management of renal cell metastases to spine are reviewed, 78% to 100% experienced pain improvement and 60% to 75% of patients demonstrated neurologic improvement (4,43,46,47). Therefore, resection and decompression with accompanying stabilization procedures are effective in management of spinal metastases.

Femur

The femur is a particularly high-risk area for pathologic fracture, which is of great concern, given the significant impact on function a fracture would cause. Pathologic lesions in the proximal femur are at high risk for fracture with minor trauma. These lesions can be managed with hemiarthroplasty or proximal femur endoprosthetic reconstructions, depending upon the extent of the lesion (36,48). There is presently no role for allograft reconstruction of the proximal femur given the reliability and good function achieved with endoprosthetic reconstruction.

Bipolar hemiarthroplasty can be used to reconstruct lesions of the femoral head and neck. This procedure is commonly performed and associated with good functional outcomes. Currently, there is debate regarding the use of cement for stem fixation. A major concern in uncemented prostheses is the possibility of local disease progression and resultant loss of fixation (36). There have been no studies to compare outcome differences in cemented versus uncemented stems. It is our practice to cement all bipolar hemiarthroplasties in the setting of metastatic disease.

Proximal femur endoprosthetic reconstruction affords the surgeon the ability to achieve wide margins for local control while providing the patient with a functional hip (49). The resection of abductor musculature, however, puts the patient at increased risk for prosthetic hip dislocation. Capsular reconstruction with Gore-Tex graft or Mersilene tape may help to stabilize the prosthetic head within the native acetabulum and decrease the risk of dislocation. If the hip abductors are resected as part of the oncologic procedure, a Trendelenburg gait is unavoidable, and the patient should be informed of this prior to the procedure. If the abductor tendon is preserved, attachment to the proximal portion of the prosthetic stem can be attempted; however, function of the repaired abductor mechanism is unpredictable.

Whether a proximal femur is managed with hemiarthroplasty or proximal femur endoprosthesis, patients are allowed to weight bear as tolerated immediately, allowing them the opportunity for return to independent function as soon as possible.

Distal femur lesions are best managed with resection and distal femur endoprosthetic reconstruction with a rotating hinge knee (Figure 7) (50). Maintenance of the extensor mechanism is usually possible and is essential to a functional extremity. Distal femur reconstructions are historically durable and reliable and would allow the patient to return to full weightbearing immediately, compared to an allograft or allograft-prosthetic reconstruction.

Diaphyseal lesions of the femur can be addressed with a variety of techniques. Resection and reconstruction with either intercalary allograft (assuming no radiation therapy is planned) and intramedullary fixation or prosthetic intercalary segment is acceptable. If the lesion is more proximal or distal, reconstruction can be combined with proximal or distal endoprosthetic reconstruction.

Total femur resection and reconstruction with an endoprosthesis is rarely used but should be included in the surgeon's armamentarium of techniques for addressing complicated or very extensive lesions.

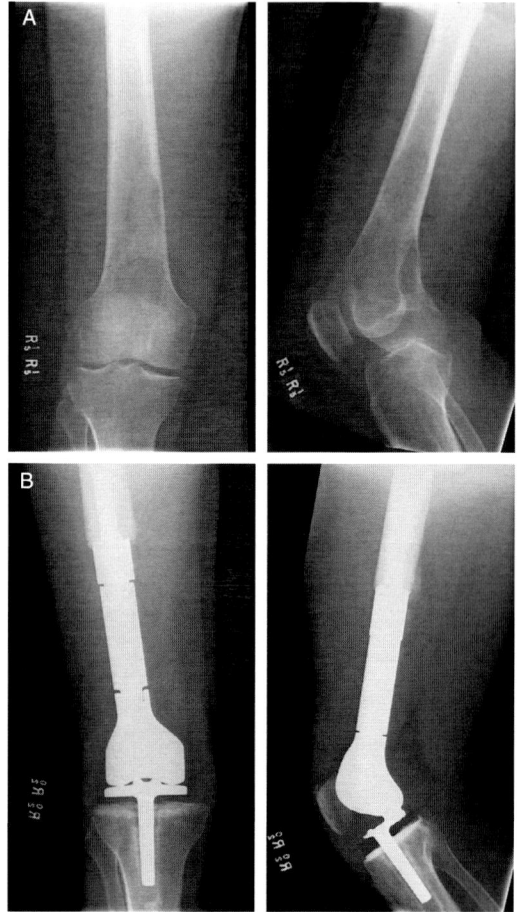

FIGURE 7

Anteroposterior and lateral radiograph (A) of the distal femur of a patient with 1-year history of knee pain. Work-up demonstrated a primary kidney cancer and single osseous metastasis. Resection of the metastatic lesion and reconstruction with distal femur endoprosthetic was performed (B).

Tibia

Lesions of the tibia, much like the femur, are at significant risk of fracture given the weightbearing nature of this bone.

Lesions involving the proximal metaphysis or diaphysis can be resected and reconstructed with an endoprosthetic proximal tibia (51,52). The unique challenge of these procedures is reconstruction of the extensor mechanism. It is well established in oncologic reconstruction of this region to maintain a portion of the patellar tendon and its attachment to the patella while using a medial gastrocnemius rotational flap to reconstruct the extensor mechanism. This necessitates immobilization with the leg in full extension for 6 weeks to allow for soft tissue healing, but the patient is allowed to resume full weightbearing immediately.

More distal lesions are less common; when they do occur, resection and reconstruction are a challenge. Wide resection in this area is difficult because of the proximity of neurovascular structures. Reconstruction is a challenge because of the small soft tissue envelope along with there being no good solutions for reconstruction of the distal tibia. In this situation, a below knee amputation would be a means of achieving a wide resection. Radiation alone or intralesional therapy with placement of cement and supportive internal fixation may be a better option than amputation. Therefore, treatment of distal tibia lesions should be individualized based upon functional status and life expectancy.

■ CONCLUSIONS

In contrast to metastatic disease from other carcinomas, treatment of osseous metastases in kidney cancers pose challenges in local control, maintenance of function, and pain control to treating physicians and surgeons. Efforts by many throughout the recent years have clarified treatment strategies to best care for these patients. Future advances in the medical management of systemic disease will help to improve long-term survival. Currently, the best outcomes are afforded to patients with solitary bone lesions who undergo wide resection and stable reconstruction.

■ REFERENCES

1. Skinner DG, Colvin RB, Vermillion CD, et al. Diagnosis and management of renal cell carcinoma. A clinical and pathologic study of 309 cases. *Cancer.* 1971;28(5):1165–1177.
2. Takashi M, Nakano Y, Sakata T, et al. Multivariate evaluation of prognostic determinants for renal cell carcinoma. *Urol Int.* 1993;50(1):6–12.
3. Lin PP, Mirza AN, Lewis VO, et al. Patient survival after surgery for osseous metastases from renal cell carcinoma. *J Bone Joint Surg Am.* 2007;89(8):1794–1801.
4. Jackson RJ, Loh SC, Gokaslan ZL. Metastatic renal cell carcinoma of the spine: surgical treatment and results. *J Neurosurg.* 2001;94(1 suppl):18–24.
5. Jung ST, Ghert MA, Harrelson JM, et al. Treatment of osseous metastases in patients with renal cell carcinoma. *Clin Orthop Relat Res.* 2003(409):223–231.
6. Fottner A, Szalantzy M, Wirthmann L, et al. Bone metastases from renal cell carcinoma: patient survival after surgical treatment. *BMC Musculoskelet Disord.* 2010;11:145.
7. Takashi M, Takagi Y, Sakata T, et al. Surgical treatment of renal cell carcinoma metastases: prognostic significance. *Int Urol Nephrol.* 1995;27(1):1–8.
8. Breau RH, Blute ML. Surgery for renal cell carcinoma metastases. *Curr Opin Urol.* 2010;20(5):375–381.
9. Escudier B, Eisen T, Stadler WM, et al. Sorafenib for treatment of renal cell carcinoma: Final efficacy and safety results of the phase III treatment approaches in renal cancer global evaluation trial. *J Clin Oncol.* 2009;27(20):3312–3318.
10. Motzer RJ, Hutson TE, Tomczak P, et al. Overall survival and updated results for sunitinib compared with interferon alfa in patients with metastatic renal cell carcinoma. *J Clin Oncol.* 2009;27(22):3584–3590.
11. Golimbu M, Al-Askari S, Tessler A, et al. Aggressive treatment of metastatic renal cancer. *J Urol.* 1986;136(4):805–807.
12. Simon MA, Bartucci EJ. The search for the primary tumor in patients with skeletal metastases of unknown origin. *Cancer.* 1986;58(5):1088–1095.
13. Rougraff BT, Kneisl JS, Simon MA. Skeletal metastases of unknown origin. A prospective study of a diagnostic strategy. *J Bone Joint Surg Am.* 1993;75(9):1276–1281.
14. Leong NL, Anderson ME, Gebhardt MC, et al. Computed tomography-based structural analysis for predicting fracture risk in children with benign

skeletal neoplasms: comparison of specificity with that of plain radiographs. *J Bone Joint Surg Am.* 2010;92(9):1827–1833.

15. Snyder BD, Hauser-Kara DA, Hipp JA, et al. Predicting fracture through benign skeletal lesions with quantitative computed tomography. *J Bone Joint Surg Am.* 2006;88(1):55–70.

16. Benson MA, Haaga JR, Resnick MI. Staging RCC. What is sufficient? *Arch Surg.* 1989;124(1):71–73.

17. Blacher E, Johnson DE, Haynie TP. Value of routine radionuclide bone scans in renal cell carcinoma. *Urology.* 1985;26(5):432–434.

18. Campbell RJ, Broaddus SB, Leadbetter GW, Jr. Staging of renal cell carcinoma: cost-effectiveness of routine preoperative bone scans. *Urology.* 1985; 25(3):326–329.

19. Seaman E, Goluboff ET, Ross S, et al. Association of radionuclide bone scan and serum alkaline phosphatase in patients with metastatic renal cell carcinoma. *Urology.* 1996;48(5):692–695.

20. Lindner A, Goldman DG, deKernion JB. Cost effective analysis of prenephrectomy radioisotope scans in renal cell carcinoma. *Urology.* 1983;22(2):127–129.

21. Middendorp M, Maute L, Sauter B, et al. Initial experience with 18F-fluoroethylcholine PET/CT in staging and monitoring therapy response of advanced renal cell carcinoma. *Ann Nucl Med.* 2010;24(6):441–446.

22. Nakatani K, Nakamoto Y, Saga T, et al. The potential clinical value of FDG-PET for recurrent renal cell carcinoma. *Eur J Radiol.* 2009, doi10.1016/j.erad2009.11.019.

23. Oyama N, Okazawa H, Kusukawa N, et al. 11C-Acetate PET imaging for renal cell carcinoma. *Eur J Nucl Med Mol Imaging.* 2009;36(3):422–427.

24. Halperin EC, Harisiadis L. The role of radiation therapy in the management of metastatic renal cell carcinoma. *Cancer.* 1983;51(4):614–617.

25. Tobisu K, Kakizoe T, Takai K, Tanaka Y, Mizutani T. Surgical treatment of metastatic renal cell carcinoma. *Jpn J Clin Oncol.* 1990;20(3):263–267.

26. Tobisu K, Kakizoe T, Takai K, et al. Prognosis in renal cell carcinoma: analysis of clinical course following nephrectomy. *Jpn J Clin Oncol.* 1989; 19(2):142–148.

27. Les KA, Nicholas RW, Rougraff B, et al. Local progression after operative treatment of metastatic kidney cancer. *Clin Orthop Relat Res.* 2001(390):206–211.

28. Manke C, Bretschneider T, Lenhart M, et al. Spinal metastases from renal cell carcinoma: effect of preoperative particle embolization on intraoperative blood loss. *AJNR Am J Neuroradiol.* 2001;22(5):997–1003.

29. Barton PP, Waneck RE, Karnel FJ, et al. Embolization of bone metastases. *J Vasc Interv Radiol.* 1996;7(1):81–88.

30. Chatziioannou AN, Johnson ME, Pneumaticos SG, et al. Preoperative embolization of bone metastases from renal cell carcinoma. *Eur Radiol.* 2000; 10(4):593–596.

31. Bowers TA, Murray JA, Charnsangavej C, et al. Bone metastases from RCC. The preoperative use of transcatheter arterial occlusion. *J Bone Joint Surg Am.* 1982;64(5):749–754.

32. Sun S, Lang EV. Bone metastases from renal cell carcinoma: preoperative embolization. *J Vasc Interv Radiol.* 1998;9(2):263–269.

33. Althausen P, Althausen A, Jennings LC, et al. Prognostic factors and surgical treatment of osseous metastases secondary to renal cell carcinoma. *Cancer.* 1997;80(6):1103–1109.

34. Mirels H. Metastatic disease in long bones. A proposed scoring system for diagnosing impending pathologic fractures. *Clin Orthop Relat Res.* 1989(249):256–264.

35. Biermann JS, Holt GE, Lewis VO, et al. Metastatic bone disease: diagnosis, evaluation, and treatment. *J Bone Joint Surg Am.* 2009;91(6):1518–1530.

36. Weber KL, Randall RL, Grossman S, et al. Management of lower-extremity bone metastasis. *J Bone Joint Surg Am.* 2006;88(suppl 4):11–19.

37. Damron TA, Morgan H, Prakash D, et al. Critical evaluation of Mirels' rating system for impending pathologic fractures. *Clin Orthop Relat Res.* 2003(415 suppl):S201–S207.

38. Fuchs B, Trousdale RT, Rock MG. Solitary bony metastasis from renal cell carcinoma: significance of surgical treatment. *Clin Orthop Relat Res.* 2005;(431):187–192.

39. Kollender Y, Bickels J, Price WM, et al. Metastatic renal cell carcinoma of bone: indications and technique of surgical intervention. *J Urol.* 2000;164(5):1505–1508.

40. Russo P. Renal cell carcinoma: presentation, staging, and surgical treatment. *Semin Oncol.* 2000; 27(2):160–176.

41. Baloch KG, Grimer RJ, Carter SR, et al. Radical surgery for the solitary bony metastasis from renal-cell carcinoma. *J Bone Joint Surg Br.* 2000;82(1):62–67.

42. Frassica FJ, Frassica DA. Evaluation and treatment of metastases to the humerus. *Clin Orthop Relat Res.* 2003;(415 suppl):S212–S218.

43. King GJ, Kostuik JP, McBroom RJ, et al. Surgical management of metastatic RCC of the spine. *Spine (Phila Pa 1976).* 1991;16(3):265–271.

44. Patchell RA, Tibbs PA, Regine WF, et al. Direct decompressive surgical resection in the treatment of spinal cord compression caused by metastatic cancer: a randomised trial. *Lancet.* 2005;366(9486): 643–648.

45. Sundaresan N, Rothman A, Manhart K, et al. Surgery for solitary metastases of the spine: rationale and results of treatment. *Spine (Phila Pa 1976).* 2002;27(16):1802–1806.

46. Sundaresan N, Scher H, DiGiacinto GV, et al. Surgical treatment of spinal cord compression in kidney cancer. *J Clin Oncol.* 1986;4(12): 1851–1856.

47. Giehl JP, Kluba T. Metastatic spine disease in renal cell carcinoma—indication and results of surgery. *Anticancer Res.* 1999;19(2C):1619–1623.

48. Damron TA, Sim FH. Surgical treatment for metastatic disease of the pelvis and the proximal end of the femur. *Instr Course Lect.* 2000;49:461–470.

49. Sim FH, Frassica FJ, Chao EY. Orthopaedic management using new devices and prostheses. *Clin Orthop Relat Res.* 1995(312):160–172.

50. Bickels J, Wittig JC, Kollender Y, et al. Distal femur resection with endoprosthetic reconstruction: a long-term followup study. *Clin Orthop Relat Res.* 2002(400):225–235.

51. Eckardt JJ, Kabo JM, Kelly CM, et al. Endoprosthetic reconstructions for bone metastases. *Clin Orthop Relat Res.* 2003;(415 suppl):S254–S262.

52. Kelly CM, Wilkins RM, Eckardt JJ, et al. Treatment of metastatic disease of the tibia. *Clin Orthop Relat Res.* 2003;(415 suppl):S219–229.

Index